Transformation and Recovery:

A Guide for the Design and Development of Acupuncture-Based Chemical Dependency Treatment Programs

Alex G. Brumbaugh

Stillpoint Press   *Santa Barbara, CA*

PUBLISHED BY:
StillPoint Press
133 East De la Guerra Street, #362
Santa Barbara, CA 93101

ISBN 09639791-0-8

Printed and bound in the United States of America.

Distributed foreign and domestically by Stillpoint Press

$39.00

Ordering information: 805-681-0070

CONTENTS

This book is dedicated to the memory of Fr. Mark Pemberton

Acknowledgments

This book grew out of several years of continuing dialogue with countless friends, colleagues, teachers and students to whom I am greatly indebted. I am most grateful to Mark Sherwood for his steadfast support, and to Laurel Weinheimer and all the staff of Project Recovery; to other colleagues in California, especially Carol Taub, Faith Cavalier, and Carol Crump for their support and contributions to this book; to Jumbe Allen, Matu Felliciano, Cally Haber, Karen Jobst, Linda Matheis, and to Leo Batson and all the people at Central Coast Support Services, and the other members of NADA-California.

So many of the ideas in this book have been inspired by my teachers and mentors Belle Muschinske and Michael Smith, and by the seminal ideas and nurturing frontier work of Pat Culliton, Pat Keenan, Ana Oliveira, and the authors Anne Wilson Schaef and Morris Berman. I am especially indebted as well to Penny Jenkins, and to the Santa Barbara Council on Alcoholism and Drug Abuse, for supporting me and for believing in Project Recovery, and to Victor Kogler and Peter Francuch at the Santa Barbara County Drug and Alcohol Program for opening doors. Special thanks to Ruth Ackerman, founder of Project Recovery, for her personal support and for her substantial contributions to sections of this book, and of course to JoAnn Hickey for making the initial connections! Many thanks to Kate Black, Muin Daly, Steve Pearce, and Gordy Coburn, for giving me the inspiration to finish, and for their thoughtful reviews and editing of the manuscript, and to Robert Catherina for all of his generous technical support, to David Eisen, for shedding early light and intelligence for me on this field, and, to Jeannie Reardon for supporting the Romantic spirit!

Most special gratitude to Laurie Avila for her boundless, thoughtful support, and for providing the loving final touches.

A Note on the Organization of this Book

This book is divided into three major parts. Each part, and the extensive appendices, while related, can best be seen from a practical standpoint as four different books with different purposes.

Part I, "The Landscape," has the premise that addiction as it has become manifested in our cultural consciousness is a uniquely Western phenomenon, afflicting not only individuals, but institutions as well. The introduction of acupuncture as a healing modality in the treatment of addiction brings a fresh and instructive perspective to this systemic problem. Drawing upon a wide range of literature, this section is a reexamination of the pathology of addiction from this emerging systemic perspective, and offers a way of understanding why acupuncture has proven to be successful as a complement in chemical dependency treatment.

Part II, "Treatment and Recovery," is a practical clinical guide to both conventional Western chemical dependency treatment modalities and to ways in which acupuncture can interface with each of these modalities. Highlights of this section are descriptions of the more discreet psychological and social mechanisms of acupuncture-based treatment, the pharmacological actions of the principal drugs of abuse, and an analysis of the efficacy of the Twelve Step programs.

Part III, "Acupuncture-Based Program Funding and Design," is largely a "nuts and bolts" manual on program start-up and management, with emphasis on funding sources, budget development, and staffing issues. The final chapter in this section is a vision for the future expansion of acupuncture-based chemical dependency treatment into the public health arena.

The Appendix section contains technical and research abstracts as well as a compendium of diverse resources that will be helpful as references in the various phases of program development and management.

Introduction

Robert Olander, the Director of Chemical Health for Hennepin County, Minnesota, has predicted that acupuncture is going to revolutionize the way we do alcohol and drug therapy in this country. Those of us fortunate enough to work in this special emergent field have come to share that optimistic prophecy. In just the past few years, acupuncture treatment for chemical dependency has been integrated into hundreds of drug and alcohol programs internationally. It pervades treatment services in such diverse places as Miami; Minneapolis; New York; Saudi Arabia; Budapest, Hungary; Katmandu, Nepal; Portland, Oregon, and Santa Barbara, California. Successful applications are also being discovered in non-treatment settings such as jails and shelters. Acupuncture interfaces successfully with methadone and hospital detoxification, social model recovery, intensive perinatal residential or day treatment services, and mental health programs. Clinical research has found the same simple protocols to be effective with a variety of major drugs of abuse, such as alcohol, cocaine, and the opiates.[1] The current federal administration has expressed specific interest in acupuncture due in part to its immensely successful application in the Miami/Dade "Drug Court," with which Janet Reno was affiliated as Dade County State's Attorney before becoming the United States Attorney General.[2]

This book began in response to the dozen or so monthly calls I began to receive as a program director asking for information on how to start acupuncture programs. I saw the need for a single volume that would provide a manual on program design and development for acupuncturists as well as for chemical dependency and other health or social service professionals. It grew, by natural implication, to serve as a primer for both the Chinese medical practitioner or acupuncturist who has little or no knowledge of the substance abuse field, and for the substance abuse professional who has little or no knowledge of Chinese medicine or acupuncture.

I have made much effort to satisfy both of these audiences. At times, it may seem a bit disorienting, as though we were in a room filled with substance abuse professionals ardently discussing the issues germane to us, and were suddenly joined by a group of Chinese medical practitioners who wished to be included in our conversation. This challenge, or the converse, clearly raises communication, informational, and semantic problems. And yet, in a treatment age in which linkages among disparate entities is increasingly a measure of competence, this may not be such an inappropriate challenge!

However, this book is more than a "two-books-in-one" primer on two heretofore unrelated fields. The whole is greater than the sum of its parts. In an optimum setting, acupuncture and conventional treatment do not simply exist side by side. They are integrated, synergistically linked, and a new and unique system of care emerges.

There are two ways, in other words, of adding acupuncture services to a conventional treatment continuum. The first, and more tempting, is to *attach* an acupuncture component to existing services. This will benefit clients, but it will not be the most efficacious use of acupuncture. For the full benefits of the acupuncture component to be realized, acupuncture itself must come to form the *foundation* for all of the other program services. This position requires that the acupuncture be a "barrier free" core service, offered daily, on demand, without screening for motivational or other requirements. Ideally, other program services are available on site, including expanded general Chinese medicine. These other services may be mandated or may not, but the acupuncture forms a baseline activity to which clients may return regardless of how they are doing. In this sense, the program in general comes to have the same horizontal flexibility as a Twelve Step meeting, where benefit does not depend upon assessment, length of sobriety, patterns of use, social or medical history, or even motivation.

It is here that acupuncture has the potential to revolutionize alcohol and drug therapy. It serves to make treatment *accessible* on a new level, thus addressing many of the conventional barriers to treatment. More important, it has the ability to make the treatment process *client centered* rather than *program centered*, placing the ultimate responsibility for recovery with the client, which is of course where it must lie if successful recovery is to be achieved. The presence of acupuncture, hence, *redefines* treatment.[3] It alters and enhances the basic clinical posture of ancillary services, and the ancillary services in turn support the acupuncture, making it far more successful than it would be if practiced in isolation.

In a broader systemic interface, the demands of the Western drug treatment setting have had a challenging and transformative impact on traditional Chinese medicine. The acupuncture protocol used in this setting, especially for detoxification, is a specialized hybrid form of acupuncture with roots in European as well as Chinese medicine. It is a protocol that does not involve traditional Chinese medical diagnosis in the early phases of recovery. This fact has raised objections on the part of many Chinese medical practitioners who fear that such a specialized form of acupuncture, broken off, as it were, from the larger clinical body of knowledge that is Chinese medicine, may have a negative impact upon the ultimate acceptance of Chinese medicine in this culture.[4] However, the panoply of physical and emotional disharmonies and syndromes that typically lie just beneath the clinical surface of acute chronic drug addiction and alcoholism are precisely those disharmonies with which traditional Chinese medicine has found its greatest clinical success, and with which Western public health has become baffled.[5] Substance abuse treatment, therefore, has the potential of providing Chinese medicine a long-awaited entry into public health and general medicine in the West.

There is an inverse phenomenon as well because acupuncture has the ability, as we have suggested, to transform conventional Western drug and alcohol treatment, to carry it to new and higher ground: seen as a method of outreach, or as an entry to treatment, it has the ability to reach far larger numbers of clients, far more cost effectively, than any traditional Western modality; it provides a drug free, physically supportive, portable, and flexible treatment option for any substance abuser in any phase of recovery; it provides a foundation for enhanced counseling and case management by making clients more psychologically available for these services; it increases client retention by providing unique support to clients in the early relapsing phase and through its special efficacy with resistant populations, and it makes the symptoms of acute withdrawal manageable in settings where they would otherwise require Western medical supervision.

Therefore, while portions of this book are necessarily covering familiar ground, this ground is being covered from a new perspective. Chinese medicine, and the philosophy upon which it is based, beyond its clinical application, provides a new "looking glass" for examining the problems of systemic addiction in modern Western culture.

The basic acupuncture protocol used in the chemical dependency setting is deceptively simple. It is a five-point auricular (ear) protocol administered in a non-verbal group setting. The only limitations upon group size are the number of acupuncturists and the number of chairs available. The treatment takes about forty-five minutes. It is scheduled daily, in the same one-day-at-a-time rhythm as recovery, with no appointments required. The vast majority of all of the research published to date concerning the efficacy of acupuncture in the treatment of chemical dependency has been based upon the protocols developed by the National Acupuncture Detoxification Association (NADA). NADA's function is to establish professional standards for this work, and to provide education and support to program planners and practitioners.

One of the primary lessons that NADA has learned in the application of acupuncture to the problem of chemical dependency is the familiar axiom that *a little knowledge is dangerous*. The fact is that many acupuncture chemical dependency treatment efforts have started and failed. This has been a set-back, not only for the individual programs, but for the growing field as well. The greatest mistake we can make is to begin programs that ignore the principles that make acupuncture so successful in chemical dependency treatment. It is in the interest of chemical dependency professionals that acupuncture program components be incorporated in light of the wisdom of our past experience. And, it is in the interest of all practitioners of Chinese medicine, regardless of their areas of specialty, that the profession become educated about all aspects of chemical dependency. Colleges of Oriental medicine are as lacking in chemical dependency curriculum as their Western counterparts. Traditional Chinese medical texts are silent on the subject of alcoholism and drug addiction. Chinese medicine as an institution is at risk of making the same mistake that Western medicine has made, denying the role that these complex pathologies play in the syndromes that are seen in the private medical practice. Many acupuncturists have had the experience of treating someone, a cocaine addict or an alcoholic, for example, in their private practice, who responded well to treatment of the presenting symptoms, reported relief, likely expressed gratitude, and then never returned because of the of the practitioner's lack of understanding of these complexities.

NADA has learned that acupuncture loses its effectiveness in the treatment of addictions when used in a vacuum and to the exclusion of other treatment and recovery modalities. Many Chinese medical practitioners in private practice can attest to this fact. Practitioners who execute treatment in a vacuum, ignoring the psycho-social and spiritual complexities of the pathology we call addiction, not only do a disservice to the client but also to the profession. For here is produced another case in which the client will say, "I tried acupuncture and it didn't work."

At the same time, we must hasten to add that acupuncture is not a panacea. A thorough knowledge on the part of the acupuncturist of chemical dependency and recovery does not guarantee success. This is not a success-prone population, and there is a great deal of frustrating clinical failure in working with this population, regardless of the modalities that are used. Traditional Western chemical dependency treatment, unassisted, is a rather bleak landscape. Its proven effectiveness depends most upon clients remaining in treatment for a long time,[6] and yet treatment drop-out is too often the norm. Some long term follow-up studies have found that even lengthy treatment stays ultimately produce low success rates.[7]

The Twelve Step recovery programs, which are based on the principles of Alcoholics Anonymous, have few good outcome studies due to the anonymity factor and other inherent research problems.[8] These programs have a plenitude of anecdotal testimony as to their success, however, and have been integrated in one way or another into virtually all Western alcohol and other drug treatment settings. But the consensus among people in the treatment field and in recovery is that *the majority of addicts and alcoholics will die as a direct or indirect result of their disease.*

Help is needed, and acupuncture has much to offer.

But more than clinical help is needed in the contemporary landscape of addiction and recovery. In fact, the emergence of acupuncture in this field is part of a larger social movement toward viewing addiction and recovery from an increasingly systemic point of view. The phrase "paradigm shift" is often used in this regard, having indeed become something of a cliché. This book seeks to explore this new landscape in an attempt to provide a context for understanding addiction and recovery from this new emerging world view. Because of the endemic,[9] systemic complexity and breadth of the addiction malaise in Western culture, of which chemical dependency is only one of the more glaring symptoms, this book ranges beyond substance abuse and acupuncture applications in an effort to discover the tap root of this malaise.

This new frame of reference leads to an intriguing discovery. As acupuncture enables substance abuse treatment to assume a more client-centered and recovery-centered organizational posture, our client base begins to expand in a unique way. We find that we have more to offer than help for our chemically dependent clients. Because addiction exists on an *institutional level* as well, our clients come to include the criminal justice system, the social service system, the public and private mental and general health care systems, and the chemical dependency treatment establishment itself.

In that this is true, we find that the challenge before us is great indeed. Just as professional ethics require professional care givers to educate themselves thoroughly before providing treatment for any disorder, we too have the challenge of educating ourselves thoroughly before approaching these other "clients." This is not only an ethical requirement, but a political one as well. It will not serve us well to contact our local judges, probation officers, county jailers, legislators, mental health professionals, local chemical dependency program directors, and so on, with the good news of the effectiveness of acupuncture until we have learned their language and have come to a keen understanding of the issues that afflict the institutions and systems in which these individuals function. We need to cultivate as much empathy for these agencies and institutions as we do for our other clients. This cultivation requires that we find a place of understanding of the "pathology" that afflicts them.

Our task requires great patience. These institutions and systems, like our other particularly needy potential clients, are in denial that they have a problem. To paraphrase the research psychiatrist Mindy Fullilove, speaking at a recent NADA conference, *that portion of society which views itself as non-addicted is the greatest difficulty.*

Traditionally, Chinese medicine has been heralded as most effective in the area of *prevention*, and its application to the problem of addiction is no exception. When we speak of addiction, effective primary prevention requires *institutional change*. We have learned in our work that the transformation and healing of addictive institutions is the primary purpose and highest use of acupuncture in the treatment of addiction.

This is new information. We are on a frontier.

PART I   THE LANDSCAPE

*The vast literature on alcoholism is
with few exceptions an apology for
not being able to do much about it.*

Eric Berne

Among the more penetrating human challenges of working in
or thinking about the field of addiction and recovery is that we find
ourselves truly on a vast frontier. We are entering upon a
landscape that has not been accurately mapped.

One has perhaps seen replicas of the quaint and inaccurate
maps of the globe and of unexplored land masses that were actually used by Western explorers from the fifteenth through the
nineteenth centuries. The earliest maps of the North American
continent, for example, which were based upon earlier explorations
(and even more perhaps upon presumptive and wishful thinking,
and an explorer's arrogance), often depict a mythical river, named
"Buena Ventura," which would provide the hoped for all-water-
route through the continent's interior from the Atlantic to Pacific
oceans.

Two things are important in this phenomenon of inaccurate
map-making. First, it made exploration in general an enterprise
characterized by unfolding disappointment after disappointment
that things weren't where they were supposed to be. The territory
didn't fit the map. That disappointment imposed, after a time, a
certain emotional perseverance on the explorers who persisted in
the work. Perseverance was imposed, and humility, because there
came for them the implicit knowledge that they were transition
figures in this drama of exploration and discovery, that they would
likely never live to see the precise form and shape of the lands they
were mapping. That satisfaction of completion would have to be
left to later explorers and cartographers. We might say that, in order to survive, both emotionally and physically, these explorers

had to be content to live in the *process* of exploration rather than in the *outcome*.

Second, it is important to recognize that these awarenesses didn't keep them from making maps. The maps they continued to make, based upon incomplete information, and though consequently inaccurate, were invaluable in the frontier process, providing the sole beacons for subsequent exploration. These early frontier-folk were obliged, therefore, whether consciously or unconsciously, to embrace their own imperfections and limitations in order to survive. The maps they left may appear, in retrospect, arrogant in their presumptuousness. Yet the courage to make them allowed subsequent exploration to take place, and ultimately, accurate maps to be drawn.

It is important to note that maps are never the same as the lands they depict, regardless of their technical accuracy. They are depictions only, rough guides. Elevation coding by color on a flat surface, no matter how "accurate," can never capture the splendor of the Rocky Mountains, or the breath-taking expanse of the Great Plains. Confusing a map for the territory it is meant to represent is to be beguiled by symbols. For the traveler, particularly an explorer, this conclusion can, of course, be disastrous.

Therefore, we realize that our map-making efforts in the field of addiction and recovery are best tempered with humility, with an understanding that we cannot ultimately know this reality by means of our maps, and that we who enter this field are transition figures on a landscape whose true dimensions and nature we may not live to see in any totality.

And we must make the maps just the same, knowing that the terrain we attempt to describe is likely much more complicated, and possibly even less so, than what we perceive and attempt to describe at the present time. We trust that those who follow will find these maps useful - and will likely smile at their inaccuracies.

Although we speak in *metaphor*, and will continue to use metaphor as a vehicle of understanding throughout this book, we should not forget that metaphors, like maps, are not the realities they represent. They are *stories about* that reality. The impact of addiction and recovery, on the other hand, is not metaphor. It is the reality, the landscape of late twentieth century America which increasingly demands attention if we are to survive as a culture and a race.

There are other reasons for beginning this journey with humility. People who work in the field of addiction and recovery have been said to have a "neurotic need" to help others. A more helpful frame for this idea was suggested by psychologist Herbert Gravitz,[10] who has called people in the helping profession *wounded artists.* It is likely that people working in this field would be, in saner times, painters, poets, architects, novelists, sculptors, weavers and potters. But for their woundedness, they would be working with material other than human relationships.

We were, according to Gravitz, wounded in relationship, and we must therefore be healed in relationship. We help in order to heal. It is important, he notes, to keep one foot in our woundedness and one foot in our own recovery. The arrogance that comes with forgetting this is an anathema to effectiveness on any level and can cause us to hurt further those we would help.

Wise frontier explorers, exhilarated at their prospects, have two necessary tasks before their journey may commence. The first is to study extant maps. The second is to establish a center, a base of operations from which they will draw essential supplies and sustenance and to which they can return as a baseline reference for where they are.

In this first section of our book, these are our two objectives: examining extant maps, and establishing a center. We will examine the psycho-historical and cultural landscape of the phenomenon of Western addiction in rather broad strokes. In pathological terms, this will be a journey through the addictive *system*, from branch to root. We will find this system, as the book *Alcoholics Anonymous* describes alcohol itself, "cunning, baffling, and powerful." [11] The addictive system is seductive as well, inviting us in, occluding reason, covering and displacing our best intentions.

Drawing upon what we know of addiction *recovery* as a system, we will seek a place to stand in order to gain perspective, a center which will empower us to act.

The metaphor that is sometimes used to illustrate the problem of describing or defining addiction is that of four or five blind men trying to describe an elephant. Each has hold of a different part of the elephant's anatomy, and so each is describing an apparently quite different animal, though each description is, from its own vantage point, accurate.

Similarly, many terms and variations of terms are used to describe the process of addiction.[12] The preferred term depends on the agency, and upon the point of view, whether medical, social, psychological, or legal, and further upon various philosophical and insurance issues. Pervading this confusion is the culture's moral abhorrence of the addict's intoxicated behavior, engendered perhaps by the culture's abhorrence of euphoria and altered mood states in general. The resulting historical ambivalence toward drug use in this country, coupled with racism and with ethnic and gender oppression, has driven our social attitudes about drugs as well as our national drug policy.[13] The latter, that began in the late 19th century with laws against Chinese opium dens, became crystallized by the Harrison Narcotics Act of 1914,[14] in which addictive drug use was defined as a matter of legal volition rather than an involuntary disease state, and culminated with the recent military paradigm of the "War on Drugs." Throughout this history, the legal and medical (primary disease model) definitions have been in conflict.[15]

Does the locus of control in addiction lie in the addicted one, or in that to which he or she is addicted? Or, in something else? In the semantically shifting terminology used to describe the phenomenon, the problem of volition is dominant.

Systemic addiction is an implication of the philosophy of Western Rationalism, and is *inherent* in the institutions and disciplines which grew from that philosophy.[16] One of the dominant features of the linear philosophy of Rationalism is that it has little tolerance for paradox. The principle of *yin* and *yang*, which pro-

23

vides the philosophical basis of traditional Chinese medicine, is, in fact and in spirit, a foreign concept to Western Rationalism.[17] Therefore, much of the problem in defining addiction arises from the Western inability to reconcile the paradox of where the locus lies, and from the philosophically obsessive desire to have it one way or the other.

"The elephant," it wishes to insist, "is trunk, *period.*"

In its Latin etymology, the word "addiction" comes from the root *dict*, which means "to speak," and the prefix *ad*, which means "yes." In a pure semantic sense, this implies volition, or *will*, since the seat of speech is within the speaker. It is a prophetic irony that in the very inception of the term we find the problem of volition, for the first recorded usage of the word is found in Roman law, describing the state of being *legally bound over*. The term was later expanded to include the status of subjugation, enslavement, or indenture, and it began to be used in 12th-century literature to apply to people bound over to such varied things as vice, virginity, and, inevitably, alcohol. So, one "speaks yes" to that to which one is involuntarily bound. Thus, the problem of the *locus of control*, both in semantics and in reality, is at the center of the concept of addiction. The term addiction was used medically and applied to pathological drug use early in the 19th century, and, by the mid-19th century, received substantial attention in the medical literature, particularly in regard to opium.[18]

The original and continuing medical definition of addiction requires two conditions: *tolerance* and *withdrawal*. Tolerance might be described as the changes or adjustments the body makes in the presence of the addictive chemical. We can describe this holistically as *the homeostatic efforts of the body to achieve balance in the presence of the drug*. The mechanisms of tolerance are not well understood, and there is disagreement as to whether tolerance occurs at the "site of action" in the calibrating biochemical mechanisms of the brain, or whether it is a function of liver enzyme production. Both are likely involved, and in either event, the effect is that increasing amounts of the drug are required to achieve the same effect.

Withdrawal is the physiological response of the organism when the addictive agent is suddenly removed. Sometimes called "abstinence syndrome," withdrawal might be described as a "rebound," the *homeostatic efforts of the body to achieve balance in the sudden absence of the drug.*

Western science is prone to becoming locked into its own definitions. Being locked into this one prevented for a long time the acknowledgment of the addictive potential of nicotine and cocaine, arguably the two most addictive drugs known. Nicotine does not produce classic tolerance, and cocaine produces no classic "physical" withdrawal symptoms. Nonetheless, this classic definition is still used, and indeed it has a measure of clinical usefulness.

Though alcoholism in particular has been addressed in the medical literature as a "disease" since the early 19th century, for the vast majority of its history in the West, alcoholism has been viewed as a moral failing, a weakness of character (*i.e., will*). A particularly keen focus of alcoholism as a moral failing has been directed at women.[19]

The 1939 book *Alcoholics Anonymous* characterized it as an "illness," citing medical authorities of the day.[20] The "primary disease concept of alcoholism," though endorsed by the American Medical Association since 1956, has come under continuing attack. Some of the opponents argue that alcoholism/addiction is a *behavior* and hence subject to control of the user, or that it is at least not a *primary* disease but *a secondary symptom of a more primary behavioral, emotional, or mental disorder.* While *Alcoholics Anonymous* avoided defining alcoholism, they went to the heart of the issue of volition by describing alcoholics as people who had lost the ability to *control* their drinking.[21] Moralizing critics have, of course, charged that this allows the so-called alcoholic to absolve him or herself of responsibility for the condition/behavior.[22]

Beyond this moral controversy, as the medical and insurance industries have taken increased control over the treatment field, the disease concept has come under more recent attack. The debate is summarized in the article, "Disease - Pro and Con",[23] by Herbert

Fingarette and Jess W. Bromley, M.D. Bromley defines any disease state as having a particular combination of the following four conditions:

1. An etiologic agent
2. An etiologic process.
3. A lesion.
4. A syndrome.

According to Bromley, when any two of 1, 2, and 4 is known, a disease is confirmed. If only a syndrome is perceived, it is taken to be evidence of a "disease on probation." Against this criteria, Bromley argues, alcoholism (and we can say, by extension, other drug addiction) qualifies as an authentic disease.

When we apply this primary disease model to the phenomenon of alcoholism or other drug addiction, some curious things happen. The etiologic agent, of course, would be the drug itself, the "invading pathogen." In forcing addiction into this frame, we shift focus from the individual to the chemical, from inside to outside. If we build a model of understanding from this premise, we are required to acknowledge the anomaly that for many individuals - in fact, for the vast majority - the substance alcohol is *not* addicting and is used without pathological consequence. There is some truth in the A.A. folk wisdom that if you are an alcoholic, you are an alcoholic regardless of how much you drink; if you aren't an alcoholic, you can't drink enough to become one. And even the most inherently addictive other drugs, such as nicotine and morphine, are used without pathological consequence by statistically significant numbers of people.

Reductionism is characteristic of Western science and philosophy, and by reducing addiction in this case to an emphasis on the chemical, we open up two complex questions: (1) why are a statistically significant number of individuals apparently "immune" to addiction to these admittedly toxic pathogens, and (2) if the problem is the substance, why do addicts and alcoholics characteristically and almost universally relapse after the etiologic agent is removed?

In applying this rational, Western, medical, reductionist, "hard science" definition of Bromley's to alcoholism and other chemical addiction to see if addiction in fact passes this "disease test," it is interesting to use the philosophy of Alcoholics Anonymous as a counter-reference. As a historical phenomenon, A.A., which began in 1935, can be seen as a non-rational, *countercultural reaction* against the failure of the three dominant rational systems of the day - medicine, psychology, and religion - to offer any effective treatment for alcoholism. Although A.A. has played a significant role historically in the acceptance of alcoholism as a disease, A.A. characterizes alcoholism, as we have said, as having lost the ability to *control* one's drinking. The locus of attention here shifts from the etiologic agent alcohol back to the center of inner volition. Therefore, while A.A. has defined alcoholism as an illness, the illness does not find its referents outside (in the agent), but inside the subject.

Having defined control as the centerpiece of the malady, it is rational to infer that the cure or antidote is, of course, control, and this is precisely the tact that Western treatment has historically taken, without much success. A.A., however, as we have said, is a non-rationalist paradigm, so it takes the case in the opposite direction, away from increasing efforts at control, and toward a state of *powerlessness*, of surrender to the "external substance." (Step One of A.A.'s Twelve Steps is that "We admitted we were powerless over alcohol - that our lives had become unmanageable." [24])

A.A.'s answer to the first anomaly, "why are a statistically significant number of individuals apparently immune to ingestion of these admittedly toxic pathogens" is that, clearly, they are not alcoholics (/addicts). Alcoholism here is implicitly a condition that preexisted ingestion of the substance. Its answer to the second question, "why do addicts and alcoholics characteristically and almost universally relapse after the etiologic agent is removed? " is because, conversely, they *are* alcoholics, alcoholism (/addiction) being a condition that exists before ingestion and beyond abstinence.

It is all, according to A.A., "an inside job," and, it has surprisingly little to do with the substance alcohol. The book *Alcoholics Anonymous* is not about alcohol; nor is it about how not to drink (*i.e.*, control). Instead, it is about how to *live*. Alcoholic drinking is seen as a symptom of a *living problem*, manifested in the issue of *personal power*. A.A. states: "Lack of power, that was our dilemma." [25] We will have a good deal more to say about this later.

From the Rationalist perspective, the two anomalous questions we have raised begin to be addressed as we consider the second disease criteria, the *etiologic process*. The etiologic process involves two branches of Western medicine: *epidemiology*, or how the agent comes into contact with the patient, and *pathogenesis*, or what happens once the contact is made. The path of epidemiology, when applied to substance addiction, leads away from the hard science of medicine and toward the softer sciences of psychology, sociology, anthropology, economics, and politics. Though softer sciences, it is important to note that these are not different paradigms. A case can be made that in modern Western culture, if medicine is the *temple*, these other disciplines are its outlying parishes.

Pathogenesis, on the other hand, leads from the hard science of medicine to the even harder and more reductionist fields of *pharmacokinetics* and *pharmacodynamics*, where we become involved with the highly compartmentalized issues of drug distribution, absorption, and elimination.

The third disease criteria in Bromley's model is the *lesion*, referring to the focus or damage at any of multiple levels and the consequences of this damage. Structural, biochemical, physiological, and behavioral elements are all taken into account.

The fourth criteria is the *syndrome*: a collection of symptoms and signs that regularly occur together which can either be noted by the diagnostician or complained about by the patient.

It is a reality, by whatever paradigm, that even the periodic use of psychoactive drugs produces both lesion and syndrome. By this Western definition of disease, alcoholism and other drug addiction seem to indeed qualify, anomalies notwithstanding. Why, then, does the "primary disease model" continue to be questioned?

The spokespersons for one school of criticism include philosopher Herbert Fingarette[26] and psychologist Stanton Peele.[27] Not surprisingly, they go to volition as a point of attack, citing research indicating that so-called "alcoholics" do in fact control, regulate, and modulate their drinking, often "maturing out" into patterns of "social drinking" without the benefit of intervention or treatment.[28] Such "spontaneous remission" is also held to be true of a statistically significant number of opiate users over time.[29]

According to these critics, drug use - even heavy, extended, and regular drug use - is a *behavior* and not a disease. And it is a behavior for which people should be held accountable, both morally and legally. They argue that the disease model abrogates responsibility ("I can't help it that I drink; I'm an alcoholic.") and fuels the very lucrative medical treatment establishment ($35,000 is not an unusual insurance-billable fee for standard thirty-day medical model alcoholism or cocaine treatment). Due as much to clinical experience as to this philosophical attack, these traditional intensive inpatient medical-model treatment programs are becoming less popular, especially with insurance companies, and have acquiesced to the fact that extremely few chronic alcoholics and addicts require medically supervised treatment during the extended acute phase of withdrawal - especially those alcoholics still functional enough to have this extent of private insurance coverage!

And so, these Rationalists of the behavioral school have found justification for their arguments.

Moreover, just as the "primary disease model" is under attack from the "rational right," it is also criticized by what we might call the "holistic left" as well. If we follow an etiologic path from the branch to the root of the addiction malaise, we can find arguments, as we have suggested, that addiction is an inevitable implication, and hence a by-product of, Western Rationalism itself. From this view, addiction is far more a cultural, philosophical, existential dilemma than a medical one. In 1970, Ernest Kurtz, an American Historian, wrote the first "outsider's" history of Alcoholics

Anonymous. He named his book *Not-God*.[30] The title comes from the quintessential discovery for the alcoholic, during the early phase of recovery, that the addicted self, the ego, the old seat of conscious attention and volition, is "not-god." Paramount to the rigid addictive system is that it *thinks* it is God. Likewise, Cartesian Rationalism and the patriarchal institutions of medicine, psychology, and philosophy which it has spawned, have, as their central flaw, the notion that they are omnipotent and omniscient. *Cogito ergo sum*, wrote Descartes; "I think, therefore I am." [31] From this premise, the seat of discursive knowing (*mind*) is the exclusive referent for the reality of one's existence.

Kurtz spoke of the America of the late 19th and early 20th centuries, from which Alcoholics Anonymous emerged, as *modernity*. It is his view that modernity (an historical period generally identified as beginning in the early 1600s with the development of Cartesian Rationalism) was characterized, particularly in America, by a fundamental obsession with *rationalization* and *control*. Because of the "thirst and quest for more rationalization and control," he wrote, "[and the] final impossibility [of either], the very *identity* of modernity, in modernity's own terms, revealed itself as inherently addictive." [32]

According to this frame of understanding, alcoholics and addicts might best be understood as individuals who are unable to adapt successfully to an inherently addictive society. Intoxication is a search for a more holistic state of consciousness in a severely non-holistic cultural environment. Using this frame of understanding, addiction is a disease all right, but its roots are not in the individual, and certainly not in the chemical, but in the social milieu of *modernity*.

This model transforms our current exercise of attempting to rationally define or describe addiction into something very curious indeed: what we are looking *at*, we are looking *with*!

Turning this self-defining element of the addictive system in on itself, we can produce the following:

Application of Disease Criteria to Systemic Addiction:

Etiologic agent:

Western Exclusionary Rationalism

Etiologic process:

Western education, media, politics, religion, science, social science, the patriarchal dysfunctional family system, etc.

Lesion:

Racial, ethnic, and gender oppression, violence, ecological imbalance, greenhouse effect, endangered species, economic depression, dysfunctional political systems, etc.

Syndrome:

Endemic addiction (pathological use of substances [drugs, food] and activities [spending, indebtedness, sex, relationship, work, etc.]), powerlessness, obsession with control, repressed rage and trauma, pathologically manipulative behavior, dishonesty, depression, anxiety, intense craving (for wholeness), denial, compulsive need to define, reduce, and compartmentalize things in order to "understand" them, etc.

This configuration of the problem, of course, gives a decidedly different turn to the primary disease concept. Mood-altering-seeking behavior, given this paradigm, can be better understood as a survival strategy of sensitive people trying to adjust to the insensitive (inherently addictive) world view of modernity.

Now, this "Rationalism-bashing" exercise may be amusing and even fruitful, and (as with addiction) it is seductive as well, and there is danger of missing the point. Western Rationalism is no more inherently "evil" than alcohol, sex, work, or the coca leaf. *Blaming* Rationalism for the addictive system is as pointless as blaming alcohol for alcoholism. Recovery is not about prohibition; it is about getting beyond blame, getting beyond scapegoating, getting past whose fault it is. If we get stuck in the blame, we fall into the reductionist trap again. To find the touchstone of recovery, it is necessary that we accept our anger and outrage, and that we ultimately move away from the blame to a different paradigm of understanding. From this vantage point, we can begin to see the "stuff" of addiction - drugs, sex, science and technology, etc. - for what they are: simply "not God."

It is, of course, precisely because Chinese medicine represents, like Alcoholics Anonymous, a different world view, a different paradigm, that it has the capacity to revolutionize addiction treatment. This different paradigm is a world view in which "mind" and "body" are not distinct entities; in which "opposites" are seen as complementary rather than competing; in which there is a seamless whole of human organism and environment, and in which "body" (life) is seen as *process* rather than static "stuff" like marrow and eyeballs. Its importance in treatment and recovery is that the medium (modality) becomes the message. It provides a philosophical place to stand outside of the addictive paradigm. It speaks intrinsically to principles of healing rather than to means of further rationalization and control.

However, before we move into this "paradigm shift," which is where recovery lies, let us continue our semantic journey through attempts to define addiction from the Western perspective. This is the language we need to learn and integrate into our own work if we are to be effective. And the art of doing this work is the art of maintaining a foothold in a recovery paradigm while at the same time interfacing on multiple levels with the addictive system. This manifests as the art of speaking two (or more) languages fluently and not forgetting who and where we are.

Failing to meet this challenge, we will be as leaves on a raging river.

Defining Terms

The currently common phrase used by professionals to describe drug addiction from a treatment perspective is usually *chemical dependence*. In a classic sense, *addiction* is a strictly medical term. Chemical dependence, now favored, is more of a psychological term, with emphasis away from pharmacology and toward a psychologically dependent relationship. In order to satisfy pharmacological considerations, however, chemical dependence is generally seen as having two elements: *psychological dependence* and *physiological dependence.* Psychological dependence implies a choice: the user has control, but his or her entire life revolves around use of the drug. Physiological dependence, on the other hand, is seen as a property of the drug.

We can see the drawing of this distinction as both an amplification of mind/body dualism,[33] and as an attempt to reconcile the inside/outside paradox of drug addiction.[34] This is what Western science does when faced with a paradox; it expands the definition to try and embrace linear consistency, and, paradoxically, reduces the process it is looking at.

To state the same premise from the standpoint of Western diagnosis, we can say that there are two basic models of chemical dependency: the *medical/pharmacological model* and the *social deviance model.* In the "real world" of Western treatment, these two are usually combined, with the emphasis depending upon the treatment methods being used at a particular agency.

The medical/pharmacological model draws its specific clinical definitions from the *Diagnostic and Statistical Manual of the American Psychiatric Association* (APA), *third edition revised* (DSMIII-R). This manual, whose definitions and language are used for insurance billing and state licensure/certification standards compliance, distinguishes between substance *abuse* and substance *dependence,* but the essence of the definition given by the APA is a *pattern of pathological use with impairment of social or occupational functioning and duration greater than one month.* "Pathological" means *out of control or damaging to the individual.* The criteria for establishing pathological use include the following:

1) Intoxication throughout the day.
2) Inability to cut down or stop use.
3) Repeated efforts to stop or control use.
4) Restricting use to certain times of the day.
5) Social/occupational dysfunction.

Practically speaking, this is a limited definition because people for whom drug use has progressed sufficiently to yield these symptoms (which are required for insurance billing), and who arrive for treatment at expensive hospitals, have generally lost the jobs that provide the level of insurance required to pay for treatment.

Paradox upon paradox!

In part, the renewed clinical emphasis upon "dual diagnosis" has come about because of insurance considerations. Often, people who have the insurance coverage that makes them eligible for private treatment for chemical dependence haven't progressed in their "disease" enough to meet the required diagnostic criteria required for third party billing. Thus, they will often be diagnosed as having a *psychiatric* illness as well, such as borderline personality disorder, depression, *etc.*, in order to justify third party payment for their treatment. This phenomenon exists quite apart from the realities of dual diagnosis among homeless and other disenfranchised populations who have no private insurance.[35] (See Appendix XII, Section B, for additional information on dual diagnosis.)

There are other diagnostic problems inherent in addiction. Because of drug addiction denial in the Western medical profession (Md.'s are the profession at the highest risk for drug addiction), and because of the social stigma attached to drug addicts, many Md.'s don't believe that the people they see are drug addicts. Therefore, addiction is often undiagnosed, or mis-diagnosed as work-related stress, hysteria, depression, and so on. There is a cliché in Alcoholics Anonymous, particularly among females, that for the last few decades, alcoholism was diagnosed by physicians as a "Valium deficiency." [36]

The second way of framing chemical dependence is by the *Social Deviance model.* As the medical/pharmacological model wanes due to the problems listed above, this way of framing addiction becomes more commonly used, and the diagnosis in this case would be made not by a physician but more likely by a clinical psychologist, counselor, or social worker. The criteria for making a chemical dependence diagnosis using this model would include:

1. Use of any prohibited drug.
2. Use of a therapeutic drug for a non-therapeutic purpose.[37]
3. Intentional taking of prescribed drugs in excessive amounts.
4. Excessive use of licit drugs.
5. Combining two or more drugs to intensify a high.

Any one of these criteria is a basis for a diagnosis.

Social deviance, then, means getting out of what is socially acceptable: a violation of the social parameters of behavior. How the use began (etiology) is not a central criteria. For example, the Supreme Court has ruled that sacramental use of peyote among Native Americans is unacceptable, therefore such use is socially deviant by definition.

The notion of social deviance leads to a third model, the *Legal model*, which has nothing to do with addiction or chemical dependence but speaks rather to substance *abuse*, defined here as *any* use of an illicit substance (see Appendix I, Section B, for a classification of illicit substances), and any *illicit* use of a licit substance (such as driving under the influence). Interestingly, and for good reason, much of the funding (and support) for acupuncture programs in the United States comes not from traditional chemical dependence sources but from the criminal justice community (see pp. 184-195, and Appendix V).

Substance abuse, a phrase widely and loosely used, contains within itself a curious enigma. It clearly has a moral and legal tone. While *chemical dependence* assumes abuse, *substance abuse* itself is pejorative. The implication in *dependence* is that the *chemical* has the power, while *abuse* shifts the onus to the *abuser* and away from the morally inert chemical. Hence we see that the semantic tendency is to bend over backward to avoid the awkward situation in which personal responsibility disappears altogether. There is also more than a little "codependent" scapegoating going on here, because the argument about whether emphasis should be placed on the drug or its user conveniently obscures the fact that the addictive onus is in fact in neither one, belonging instead to the defining system itself. Besides, "substance abuse" is a *non sequitur*. For the alcoholic, it would have meaning only in the sense of something along the lines of mixing a good Kentucky whisky with canned fruit punch!

Returning to the reality of the contemporary Western treatment setting, we most often find a combining of the medical/pharmacological and social deviance models, and a diagnostic criteria applied to the client that includes the following:

1. Takes substance more than originally intended;
2. Fails in attempts to cut back;
3. Spends a lot of time taking, getting, and recovering from substance;
4. Is often intoxicated;
5. Curtails or gives up significant social activity because of use;
6. Uses despite persistent psychological or social or physical consequences;
7. Needs more and more to attain the same effect (tolerance);
8. Suffers characteristic withdrawal;
9. Takes substance to relieve withdrawal.

To complicate further these definitions, there is yet another concept that came into the clinical and popular literature in the late 1970s in Minnesota, the concept of *codependence*. Codependence derived from the original notion of "co-alcoholism" that was identified soon after the beginning of Alcoholics Anonymous. People who lived with a practicing alcoholic over time became conscious of a syndrome that was assumed to result from that relationship, a way of coping which was a reaction against the alcoholism. The wives of the early recovering A.A. men began getting together to socialize while their husbands were at their A.A. meetings,[38] and they began to recognize that they had a common experience, not only in the behavior of their alcoholic spouses, but in their own behavior. Lois Wilson, the wife of A.A.'s co-founder Bill Wilson, started Al-Anon, adopting the same Twelve Steps used by A.A..[39] The experiences and feelings that they shared were soon recognized as generally applying to anyone who lived for a prolonged period with any dependent person - hence, *codependence.* In the 1980s, Tim Cermak[40] defined codependence as a *mixed personality disorder* with the following cluster of symptoms:[41]

1. Involving one's self in the life of another in spite of adverse consequences;
2. Meeting others needs at the cost of one's own;
3. Boundary distortions;
4. Enmeshment.

This syndrome, which also involves depression, compulsivity, anxiety, and much more besides, has been widely dealt with in the popular literature. Anne Wilson Schaef[42] has taken codependence a step further by suggesting that it is at the core of all addiction, underlying the addictive process itself. She has suggested further that, while codependence has been a useful concept, it now needs to be challenged. She has recognized that the syndrome of what we have called codependence is not a product of living with a dependent person, but exists *independently* of any particular relationship. It is a syndrome, in other words, that does not require being in relationship with a dependent person, but rather predates and in fact *draws one into* such a relationship, often repeatedly. She believes that the syndrome can be more accurately understood as *relationship addiction.* Charlotte Kasl[43] believes that codependency is a euphemism for the characteristics of internalized oppression.

What do the non-substance activities to which people become addicted, such as relationships, romance, sex, gambling, spending, indebtedness, power, work, television, jogging, and so forth, have in common? In an existential sense, these are activities by which people negotiate the self/other fault or schism that they experience. They speak to subject/object relationship, revealing the dilemma of dualism that is central to Rationalist philosophy. When engaged in or used in a compulsive or addictive manner, these activities can be seen as a misdirected search for a sense of inner wholeness and a sense of outer connectedness. Since the essence of the addictive (*i.e.*, Rationalist) state is to turn off feelings, people therefore go *into* their addictions (becoming "intoxicated") in order to *feel*. In terms of the actual substrate of addiction, these activity addictions have raised an interesting pharmacological question. Since a state of intoxication can be precipitated by pleasure-inducing or sense-diverting activities as well as by chemical substances, do people in fact become addicted to chemical substances such as drugs, or do these substances act in some way as precursors or catalysts for an internal, endogenous neurochemical process that is the source of the mood alteration?

We will leave this interesting hypothesis as well as the existential and spiritual questions raised by "activity addictions" for later discussion. What becomes clear in attempting to define all of the terms used in this field is that, from the dominant Western paradigm of Rationalism, it is all very complex indeed! If we are to "grasp the elephant" in all of its *elephantness*, we are likely to need a new looking glass, a new paradigm, a new place to stand to gain a reasoned perspective.

Chinese medicine, as we have pointed out, represents such a non-Western, non-Rationalist *terra firma*. But the ancient and revised Chinese medical texts, and the curriculum of our Colleges of Oriental Medicine, do not provide much specific philosophical or clinical guidance for understanding or addressing the malaise of addiction.

We are, as we have said, in a new dimension, on a frontier with few maps.

We can indeed see that any functional description of addiction within the Western rational paradigm would have to be quite broad, covering all of the complexities of "elephantness." It might sound something like this: *addiction is characterized by physiological and/or psychological dependence upon a human activity, process, or chemical substance, and is a function of the environment, the individual, and the activity or substance to which one is addicted.*

This definition would conceivably, of course, pass as a definition for life itself! But, using it for the moment, we at least have it that addiction is an *interactive process.* This characterization of addiction has been termed the "multi-variate" model, in which there is an interplay between and among these various elements: Society <> Individual <> Substance (or activity).

There is not much humility nor perhaps even meaning in this definition. It's a bit like suggesting that "an elephant is a thing that is very big and complicated." But at least it is a map, and so let's not be too quick to throw it away. Instead, let's explore this linear, reductionist terrain to see where it leads and what insight we might gain from it, beginning with the favorite Western question (and the addict's favorite question): "*Why?* " Why do people become addicted? What is the cause of addiction/dependence potential/susceptibility?

We begin with the first element of our "multi-variate" model, society - not so much the dynamic psycho-historical notion of society implied by Kurtz's "modernity," but more the static, compartmentalized society of the social scientists. We realize that this is a potentially valuable line of reason so long as we remember that it is "not God." It is not truth, or reality, but simply metaphor, a tool. This is the proper use of all science. The value of science, psychology, social science, and of research is the assistance offered in disclosing and revealing the *process* and its aspects. The important issue, as we have said, is not to mistake the map for the territory.

Different aspects of the social environment of the individual that put one at risk of addiction can be called "social or environmental precursors of addiction," and we can say that such an environment in general is a barren, stress-inducing environment,[44] nonvalidating of health (wholeness). Such an environment is characterized by loneliness and isolation, an environment in which the individual has been cut off from what is conventionally thought of as a social support system, which we translate as external sources of validation for life-enhancing feelings and behaviors. Examples of such an environment are urban slums, war zones, prisons, schools, and primary social systems such as families which function to *alienate* rather than *validate* or reinforce living processes.

One of the primal functions of positive social support systems is to validate human *trauma*, such as loss, death, abuse, violence, homelessness, repression, or political, economic, or sexual exploitation. In 1980, the *DSMIII* first recognized *Post Traumatic Stress Disorder* ((PTSD), and a less acute form called *Post Traumatic Stress Syndrome* (PTSS).[45] PTSD is, in general, a re-living beyond memory of emotions elicited by trauma. There is a latency factor with PTSD; it gets worse if not treated. Alcohol and drugs are often used in these cases as self-medication to mask the underlying issue. When alcohol and drugs are used in this manner to mask invalidated trauma, the true addiction is perhaps best understood as addiction not to the drugs or alcohol or other "things" but to feelings: relaxation, arousal, oblivion, fantasy, sleep. The somewhat oversimplified psychological dynamic of this in the classic American dysfunctional family is: distant father + helpless mother = anger not expressed; society says "feel good," so that's what we do, using chemicals or activities to alter or regulate mood.

PTSD became publicized in reference to Vietnam veterans returning from the trauma of that war.[46] The syndrome had been called "shell shock" in earlier post-war periods. It has now been clinically recognized that *any* unresolved trauma can produce the syndrome. At the 1992 National Conference of the National

Acupuncture Detoxification Association (NADA), research psychiatrist Mindy Fullilove, reported her findings that 86% of women presenting chemical dependence at Lincoln Hospital in New York had either witnessed or been victims of violent trauma, 58% to a degree that justified a clinical diagnosis of PTSD.[47]

Another environmental factor that might be a precursor for drug dependence or addiction is *criminalization*. In a culture characterized by generational alienation - a psycho-social separation of youth culture from adult culture - any criminal, unconventional, or non-sanctioned activity will come to serve as a potential act of symbolic rebellion. American society has chosen psychoactive drug use as a premier criminal, unconventional, and non-sanctioned activity. Add to this a drug-rich environment in which drugs are widely available, and in which there are few social guidelines for proper use, and we have an environment in which drugs are likely to become a problem for youth, or indeed, for anyone who experiences themselves as alienated from the society proper.

It is of interest that even those in our society who argue for the legalization or decriminalization of drugs often miss this point. Virtually all legalization advocates concede, for example, that nicotine should continue to be legally restricted for young people since it is the most dangerous, addicting, and life-threatening psychoactive drug of abuse. The point that is missed is that, because it is illegal for people under the age of eighteen to purchase tobacco, and since nicotine is in fact the closest thing we have to a universal gateway drug for all addicts, society has made nicotine use the *first criminal act of all drug users*. Its illegal status for minors dramatically enhances its role as a convenient source of symbolic rebellion and self-initiation into adulthood. For example, for all the recent public awareness about the health hazards of nicotine, and despite the fact that cigarette sales are down among most population groups, these sales continue to rise for the most inherently alienated population in our culture: teenage females.

Historically, in contrast with modern and particularly Western (or Westernizing) culture, psychoactive drug use has been, largely, *ritual* use. When used in connection with religious ritual, customs, celebrations and rites of passage, its use is *sanctified*. The well-understood function, for example, of tobacco smoke for the native population of America was to carry prayers to the heavens for the welfare of the tribe. In this context, teenage Native Americans were not very likely to sneak tobacco off behind the sweat lodge and "party," irrespective of the "addictive potential" of the drug itself.

However, with the arguably less blessed exceptions of high school graduation, and the superficial surviving remnants of rituals such as Irish wakes, Jewish *bar mitzvahs*, stag parties preceding Anglo weddings, *etc.*, life-sanctifying drug rituals (like life-sanctifying rituals in general) have disappeared from the dominant cultural landscape of modernity. Replacing these is a cultural ambivalence about any and all drug use.

Many who advocate laws restricting drug use falsely hope that such standards of use can be *imposed*. But ritualistic regulation of drug use is by definition an endogenous social value, not an exogenous one. And, we can in fact witness endogenously sanctioned ritual drug use[48] among alienated populations such as youth "gangs," where rituals in which drug use signify entry into the alienated group. Ritual drug use here functions not to enhance or validate spiritual life in the conventional sense, but in fact to *de*value life and validate the state of alienation itself. In these cases, the drug use is not reserved for the spiritually elite - the priests or medicine men or seers - but is exacted by peer pressure to convey membership, a rite of passage into a state of non-membership in the community proper. Gangs themselves of course are ritualized behavior related to youth survival. They are also linked to the pain of youth in having been abandoned by adults whose task it is to initiate them into adulthood. This is perhaps the most devastating loss of meaningful ritual in our culture. Robert Bly often points out that in male youth gang culture, we are witnessing young people trying to initiate one another into adulthood because of this psychic abandonment.

The second element of our multi-variate model is the Individual. In examining the first element, Society, we used a sociological frame of understanding. Here, we will use biology and psychology, asking the same question: "Why? " For the answer, we will look for factors within the organism that seem to be precursors for addiction or substance abuse.

In the area of physiological or biological predisposition, there is little agreement among professionals, and they all have their research. We will begin with the area of genetics, since there is a strong research bias that genetic predisposition will become more important the more we learn about it.[49] Genetics is extremely complicated, with no exacts. There is research showing that an alcoholic mother or father predisposes their offspring to alcoholism at four to ten times the normal population, and as many as 75% of cocaine addicts have an alcoholic parent, but the correlation is not known.[50] There are a number of research avenues being taken concerning what, precisely, is likely inherited.

One theory concerns enzymes and/or enzyme deficiency. An enzyme is a protein, synthesized by cells, that induces chemical changes in other chemicals. It is a catalyst, apparently remaining unchanged itself in the process. Psychoactive drugs are broken down metabolically into non-toxic substances by the liver in an complex enzymatic process. Increased enzyme production is thought to be a mechanism of tolerance. In this enzymatic process, alcohol (C_2H_5OH) yields acetaldehyde (CH_3CHO), which yields acetic acid (CH_3COOH), which yields acetylcoa, which finally yields the non-toxic CO_2 H_2O, which the body can eliminate. The slowest phase of breakdown, from acetaldehyde to acetic acid, is induced by the enzymes that are collectively called *alcohol dehydrogenase*. It is here that genetic factors most likely play a role. One theory is that in a certain type of male (father-to-son) genetic alcoholic, the liver's inherent ability to produce alcohol dehydrogenase is abnormally high at the beginning of life, explaining this type of alcoholic's abnormally high tolerance early in his drinking career. But this inherent ability, independent of how much he may drink, declines throughout the life span to an abnormally low production level late in the drinking career. Therefore, what is inherited is a *progressive decrease in tolerance*. This is in contrast to the non-alcoholic's fairly consistent ability to produce alcohol dehydrogenase throughout his or her lifetime.

Another genetic candidate has been *tetrahydroisoquinoline* (THIQ). THIQ is an addictive substance produced in the neuron. It was initially thought to be activated only by opiate use, but researcher Virginia Davis of the University of Texas in 1964 discovered it in the brains of chronic alcoholics as well. It is now thought to be activated by a defect in the production of acetaldehyde, which may be an inherited trait. The most recent studies failed to replicate earlier ones, however, and so THIQ research remains largely speculative and unconfirmed.

Other genetic research concerns the ability to produce beta-endorphins, dopamine, and other *neurotransmitter* substances. Theoretically, endorphins, which are the body's "natural" or "endogenous opiates," act like hormones, which are body-regulating chemicals in the blood.[51] They act in a negative feedback relationship with the pituitary gland. They are a subset of a huge peptide compound released by the pituitary gland. There are ninety-one amino acids in the peptide chain; the last thirty-one, when cleaved, constitute endorphin. It is stored in the synaptic vesicle inside the neuron, and apparently released to ameliorate physical or emotional pain.[52] Rats become addicted to human endorphins as they would to an exogenous opiate.[53]

Psychoactive drugs interact with beta-endorphin and other neurotransmitter or "messenger" molecules and their receptor sites in a multiplicity of ways, and these neuronal pathways are the focus of some genetic researchers.[54] Belle Muschinske has developed a sensitivity theory of alcoholism[55] based on the premise that there are a high concentration of beta-endorphins in the limbic system, where we feel, mediating emotional as well as physical pain. It is Muschinske's theory that alcoholics have, by genetic predisposition, the receptor sites but not the neurotransmitters for which the receptors are designed. They are individuals who are hyper-sensitive. Many alcoholics describe the experience of the first drink in terms of something finally "fitting." They report "feeling whole" for the first time. We will discuss this existential sense of "intoxication" in some detail in the next chapter.

Cocaine also interacts with a variety of neurotransmitters. A principal one is dopamine. There are five dopamine receptors. One of them, the D_2 receptor, which is associated with euphoria, is formed by the al allele gene. Some research has found an excess of this gene in the blood of alcoholics and cocaine addicts,[56] although this research is currently controversial. An emerging hypothesis by the genetic research community is that genetic propensity may not be for alcoholism or other specific drug addictions but for some common phenotype connected with compulsive/obsessive behavior or "impaired control" in general.[57] Others take issue with this hypothesis, claiming that alcoholism and drug addiction are intrinsically different maladies than obsessive/compulsive disorders.[58]

The issue of individual differences in physiological drug sensitivity is of paramount interest. It is not known why certain individuals can use the most addictive substances with impunity, while others seemingly become addicted with their first exposures to the substance. It has been suggested that individuals with psychological or emotional tendencies toward drug addiction will experiment until they find things that work well.

Because of the anomalies produced by genetic research, (identical twins show differences in metabolism), the current thought is that there are different types of alcoholism/addiction, including gender (father-to-son, etc.). According to this theory, non-familial alcoholism (alcoholism with no genetic precursors) has a later onset and is more prompted by life events.

Besides genetic predisposition is the issue of fetal predisposition. We now know that exposure to psychoactive drugs causes discrete alterations in the developing neurological mechanisms, and that these mechanisms probably do not return to normal in adulthood. Therefore, since the placenta is not a barrier to psychoactive drugs, the drug-exposed fetus may theoretically be more susceptible to addiction upon later exposure to the same or similar drug.

Other intrinsic and individual physiological precursors to addiction may include such health factors as chronic intractable pain, especially low back pain, migraine, arthritis, and other forms that don't respond well to medically prescribed narcotics. These conditions place people at risk for addictive narcotic use through self-medication for these conditions.

The enterprise of looking for *psychological* factors that may predispose people to addiction is muddy water indeed, and is attended by a great deal of controversy and difficulty. In the field of psychology (an offspring of medicine and physics) we are, of course, dealing with *mind*, which is the fundamental template of Rationalism and its ultimate anomaly as well. It is also an enterprise that returns us to the central dilemma of control and volition, of which mind, in the "theology" of Exclusionary Rationalism, is thought to be the proper seat. Indeed, historically, all phenomena that Rationalism has not been able to explain in material, somatic, measurable terms has been cast off into the aberration called "mind." If, as we have maintained, the addictive process and the theology of Exclusionary Rationalism are in fact one and the same, it is the paradox of paradoxes to direct our rational attention here to ask, "why addiction? "

Rene Descartes, author of Rationalism, reached his conclusion, *cogito ergo sum*, through the process of *doubt*. He doubted his senses, the material world around him, religious faith, the reality of his organism. He concluded that the only thing he couldn't doubt was *the mind with which he was doubting*. "Mind" had to be the sole reality beyond doubt because how else could he doubt the rest? Descartes wrote, "I suppose...that all the things I see are false; I believe that none of those objects which my fallacious memory represents ever existed; I suppose that I possess no senses; I believe that body, figure, extension, motion, and place are merely fictions of my mind. I am - I exist: this is certain; but how often? As often as I think ...I am therefore, precisely speaking, only a thinking thing, that is, a mind." [59]

There are some curious yet profound implications in this reasoning. First, it is clear that, for Descartes, *mind* is the only reliable reality, the only thing that can be trusted. But there is a qualification. It can be trusted *only while engaged* in the process of *thinking*; otherwise, it is prone to weave *un*realities. Here, therefore, in the birth of Rationalism, is the incipient need for control (*i.e.*, volition). Modern science is born of Rationalism; therefore, the "science" of *abnormal psychology* is, by definition, *the study of the failure of volition or control.* Memory, dreams, associational thinking, and the stuff of the unconscious - all that is, by definition, *non*-rational - becomes at best problematic and at worst pathological. It was not, therefore, much of a leap for Freud, the father of psychoanalysis, to define mental health in essence as successful *repression* of these uncontrollable (irrational) tendencies of *mind*.[60] It was a logical extension of this "logic" to conclude, as rationalists have, that addiction is a loss of control over a substance or activity. The compulsive (pathological) state, is the state in which one has no control over when or how much.[61]

Here, the essentially political nature of modern Western medicine, in which Rationalism finds its most crystalline state, becomes salient.[62] Just as the Social Deviance model we described earlier defines substance abuse as deviation from a socially proscribed norm, so here addiction is defined as an irregularity of the proscribed state of *control.* Therefore, when the psychologist considers the etiology of addiction, it is, as Morris Berman has suggested of schizophrenia, a little like Alice entering Wonderland, a place where telling the queen that she is a bit loony is tantamount to losing one's head (see p. 70 and *n*110).

It is common for psychologists to account for the therapeutic mechanisms of Alcoholics Anonymous in the framework of attributing its success to such things as disclosure, secondary bonding, etc. However, as we have suggested earlier, A.A. has a curious and non-rational approach to the "aberration" of loss of control. Instead of requiring as a cure that the alcoholic make the rational move toward increased control (as Western treatment does), they go, as we have said, in the other direction and propose, as the antidote, *surrender.* The "cure," therefore, is *acceptance of the aberration.* In so doing, A.A. circuitously validates the inebriated state (the search for "wholeness"); Rationalism views intoxication in fact as the salient aberration. (Note that we are drawing a profound distinction between the *addictive* state and the *inebriated* state; addiction is the state of craving and obsession with control *preceding* inebriation.)

Given this perspective, it is perhaps not surprising that psychiatric disorder is a significant precursor to addiction. There is substantial Western research to indicate that the number of psychiatric disorders such as depression, character disorders (e.g. schizophrenia), and other behavioral or "learning disorders" are greater among alcoholics and their families than among the non-alcoholic population. For Western researchers the problem is, what precipitates what? It is important from this point of view to differentiate between what is called the "alcoholic" or "addictive" personality and the *clinical* alcoholic or addictive personality, a phrase used to describe those personality traits which are the logical manifestation of prolonged addictive use of the substance, traits which are, in other words, effects rather than causes.

Much of the search for precipitative or causative personality traits has been abandoned, and what remains is controversial.[63] One source of controversy is that much of the research has been done on sober members of A.A., and the mental health paradigm says that the A.A. group is by nature a different population than a clinical one. Nevertheless, the current psychological profile of the individual prone to addiction has been found by some research to be, in general, a brash personality lacking self-control. He/she is uninhibited, the "fool who rushes in where angels fear to tread." This individual tends to display the following characteristics:[64]

1. high interest in sensation seeking.
2. low self-esteem.
3. ineffective coping ability.
4. low psychological well-being.
5. ego deficiency.
6. regressive tendencies.

7. more rebellious, untrustworthy, and impulsive.

8. less self-reliant and ambitious.

These studies have been replicated. Little wonder! For these traits can be seen as the pre-addictive personality imprints of individuals who, for whatever reason, find themselves unable or unwilling to acquiesce to the addictive system. They do not accept the social, public version of reality presented by the paradigm of Exclusionary Rationalism and manifest in its institutions. They are individuals not unlike Alice in Wonderland, who, unable to reconcile her own identity in such a strange and nonsensical environment, ultimately follows the advice of the opium-intoxicated Caterpillar and reaches for a mushroom in her ardent desire to set things right!

One of the more popular writer/speakers who attempts to bring the insights of the recovery paradigm to this field of psychological predisposition is John Bradshaw.[65] Drawing upon the earlier work of Alice Miller[66] and others, it is Bradshaw's view that the developmental/psychodynamic precursors of addictive behavior are the low self-esteem and feelings of powerlessness and shame that are the legacies of being raised in a "dysfunctional" family. The psychic splitting off of the sense of self resulting from physical and sexual abuse and unvalidated childhood trauma forms the basis for addiction. Here we can again define addiction as the quest for regaining a lost sense of wholeness. Those who are the most disempowered have the highest self-destructive abuse potential. For Bradshaw, the disempowered, disowned, disenfranchised "inner child" of unresolved trauma continues to live on in the addict, outraged at having been abandoned by self. Whether one views this "inner child" as a genuine figure, or as an undeveloped aspect of self, or as archetype, or as a metaphor for the totality of one's organism (the unconscious and polarized "body" that was denied in the ascent to the disembodied mind), the addict's quest is to reclaim, through the senses, the lost part. Here, in what Bradshaw calls the "toxic shame" of pre-rational childhood, we see the passing of the Cartesian torch, the mechanism by which the legacy of

Exclusionary Rationalism is handed down generationally through the primary social institution of the family.

The third aspect of the multi-variate model is the <u>Substance</u> (or activity) to which one becomes addicted. Our question here is, if we search for the "why" of addiction, what answers are there in looking at addictive substances themselves as opposed to the society in which they are addictively used and the individual for whom they are addictive? Several experts were asked by *In Health* magazine to rate drugs as to addictive potential (November/December, 1990). Drugs were ranked on a scale of 100 to 1 based upon (1) how readily people get hooked and (2) how difficult most people find it to quit. The highest addictive potential was given to nicotine, followed closely by smoked methamphetamine ("ice") and by smoked cocaine ("crack"). Injected methamphetamine was next, followed by the benzodiazapine minor tranquilizer Valium. This was followed by Quaalude (methoqualone), Seconal (secobarbitol), and then alcohol, heroin, and oral amphetamine ("crank"). Powder cocaine was next, followed closely by caffeine. PCP (Phencyclidine) was in the medium range, and the drugs with the lowest addictive potential were ecstasy (MDMA), and the psychedelics: mushrooms, LSD, and mescaline (the psychoactive ingredient in peyote).

When we examine these psychoactive drugs as to "addictive potential," we can again use the sociological frame, discussing such things as *availability*. Availability as it relates to a drug's legal status is a concept important to both sides of the legalization debate, and also to "prevention philosophy." It is of interest that licit or illicit status seems to make a negligible difference when we compare the top four drugs in the ranking above as to addictive potential. We find the addictive potential of nicotine, the most available and legally sanctioned of those drugs listed, to rank in a similar category with crack cocaine, upon which the legal machinery of regulation and restriction has been so sharply mobilized and focused.

Still referring to the ranking by the experts above, we can also use a psychological frame and look at such things as the *primary reinforcement* potential of drugs: their ability to produce a rapid and dramatic euphoric state, which conditions the subject's likelihood to return to the experience again and again. The three most addictive drugs in the grouping, which are pharmacologically quite different, have in common the *route of administration*. All three are smoked, and smoking is the most efficient way of transporting a psychoactive substance to the site of action, the brain, which results in the quickest and most dramatic "high." In general, we can conclude that the steeper the absorption curve, the more intense the euphoria and crash, and the greater the addictive potential.

We can also go to "hard science" and use pharmacology as a frame for asking the question, "Why are some drugs more addicting than others? " And, it is to pharmacology that we now turn.[67]

We are going to limit our examination of this question to *psychoactive* drugs, drugs for which the "site of action" is the central nervous system (CNS). From a clinical perspective, however, it is important to note that while it is because of their effect on the CNS that these drugs are sought and prone to addictive use, it is not generally to their psychoactive nature that the common adverse medical consequences (the lesion) can be ascribed.

All psychoactive drugs act by gaining access to neural tissue where they alter the transmission process. While some psychoactive drugs have their effect by simulating a state of acute stress, there are many discrete differences between stress and drug-induced states. But *fear* and many psychoactive drugs elicit nearly the same physiological response.

Pharmacology comes from the Greek *pharmakon*, a word which meant originally both *medicine* and *poison*. Pharmacology includes both pharmacokinetics and pharmacodynamics. *Pharmacokinetics* is concerned with the mathematical distribution of the drug in the body. All drugs distribute differentially; some penetrate tissue easily, and others do not. Medically, this is the study of fine tuning fairly toxic drugs. *Pharmacodynamics* is the study of how much of a drug is required to get a response ("log dose response"). The dose required to elicit a response is based on the height, weight, age, sex, etc. of the user.

Other basic terms used to describe the effects of drugs are *acute, chronic,* and *latent.* Acute effects are those that occur right after the absorption into the body of a single dose. Chronic effects are those caused by continued use of the drug over time,[68] and latent effects are residual or protracted effects, those chronic effects that were originally unobserved but which become manifest after drugs are eliminated.

The length of time a drug remains in the system is measured in terms of the drug's *half-life.* The half-life is the length of time required for a drug to decrease by one-half in the body due to enzymatic breakdown and elimination by the kidneys. Five half-lives are required to ineffectiveness. Half-lives vary based upon the drug taken and the route of administration. The half-life of cocaine is one hour when taken intranasally; Valium, taken orally, is twelve hours, and smoked marijuana's half-life is three days.

When two or more drugs are taken at once, one drug may increase the effect of another. This is called *potentiation;* if one drug inhibits the effect of another, it is called *inhibition.* Addicts, naturally, go for potentiators, not inhibitors.

There are three primary factors influencing a drug's psychoactive effects. The first is *intensity.* This is not necessarily the strength of the dose, but more important the *concentration of the pharmacologically active substance at the site of action.* The second factor is *tolerance.* A drug's effects will vary greatly between someone who is "drug-naive" - who has never taken the drug before - and someone who has developed a tolerance to the drug's effects. What might be a lethal dose for one individual could be a typical dose for a seasoned addict. Note also that tolerance is a possible genetic marker for alcoholism and addiction, hence, a drug-naive subject with a genetic predisposition would have a different response than a drug-naive subject without this predisposition.

The third primary factor is the *route of administration.* There are four general routes by which drugs are administered: 1) *oral,* 2) *across mucous membranes,* 3) *inhalation,* and 4) *injection.*

Oral administration is the least effective. Drugs taken orally must pass first through the stomach, intestines, and liver, where many of their molecules metabolize even before reaching the sites of action in the brain. This is called the *"first pass effect."* That portion of the drug surviving the first pass effect then passes by way of the blood to the heart, the lungs, back to the heart, and finally to the site of action, minimizing the effects of oral drug use. An exception is alcohol, unique in that it is easily absorbed through the stomach and intestinal walls into the bloodstream.

Intranasal administration across mucous membranes typically involves "snorting," and includes "sniffing" (which is the common route of administration of amyl nitrite, glue, and gasoline). Other routes of administration through mucous membranes include sublingual, anal, genital, and urethral ingestion, which are more efficient than oral ingestion because the intestinal track is bypassed.

Inhalation is an even more efficient route of administration. If a substance is smoked, it travels first to the lungs, and then to the heart. Then the drug is distributed directly to the brain, three to five seconds following ingestion. The better the lung capacity, the more risk of damage. Cocaine is an anesthetic, and the crack Cocaine over-dose syndrome in athletes results from an enormous anesthetic jolt to the heart.

The fourth route of administration is injection. This is the most dangerous because there is no natural barrier for toxic impurities. Many intravenous (IV) "drug overdoses" are not from the drug but from other substances with which the drug has been mixed or "cut." Besides IV injection, there is subcutaneous injection, common for beginning heroin addicts, and intramuscular, which is not particularly effective because muscles are such dense tissue.

Other factors can complicate drug distribution. Some drugs stay in the bloodstream because the blood has binding sites to which some drugs inherently bind, while others do not. Some drugs, like alcohol, distribute almost uniformly to every cell. Most, however, distribute unevenly, depending upon the drug's ability to permeate various membranes. A few drugs concentrate in one or more tissues or organs. Fats attract non-polar drugs, such as tetrahydrocannabinol (THC), the active ingredient in marijuana; THC will bind and hold to fat tissue for 45 days or longer.

Drugs are eliminated by the liver and the kidneys. The liver is a very resilient organ. An individual can maintain normal life functions on 10% liver capacity. The liver has a multitude of functions, with natural detoxification is among them. Red blood cells are manufactured in the bone marrow and live 120 days. When they fragment, they die and go to the liver where they are broken down and reformed into bile (which is collected in the gall bladder, coloring feces and urine). In the process, these fragmented red blood cells, having been cleaning up for 120 days, are detoxified by the liver. When the liver is busy detoxifying alcohol or other toxic drugs, the dead red blood cells back up.

Other minor pathways of elimination are the sweat, lungs, and feces.

The liver also breaks down female hormones in men and male hormones in women. This process is arrested by chronic drug use, sometimes resulting in sexual dysfunction and gender preference confusion.

Metabolism is the complex enzymatic process by which all substances taken into the body are broken down. In the case of drugs, it is a process of chemical changes that alter the drugs and convert them to substances that can be eliminated. In this sense, detoxification is the natural process of making substances non-poisonous, with the effect of changing the configuration of the drug molecule to make it more water soluble so it can be eliminated by the kidneys. Both conjugation reactions and chemical reactions are involved, and the chemical process is rarely one step. It is usually three, four or five steps. In urine testing for drugs (*chemical assay*), it is generally not the presence of the drug itself that is detected, but rather the presence of a metabolite of the drug.

These are the primary steps by which alcohol is detoxified: **Ethyl Alcohol > acetaldehyde > acetic acid > CO_2+H_2O**. There is a rate-limiting step in every chemical reaction. The rate-limiting step in the example above is alcohol > acetaldehyde. The drug *Antabuse* (disulfiram) causes a build-up of the very toxic acetaldehyde by preventing its normal metabolism. This drug is used in treatment to control an alcoholic's drinking by eliciting vomiting when any alcohol is ingested.

Factors that affect liver metabolism include, of course, the functionality of liver. Carbon fragments from smoking affects metabolism. These byproducts of smoking induce liver enzyme production, which causes drugs to be metabolized quicker. It takes six to eight weeks after smoking cessation for the enzymes to return to normal. Liver enzyme production is also induced by alcohol, barbiturates, and dilantin (an anti-seizure drug). Metabolism is complicated when more than one drug is taken. Sometimes, drugs compete for enzymes in a random, one-on-one fashion. In other drug combinations, one drug (such as Antabuse) may have an affinity for the enzyme, in which the enzyme action depends upon gross drug concentration.

Following successful drug detoxification, the detoxified substance is carried by the blood to the kidney, where it is eliminated either through active secretion or by glomerular filtration. The kidney resembles a giant filter, while the liver more resembles a machine. They work in concert. If the kidney can eliminate a substance without breaking it down, it does. Its success decreases with age, the average glomerular filtration rate decreasing by half by age 60.

Our journey through this "multi-variate" view of addiction has left us in something of a wonderland of great complexity. It is a distinctly linear complexity, however. And even at that, we have only barely scratched the technical surface of the Western "hard edge" of addiction. There is more hard Western science ahead when we begin to look at the substrates, pathways, and mechanisms of individual drugs. In the meantime, let's try to cover ground similar to that just covered from a less linear perspective - using a different looking glass to see if we can find what the Taoists call a radical center in which to stand.

A principal map used to describe this addiction-recovery frontier process is the map of Alcoholics Anonymous (A.A.), which is the prototype of the Twelve Step programs that also include Narcotics Anonymous (N.A.), Cocaine Anonymous (C.A.), and many others addressing other substance and non substance addictions (see Appendix VI for a complete list of recovery resources). There are those who find fault with this Twelve Step map. Their criticisms include that people get "stuck" in A.A.;[69] that they are just trading one addiction for another (the Twelve Step group itself); that people in A.A. just talk about drinking all the time and never get past that; that people in A.A. notoriously abuse and validate the abuse of the drugs nicotine, caffeine, and sugar; that A.A. is exclusionary; that people use A.A. to avoid taking responsibility for their past behaviors, and that A.A. smacks of religion and of the myth of patriarchy[70] from which addiction in large part sprang.

All of these observations deserve discussion, and we will examine them at some length in later chapters. The fact remains, however, that A.A., with all of its shortcomings, is probably the best map we have to date of the landscape of recovery, so we will seek its wisdom and usefulness in spite of its shortcomings.

This metaphor of frontier is apropos for describing the process of recovery from addiction. In our introduction to this section, we suggested that frontier exploration involves the tasks of studying extant maps, and of establishing a center. In geographical frontiering, this center serves as a base of operations to which one can return for essential supplies and sustenance. It also serves as a baseline reference for keeping perspective about one's location, and for making new maps.

Recovery, likewise, is a *venturing out from a known center*. The venturing is based upon faith, in combination, of course, with somewhat accurate maps! However, the area we map in recovery is not three dimensional or linear terrain, but intra-psychic, or what is often called a "spiritual" landscape. We cannot come to an understanding of the recovery process without a careful consideration of this landscape of internal consciousness.

The first and most basic lesson in venturing into this process is the Rationalist's anathema that *truth lies in paradox.*[71] Among the first paradoxes of recovery is that while it is in essence a process of venturing out, it is, at the same time, a process of more and more profound *center-seeking*, coming to know one's center in a deeper and deeper way. There is a center-seeking and a certain mastery of the center required, and this is where the recovery journey begins. And, the center - like centers from which other frontiers are explored - is an ever-expanding one as the journey develops.

In the Twelve Step "map," the center clearly begins with one's relationship with the substance or activity to which one has been addicted. So, in the case of A.A., it is to drinking, to the substance alcohol, that the alcoholic's attention and focus is first invited.[72] This *relationship* with the substance must transform if recovery is to be achieved, and this transformation cannot occur unless drinking is placed at the center of attention in the early or transition period of recovery.

What we seek is what Thomas Kuhn has called a *paradigm shift*,[73] or what the Upanishads called a *turning in the deep seat of consciousness.*[74] From a more clinical point of view, this turning is *away* from dependence upon the substance or activity of addiction and *toward* inner healing resources,[75] or, paradoxically, away from the inner psychic state of isolation and toward outward acceptance of the tools and resources that will support recovery.

In this turning, recovery and transformation are handmaidens. The first potential "stuck point" is in hoping for one without the other. Transformation cannot occur without recovery, and recovery cannot occur without transformation. To seek recovery without transformation is to hold on to the old ideas of control; to seek transformation without recovery is to look for the "magic fix," the miracle without the "footwork." It is to continue in the belief that the solution is "out there" rather than in owning and participating in one's own life process. The "life process" to be "owned" is, in this case, the relationship with the substance of addiction.

Some recovering alcoholics report that the change in their relationship to alcohol occurs in an instant in which the obsession to
drink is lifted. It is likely that this "magic" instant arises, like
Satori in Buddhism, from a context of patience and education and
hard work over the time preceding it.[76]

By what mechanism does this gestalt switch in perception, this
"paradigm shift," happen? According to the map we are currently
following, it happens in one's induction into the so-
cial/psychological milieu that is A.A., and as a result of taking the
first three of A.A.'s suggested Twelve Steps of recovery:[77]

1. We admitted we were powerless over alcohol - that our
    lives had become unmanageable.
2. Came to believe that a power greater than ourselves could
    restore us to sanity.
3. Made a decision to turn our will and our lives over to the
    care of God *as we understood Him.*

The anthropologist Gregory Bateson, in his study of theories of
learning, became interested in the process of how A.A. works, in
what we might call its "therapeutic mechanisms." [78] He concluded
that the practicing alcoholic has but two strings on his or her gui-
tar: rigidity and collapse. The individual knows that he or she
needs to stop, or, more wishfully, *change the manner* of (e.g.
control) his or her, drinking.[79] The seat of motivation for this is
naturally perceived, of course, as *will* or conscious volition. It just
makes sense, rationally. After all, in the chronic stage, one's relationships, job, moral integrity, physical health, and so on are
greatly compromised and threatened. And so, in the rigidity phase,
the alcoholic moves toward self-imposed abstinence.

In this system of understanding, the rational and superior *will*
(mind) must take charge or control of the weak and wayward *flesh*
(body) in the classic sense of Cartesian dualism. One is divided
against one's self in an earnest life and death struggle. The importance given this struggle by the alcoholic's peers and significant
others and employer and so forth further reinforce and entrench the
position and serve to enhance the resolve of will. This state of ri-

gidity is what is called "white knuckle sobriety" in A.A.. It is a state in which victory over the substance alcohol is seen as possible *through an act of volition.*

We can see clearly that the Rationalistic view of alcoholism that we have described earlier is a view fiercely endorsed by the alcoholic him/herself. The alcoholic's contest of will implies that the substance alcohol is an external invading force (pathogen), and hence the essential focus of the battle being waged. This imbuing of the morally inert substance with anthropomorphic quality is similar to the previously discussed semantic implications of the phrase "substance *abuse*," which implies that the actually neutral chemical alcohol, and not the individual "abuser," is the object of the harm that is being done. This awkward myth becomes Kuhn's "ambiguous figure" about which a "gestalt switch in perception" is required in order that the substance alcohol may ultimately be placed in its proper position of *neutrality.*

So, our Batesonian alcoholic, in a state of rigidity, begins a trek through self-imposed abstinence, having sworn off from (and avowing victory over) the empowered enemy alcohol. Morris Berman points out that "this Cartesian paradigm isolates the alcoholic and tries to ascertain the cause which is producing the undesirable effect. (The) assumption (is one) of direct linear influence based on the model of 17th-century impact physics in which mind is explicitly conscious and external to matter." [80]

This trek is unsuccessful, according to Bateson, because the organism in its totality is a homeostatic, balance-seeking system and cannot long endure an imposed and arbitrary (mind/body) dualism of this sort.[81] In desperation at his/her discomfort, in order to relieve the pressure, the alcoholic says to him/herself, "how about a little controlled drinking? "

This too is impossible, of course, since an alcoholic, by A.A.'s definition, is one who has *lost the ability to control* his or her drinking. Thus, our alcoholic's attempts at "a little controlled drinking" fail, and he or she gets drunk and moves from the state of rigidity to the state of *collapse.* The Cartesian dualism breaks, the organism heaves a great sigh of relief, and the alcoholic again feels that he or she is at one with the physical universe. Not only does the inner dualism collapse, but the sense of isolation from self/other that accompanies addiction also collapses. The alcoholic often finds the old companionship with fellow drinkers that has been lost in abstinence.[82] Feelings and personal history can be shared with others, and pretenses dropped. What Bateson calls a "pseudo-holism" is achieved. This pseudo-holism, according to Bateson, is actually the *more correct state*! Note that we again draw a sharp distinction between the *addictive* state and the *inebriated* state, defining addiction as the state of rigidity and craving *preceding* inebriation.[83]

What is wrong with this state of pseudo-holism is, of course, that it is chemically induced. It is veiled. And the alcoholic, regardless of the degree of holistic pleasure and relief, knows that this inebriated state is the result of having ingested the drug, which further reinforces the drinking behavior and entrenches the hopelessness that gives rise to further rigidity when the drinking episode is over.

And so it becomes a closed cycle.

According to Bateson, the central wisdom of A.A. is that it provides a third alternative to rigidity and collapse, which is *surrender*. This comes quintessentially with the admission of *powerlessness* over the substance. Instead of being faced with a contest that one is to win, the alcoholic is asked to accept "defeat." [84]

This is not rational, and, as we have noted earlier, has caused skeptics to conclude that A.A. breeds irresponsibility. This conclusion derives from our impulsive fear that if this surrender is made, the seat of rational "will" and hence volition and control will fall away to the great void and be lost. This is, of course, partially true. What is false about that assumption is that "mind" (the conscious center of attention and volition located halfway between the ears and a little bit behind the eyes) is the sole locus of intelligence and power in the organism.[85] This is the unifying theological tenet of the disembodied mind. What has been forgotten is that there is, in fact, a real power greater than that precise and invented sense of self.

As Morris Berman describes, the admission of powerlessness in A.A.'s First Step "undercuts Cartesian dualism in a single stroke." When the newcomer says, at the A.A. meeting, "My name is John/Mary, and I'm an alcoholic," the dualism that has placed alcohol somehow *outside* of the personality collapses, and the alcoholism is internalized and conceded to be part of the personality. "The symmetrical battle evaporates without (the alcoholic's) getting drunk." [86]

Thus we have begun at a center of consciousness which involves the alcoholic's relationship with drinking. A.A. "newcomer meeting" experiences are dominated by what is called the "drunkalogue," in which one's drinking history (relationship with alcohol) is reviewed in ever increasing depth and detail. These stories typically reinforce the alcoholic's powerlessness, reinforcing how unmanageable one's life had become. They consequently reinforce the newly attained deeper center, and enhance the process of dissolution of the ego in its aspect of control.[87] "Reinforcement," in the classic learning sense, is an apt description of this process, since one is *relearning* one's relationship with the substance. This is a very painful process, and the center is slippery, a learning and a forgetting, usually characterized by relapses or "slips." A process that may, in the abstract, require only three to six months to "get," can therefore take several years, as the obstinate rational ego relinquishes the seat of control.[88]

This is reminiscent of the *learning-as-forgetting* in Wordsworth's "Ode: On Intimations of Mortality." It is a learning but a forgetting of the alcoholic (*i.e.*, Rationalist or addictive) state, which has, in personal historical time, been superimposed upon the pre-addictive state. In its highest sense, this is a childlike venturing out toward new growth, literally a "rebirth" of an earlier, pre-rational innocence.[89]

And the center itself can now be seen as subtly expanding beyond *relationship with alcohol* to include *relationship with self*. This is not the old "self-as-mind" in isolation,[90] but the new, deeper, emerging, reconstituted or rediscovered self. As this new self is realized, the center expands again to include its next concentric layer, *self-other*, because, in reality, things (such as self) have meaning only in relationship. Nothing exists in fact in isolation. That the alcoholic has felt him or herself to exist in isolation has been an illusion. This is manifested in step two in which the alcoholic's existential field is joined by some power beyond self (a power other than the previous "companion" alcohol).[91]

Berman assumes this power to be the unconscious, (which, in the Reichian view, is the same as *body*).[92] Subjectively, some A.A. newcomers conceive this power-greater-than-self as the A.A. group as a whole, or as God. It is in this regard that A.A. is often accused of being religious because of the use of prayer and the word "God" at most meetings. This has also earned criticism in that God, for uninitiated females and for people of color, automatically calls up the (White) patriarchal God of the sexist culture which Exclusionary Rationalism has itself produced and promulgated.[93] The fact is that many recoverers do indeed become stuck at this stage. We need to remind ourselves that this map we are describing is imperfect, and useful, and that this stage of recovery is *transitional*. We will explore this issue at depth in Chapter Seven, but the point here is that the sources of inner healing will remain inaccessible and blocked so long as the false sense of self as *controlling ego* is held. Surrender to *something* else is the homeostatic need of the moment. The vacuous and ego-dissolving state of powerlessness admitted in step one *requires* a step two of *faith in the possibility of wholeness without drugs*. There will be ample time later in recovery for a more sophisticated refinement and consciousness of the exact nature of the power to whom or to which one surrenders. As A.A. suggests, "first things first." People need to be free to negotiate these first three steps in whatever cultural framework is useful for them, hence the qualifying phrase, *"as we understood Him"*[94] following the word "God" in the Third Step.

The fundamental Cartesian dualism we described earlier of "white knuckle sobriety" - the *rigid addictive system* that springs from Exclusionary Rationalism, - is in fact a *two-fold dualism* extending from *mind/body* to *self/other*. This self/other split constitutes the foundation for the isolation that characterizes addiction. Notice that this psychic splitting off is the basis for but not the same as addiction. The unvalidated trauma with which it is associated is the precursor for addiction; addiction itself can be seen as trying to get back to the lost state of wholeness.

Historically, this self/other split also constitutes the basis for modern science, which can be seen as another *implication* of Rationalism and for which the philosophy of Rationalism provided a pedestal. At the heart of modern science was what Morris Berman calls the "myth of objectivity," in which the field of observation was seen as a process distinct from the perception of the observer. According to this myth - which has now become a *theology* - it is believed that genuine isolation is not only possible but is, in fact, the *desired* state. In scientific experimentation, for example, one seeks above all else objectivity, seeks to stand as far back from the field of observation as possible in order that all experimental variables can be isolated. In this fashion, "objective truth" can be discerned.[95]

In step two in the alcoholic's recovery, in the rejoining of self/other, is intimated the hope of *sanity* (from the Latin *sanus* which means "whole"). Carl Jung, in a letter to A.A. co-founder Bill Wilson, called the "craving for alcohol the equivalent on a low level of the spiritual thirst of our being for wholeness, expressed in medieval language: the union with God." [96] Here, at steps two and three, Bateson's "pseudo-holism" of the collapsed (drunken) state becomes a *genuine* wholeness which was the alcoholic's search all the time. This is what is meant when A.A. gently counsels the newcomer, "don't leave before the miracle happens!"

And so the center, the "turning in the seat of consciousness," the "gestalt switch in perception" or "paradigm shift," is not static, but rather a dynamic, expanding, outward-reaching process of rediscovery of an earlier truth as the new self emerges in relationship.

The A.A. historian Ernest Kurtz, whose notion of modernity we have previously mentioned, chose an apt title indeed for his book, *Not-God*. The quintessential discovery for the alcoholic in the early phase of recovery is that the disembodied mind - the addicted self (ego), the old seat of conscious attention and volition - is Not-God. Paramount to the rigid addictive system is that it *thinks* it's God. *Cogito ergo sum.*[97]

Thus the addict/alcoholic, in the venturing out from the expanding center, begins to view his/her malaise for the first time in the *context of a larger system.* The malaise is not of the addict's singular invention, but instead a function of a larger matrix. This begins with a reflection on personal history in step four: "(we) took a fearless and searching moral inventory of ourselves." [98] Properly taken, this helps the alcoholic begin to see that his or her addictive state did not occur in a vacuum, in isolation, but was conceived and grew in the context of a larger system. The addiction, genetic predisposition notwithstanding, was *learned.* It can be viewed as an inheritance or legacy of one's "inherently addictive" (or "dysfunctional") family system.

A torch was passed.

Here is perhaps the most common "stuck point" in recovery, as the traditional Fourth Step is often not seen as a container large enough to address this essential phase of establishing the context in which the addictive behavior developed. This process often gets addressed, therefore, outside of the A.A. group, in psychotherapy, or in an ancillary Twelve Step group such as Adult Children of Alcoholics (ACA), Codependents Anonymous (CoDA), Incest Survivors Anonymous (ISA),[99] or perhaps in an "inner child" workshop.[100]

This expansion of focus, which begins with the Fourth Step and moves through the next five steps,[101] can also be undergone prematurely before the alcoholic is fully centered in the new "seat of consciousness." Sometimes the material that comes up is too psychically painful to be processed, and can trigger relapse.[102] Or, the recovering person may become overwhelmed with self-pity, and get "stuck" in the seductive status of "victim" of family dysfunction or trauma.

What is required clinically at this stage is that the recovering person own and process and resolve and then move past the anger, or what we have called the "pre-cognitive rage" which is, in the dysfunctional family system, the precursor of the addictive state. Much has been written about the dynamics of unvalidated and unresolved trauma, and the consequent "psychic splitting off" of self.[103] Suffice it to say that, in the landscape of recovery, the recovering person has now moved from a position of perceiving the addictive phenomenon as having occurred *in isolation* toward seeing it as *a larger process.* One also comes to see that the "torch" of dysfunction was passed not only in one's own personal history but indeed *generationally*, for the dysfunction of one's own family of immediate origin itself grew from an earlier dysfunctional system.[104]

This can be validating for the recoverer. The great operational barrier to treatment and recovery is the social stigma which our (inherently addictive) society has placed upon addiction in general and alcoholism in particular. Clinical treatment is, in fact, in the transition stage, primarily concerned with addressing this issue of stigma which society imposes from without and which the addict endorses and imposes from within. Viewing alcoholism and addiction as *primary disease entities* is helpful in this regard. Also helpful is the view that the alcoholic or addict is a *survivor* rather than a *victim* of the precipitating family dysfunction.[105]

There is yet a further source of validation for the recovering addict, and a further source of understanding of the nature of addiction. This lies in the discovery that, just as the individual addict's dysfunction did not begin in a void but rather in the larger context of the multi-generational family, so the family itself did not become dysfunctional in a social vacuum. It drew its addictive rigidity from an even larger system of dysfunction, which is the cultural milieu which Ernest Kurtz calls "modernity."

An even larger torch, in other words, was passed, and the center of recovery naturally expands to include this largely uncharted terrain.

The family, though the primary institution and hence the primary purveyor of cultural values in society, is not the sole architect of those values. It draws them in large measure from historical and cultural systemic forces as they become manifest in science, religion, education, media, literature and the arts, political and economic institutions, and so on.

This is to say that what Anne Wilson Schaef often calls "the underground river of addiction," which is endemic in our society today, threatening the very fabric of all of the institutions mentioned above, has come about in an historical context. It is to that context that we now turn in our map-making.

Let us put our A.A. map aside, and turn to two familiar works of fiction that may provide helpful analogies or frames for understanding the themes of addiction and recovery in the field of this larger context. These two books have in common that their appeal has been to children. They also both provide images that have pervaded modern popular culture.

The first is Frank Baum's *The Wonderful Wizard of Oz*, written in 1900. 1900 marked the end of what Mark Twain called "The Gilded Age" in American history, the opulent decade of the 1890s. This period, in which the Industrial Revolution in the United States reached its zenith, was characterized by the unbridled ascent of the corporate monopoly. This was the period in which were amassed the fortunes of the Carnegies, Rockefellers, and Morgans. It was also the period of the emergence of cities and the end of the agricultural frontier. The era was accompanied by a series of Federal Presidential administrations (with notable corruption) dedicated to protecting and enhancing this prodigious growth.

This was a period, as Twain's characterization implies, overlain with gold. What lay beneath was greed and the exploitation and abuse of people and resources. The philosophical justification for these improprieties was provided in part by the tenets of the philosophy contained in the historical era of Enlightenment,[106] and by Social Darwinism, a convolution of Darwinian scientific theory in which the rich were thought to be "naturally selected" by God and consequently endowed with unlimited license to exploit the continent and all of its resources. The earlier and complementary religious belief in Manifest Destiny assisted this effort as well, by providing a platform for imperialist expansion in the Western United

States, South America, and the Far East. This phase of geographical expansion peaked with the Spanish American War of 1898 (though it has continued ideologically and politically through the present day).

This was the form modernity had taken in the 1890s. From each movement in history, there is a counter-movement, for each culture a counter-culture. The form this counter-culture had taken by 1900 included a political movement called *Populism*. Populism opposed the protectionist economic policies of the Eastern banking establishment, and the Western mining and railroad monopolies. In its inception, it had been largely a farmer's movement and a farmer's political party. Its demise as an autonomous movement came in 1912 with the election of the Democrat Woodrow Wilson, who defeated the then Third Party Progressive candidate Teddy Roosevelt and who ultimately adopted several Populist planks in his political platform. It is the fate of counter-cultures is to become occluded, absorbed, co-opted by that which they originally opposed. This is a salient aspect of the addictive system.

Populism, as a political party dominated by farmers, had found an early leader in Mary Ellen Lease, remembered for her advice that "farmers should raise less corn and more hell." The party was strongest in such states as the Dakotas and Nebraska and Kansas and Wyoming. These states were also among the first to grant women's suffrage, and so we find early feminist strains in this counter-cultural movement.

Frank Baum, the author of *The Wonderful Wizard of Oz*, lived in North Dakota, and he was a Populist. In fact, *The Wonderful Wizard* has been given a political reading by some critics in which the wicked witches represent respectively the banking interests of the East and the mining interests of the West (the demand for the free and unlimited coinage of silver was a central Populist theme).

Also of relevance is that in the history of children's literature in general, *The Wonderful Wizard of Oz* can be seen as among the first children's books in which the *inner world of the child* was given free reign, was seen as legitimate and valid thematic material in its own right. Included in this revolution in children's literature are Lewis Carrol's *Alice's Adventures in Wonderland* (1865) and *Alice Through the Looking Glass* (1872), and some of Beatrix Potter's work written between 1900 and 1910. Most children's stories before that time, and many since, were *pedantic* in nature. They were designed primarily to instruct rather than entertain. Their tacit goal was to teach children how to be more "grown-up" (rational), either by way of a "moral" at the end, or by some other more or less subtle means of fear and manipulation. In this sense, both Dorothy in *The Wizard* and Alice in *Wonderland* validate the child's pre- or non-rational paradigm.

Coincidentally perhaps, *The Wonderful Wizard of Oz* was written while the first federal laws against narcotics were being enacted. These laws limited the manufacture and sale of opium. Opium, of course, derives from the poppy, and, in the book, it was a field of poppies that represented the last of a number of barriers that the Wicked Witch of the West placed between Dorothy and the Emerald City of Oz.

The poppy field proved an ineffective barrier, however, because, as Emily Dickenson had written a few decades earlier, "narcotics cannot still the tooth / that nibbles at the soul." And, it could certainly be said, in the Jungian sense, that Dorothy and her companions were "soul-searching." What the Tin Woodsman, the Scarecrow, and the Lion each sought in the Emerald City - what they "thirsted for" - was that part of themselves that was "missing" - to fill the inner ("split-off") emptiness: respectively, a heart, a brain, and courage. What Dorothy sought was home. Her center.

When they arrived after great trials in the Emerald city and were at last admitted to the inner chamber of the great (patriarchal) Wizard of Oz, whom they hoped would restore them to wholeness and grant their wishes, they would learn the first great lesson of recovery from addiction, that, as we have said, *truth lies in paradox.* They would learn another great lesson as well (which is itself perhaps *the* fundamental paradox): *what they were looking* for *they were looking* with.

Put another way, "God" was hiding in the last place they would have thought to look - not behind the curtain in the Wizard's chamber manipulating the magic machine, but *inside* of them! What Dorothy's companions most desired (and thought they lacked), they already had. Through Baum's marvelous irony, it had already been revealed that it was the Woodman's stout heart, the Scarecrow's superior intelligence, and the Lion's great courage that had delivered the group more than once from harm's way. And while the Wizard, by his own admission, was a very bad wizard, he was not a bad man. And, he was a very good teacher (or, we could say, a good *sponsor*), for he was able to convey to each of these three searchers that the thing they most sought was something they already had. And so they learned, to turn it around, that the "fix" was not "out there."

Of course, it takes Baum's Goddess archetype Glinda, the Good Witch of the North (Mary Ellen Lease?), to reveal to Dorothy that she doesn't have to worry about getting back to Kansas because she never really left at all. She is not to be beguiled by all of this glitter ("somewhere," as Hollywood later embellished, "over the rainbow"), nor by the empty authority of the charlatan Wizard, whose power was based upon misrepresentation. Her true happiness and bliss instead lay in her own backyard.[107] But the "home" to which she returns is not the dysfunctional (distant father + helpless mother = anger not expressed) adoptive-family in Kansas. If we view her companions as representing unaccessed parts of herself - courage, love, and wisdom - the "home" to which she may now return, initiated, is her true and whole self. As A.A. folk wisdom would later declare, "it's an *inside* job." The lessons for the Oz travelers, of course, do not come magically, but are hard won through the process of securing the (magic) broomstick of the wicked witch of the West.

Thus we have, in *The Wonderful Wizard of Oz*, written thirty-five years before the inception of Alcoholics Anonymous, a counter-cultural response to the form that modernity had taken in 1900, and a profound and revolutionary recognition and validation of the pre-rational consciousness of the child. We offer it here as a *pre-recovery metaphor*, a partial map of the center of recovery consciousness. The degree to which it has survived and flourished in popular culture is testament to the resonance of its transcendent motif.

We are developing the case that recovery from addiction represents a *paradigm shift.*[108] "Paradigm" is a word we have been using to describe both the addictive and the recovery systems. A paradigm, according to research psychologist Julian Silverman, is simply "the way we organize data to look at a problem." [109] This is a very significant concept, particularly if one is a research psychologist! - for it is easy to see that the way in which one organizes data to look at a problem in psychology will have a profound impact upon the *conclusions* one draws. Silverman's research was at Agnew State Mental Hospital in San Jose, California, in the late 1960s and early 1970s, before such facilities were closed, relegating the responsibility for their patients from the state to local communities.

The specific problem under discussion for Silverman and his colleagues at that time was schizophrenia. In this field of research psychology, the paradigm that was "shifting" in the late 1960s was away from the view that schizophrenia and acute psychotic reaction were pathologies or "illnesses" in the classic sense, and toward the view that these were symptoms of acute, stress-induced learning experiences. What was occurring, from the point of view of this new paradigm, was that the essentially sane subject was in a process of adaptation to an essentially *in*sane society.[110] These ideas came to be expressed most eloquently perhaps by the psychiatrist R.D. Laing,[111] and of course were popularized in Ken Keysey's *One Flew Over the Cuckoo's Nest.*

Gregory Bateson, whose work with early alcoholism recovery we have already discussed, also became involved in this paradigmatic shift in the assessment of schizophrenia. But a larger theme of his work was in the nature of paradigms themselves. His work contributed to a significant illumination of what we have described earlier as the scientific "myth of objectivity."

Bateson's initial awareness in these matters came from his field work in anthropology, studying non-industrialized native cultures. The classical scientific premise in this sort of work was that, as an objective observer, one could derive knowledge about a culture's customs, beliefs, and so on. As his work developed, Bateson became aware that his presence among these people as an "outside observer" was influencing the behavior he was observing, making objectivity impossible. Moreover, he became aware that, no matter how consciously he tried to be objective, his own cultural values and beliefs acted as a screen, influencing his conclusions. These conclusions, therefore, rather than being objective, were inescapably *subjective*. He was viewing the field through a "looking glass" that he was unable to take off. He realized, in other words, he could not remove himself entirely from the field of observation, either inwardly or outwardly. True objectivity was in fact an impossibility.[112]

The paradigm of scientific objectivity so pervades consciousness, however, that the illusion appears real. Rationalist conditioning causes us to repress the reality of participation between the observer and the observed, the reality that one is *in* and hence also *of* the field, and can never move back far enough to be "outside looking in."

One way to demonstrate this is by Bateson's following illustration, a variation of "Epimenides' Paradox," also called the "Liar's Paradox." [113]

```
┌─────────────────────────────────────┐
│     All Statements within this frame │
│            are untrue.               │
└─────────────────────────────────────┘
```

The rational intellect, trained in the paradigm of modern science, rebels at this configuration. It becomes, the longer one studies it, the same order of nonsense riddles that made Alice so crazy in her adventures in Wonderland. The question is, *where* is the craziness, the insanity, the nonsense? Is it in the field, in what one sees "through the looking glass? " Is it in the statement in the box, or is it in the "eye of the beholder? "

One recalls the *magus* figure in *Alice in Wonderland*, the perched caterpillar blowing smoke rings (of, not coincidentally, opium). Alice shares with the caterpillar her confusion, and seeks answers to the many questions she has. The caterpillar responds with the unsettling, "*who* are *you*? "

"Who? " indeed. If one tries to define oneself by external, conventional, objective, rational referents, all comes up nonsense. Alice's attention is directed by the wise (though somewhat stoned) Caterpillar to where the answer lies, which is, as it was for Dorothy, within herself.

To our riddle, the intellect seems to demand the answer to a very simple question: Is the statement in the box true or untrue? Where is the data needed either to refute or validate the statement?

Two things are important here. First, this configuration violates a tacit rule of modern science that people generally learn in about the seventh grade (the same grade Alice may have been in when she fell down the rabbit hole). This rule is so well integrated into our consciousness, and into our perceptual processes, that we have forgotten (unless, perhaps, one is a mathematician or logician) that it's a made-up rule. It is an *axiom*, a rule of science we are asked to accept as true so that we can perform certain mathematical or other functions. It is an organizing principle imposed by Rationalism. One has mistaken it for a certain order of reality. Such is the implicit nature of paradigms.

The forgotten rule or axiom in this case is: *"The class is not a member of itself."* [114]

To illustrate, if we change the configuration to:

All Statements within this frame are untrue:

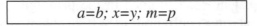

$$a=b; \ x=y; \ m=p$$

...then the intellect heaves a sigh of relief, not minding at all that *this* configuration is every bit as nonsensical as the first one. Not a whit more data or "reality" can be drawn from this proposition than can be drawn from the first. However, it *works* for us because it complies with the forgotten rule illustrating that the problem with the first configuration is that "what we are looking at, we are looking with." We impose upon it a paradigm that *makes* it nonsensical.

Second, it is important in this exercise to illustrate the relationship of the Western scientific paradigm with what we have suggested is the first lesson of recovery, that truth lies in *paradox*. Western science abhors paradox. The linear Rationalist view is an either/or, black-or-white way of looking at the world. This rebellion against paradox can actually be *felt* when one contemplates our puzzle. The truth is that the statement is true, and the truth is that the statement is untrue. The answer is, "yes," to both questions.

Someone as culturally conditioned to classical Chinese philosophy as a Westerner is to Rationalism would not have difficulty resolving this apparent contradiction, since Chinese philosophy is of course based upon a systemic coincidence of complementary "opposites" as being implicit in all things.[115] These divergent but mutually inclusive fields, represented as *yin* and *yang*, each contain an element of the other and form the seamless whole that is the non-linear universe, a universe in which the statement in the box, due to the larger matrix of which it is a part, can be both true and false at the same time.

Recovery is also a non-linear paradigm, a paradigm of integration and inclusion. It seeks completion and wholeness through acceptance of the process of interconnectedness. Addiction, on the other hand, is a paradigm of imposition and exclusion, a systemic denial of alternate or complementary truths. It seeks perfection through compartmentalized disembodiment, which brings us to the second book which will be helpful in framing our discussion. *Frankenstein; or the Modern Prometheus*, was written in 1816 by Mary Wollstonecraft Shelly. Mary Wollstonecraft, two years before writing the novel, had become the sixteen-year-old bride of the poet Percy Bysshe Shelly. In the summer of 1816, Mary and Percy were vacationing at Lake Leman near Geneva Switzerland at the home of Percy's friend and fellow poet Lord Byron. For entertainment, they had been reading German ghost stories aloud, and, in the spirit of a parlor game, had conspired each to invent a ghost story or phantasmagoric tale to see who could frighten whom the most.

Percy Shelly's contribution to this game is lost to the literary ages. A fragment of the story Byron made up eventually found its way into the end of his "Poem of Mazeppa." Mary's story, conceived in a "dreamlike state," became *Frankenstein*. It was one of the best-selling novels of the 19th century, produced on stage numerous times before Frankenstein's monster became an abiding image in countless Hollywood films.

From whence did an eighteen-year-old English girl on the eve of industrialization conceive what she herself called this "hideous progeny? " Mary and her husband Percy, along with Byron and their other literary friends, were immersed in the English Romantic movement. This was a counter-cultural literary and philosophical movement begun in Germany in the late 18th century. Like Populism in America seventy-five years later, Romanticism was a historical reaction against the form that modernity had taken in England and Europe at the beginning of the nineteenth century.

To characterize this cultural milieu against which the Romantic movement was formed, we return again to the "theology" of modern science, and to the Cartesian Rationalism from which it sprang. Modern science began with the Copernican hypothesis early in the 16th century that the earth was not the center of the universe, and it was crystallized by the end of the 17th century with the "scientific method." [116] It included most prominently Galileo, Isaac Newton, Rene Descartes, and their philosophical proponent, Francis Bacon. As we have seen, Descartes' "doubting" philosophy of Rationalism, formulated in 1619 (see p. 46), which formed the basis for modern science, was in turn based upon a fundamental dualism: the separation of *body* and *mind*, and of *self* and *other*. Rationalism has been called by Morris Berman a philosophy of "non-participation,"[117] which we have described as the "myth of objectivity."

Carl Jung said that "one of the chief factors responsible for psychological mass-mindedness is scientific Rationalism, which robs the individual of his foundations and his dignity." [118] Of even greater import perhaps is the spiritual loss in this system of the possibility of a personal relationship with God. According to the

tenets of this Rationalist theology, the Universe (and hence nature), resembles a huge machine, understood through an application of the principles of mechanics. The universe, then, by rational
implication, is lifeless, "disenchanted." God, if there is one, is
thought to reside not *in* the machine He has created but somewhere
outside of it, "sitting back," as James Joyce would write in *Portrait
of the Artist as a Young Man*, "paring His fingernails" in a chilling
combination of omnipotence and profound indifference. As E. A.
Burt noted in *The Metaphysical Foundations of Modern Physical
Science* in 1932, "The 17th century, which began with the search
for God in the Universe, ended by squeezing Him out of it altogether."

Robert Bly wrote that this Rationalistic, mechanistic view,
which he called "The Old Position," held "the conviction that nature is defective because it lacks reason." Descartes' ideas, he went
on to say, "act so as to withdraw consciousness from the non-hu-
man area, isolating the human being in his house, until, seen from
the window, rocks, sky, trees, crows seem empty of energy, but
especially empty of divine energy." [119] This sense of isolation led
the English poet A. E. Houseman to write, "I a stranger and
afraid... in a world I never made." And so, a dream-like darkness
falls upon the earth - what Matthew Arnold would later call, in his
poem "Dover Beach," a "darkling plain."

A further centerpiece of the philosophy of Rationalism is
control, which we have earlier defined as the hallmark of addiction. (see p. 24) According to Francis Bacon, an early English
spokesman for the Rationalist movement, the goal of science was
knowledge that could be used "to dominate and control nature,"
"hounded in her wanderings," "bound into service," and made a
"slave," and "put in constraint" to "torture (from her) secrets." [120]
Repression of the feminine was of course implicit in the repression
of nature. Robert Bly points out that in the male psyche, attitudes
toward women are usually the same as those toward the earth and
the unconscious.[121] Thus we have, under the White male-dominant
system of Exclusionary Rationalism and scientism, a profound link
between feminism and ecology. As Carolyn Merchant has said,

"the image of the earth as a living organism and nurturing mother served (in the Middle Ages) as a cultural constraint restricting the actions of human beings. One does not readily slay a mother, dig into her entrails for gold, or mutilate her body." [122]

There is a profound ethnic, racial, and political link with Exclusionary Rationalism as well. Historically, this paradigm, which was to provide the theological basis for the crystallization of the modern patriarchy, gave philosophical impetus to the Colonial period of European history which resulted in the imperial conquest and economic exploitation of the "unexplored regions" of the globe. What we now call the "Third World," peopled by the non-Anglo races of the earth, became lifeless objects, often enslaved, and an extension of the divineless, disenchanted landscape.[123] And so it was against this paradigm and its emerging dominance that the Romanticism of Mary Shelly's time was an expression.

As to Mary's own personal history, we have a modern dysfunctional family. Her grandfather on her mother's side was alcoholic. Her father, according to Samuel Cooleridge, "drank little and rarely smoked a pipe" but *ate* to excess.[124] The vision which drove his life was that perfection could be achieved, and it could be achieved by use of the intellect alone.[125] In counterpoint, Mary's mother (who died ten days following Mary's birth) was the first Anglo Saxon feminist to gain notoriety, with her book *A Vindication of the Rights of Women* in 1792. And she was a true feminist, advocating not that women should aspire to the status of men, but that their strength lay in their femininity.

Mary wanted to write a story that would "speak to the fears of our nature." [126] Her forlorn hero, Victor Frankenstein, who would become the prototype for a thousand Hollywood mad scientists, was a tinkerer, an inventor, a "hounder of nature in her wanderings," possessed with the idea of creating a man, of infusing life into lifeless parts. His fatal flaw of egotism is that "he forgets his 'natural' bonds to the people he loves and to nature in the frenzy of his work." [127] Among those he abandons is his fiancé Elizabeth, whom he had passionately loved ("Till death she was to be mine only."). Mary Shelly portrays the childhood sweetheart Elizabeth as the epitome of the idealized feminine: docile, good-tempered, "gay, playful, and lively, with animated feelings," "strong and deep of disposition," and "uncommonly affectionate."

In perhaps the most chilling scene in the novel, Victor has begun to suspect that the nameless Monster, whose creation he has just completed, is not quite the model of perfection he had intended. He begins to have self-doubts. He retires to his room and falls on his bed in a fretful sleep. He dreams that Elizabeth, his fiancé, from whose love he has strayed in this ill-fated enterprise, is returning to him. In his dream, she comes into his arms, but as he is embracing her, she transforms into the corpse of his dead mother! He awakes in terror from the dream and looks up into the face of the Monster (at whose hands Elizabeth will in fact die on their wedding night).

Following the nightmare, Victor flees, and writes:

> *Like one, that on a lonesome road*
> *Doth walk in fear and dread,*
> *And having once turned round walks on*
> *And turns no more his head*
> *Because he knows, a frightful fiend*
> *Doth close behind him tread.*

The transcendent motif in *Frankenstein* is that Victor and his Monster are not ultimately two distinct entities. They are one, and the Monster is simply a metaphor for Victor's unowned, repressed self - his projected, rigid, perfection-seeking Rationalism.[128] This is the same "shadow theme" Robert Lewis Stevenson would develop sixty years later in *The Strange Case of Dr. Jekyll and Mr. Hyde*.

It is a mistake to objectify Frankenstein's Monster, to view his identity as distinct from his creator. And, just as in Mary's book the Monster is in reality a metaphor for Victor himself, so too the addict "out there" in our culture is a manifestation of who we are inside. We live in, are products of, the addictive paradigm. As Anne Wilson Schaef has said, "it is in the air we breath."

Frankenstein provides, from the mind of an eighteen-year-old girl in 1816, an apt pre-addiction metaphor. Her "frightful fiend" treading "close behind" has now overtaken us, haunting us in our waking dreams, filling not only our courtrooms and prisons and jails and inner cities, but our highest offices of government and commerce as well. "He" is our reflection, our shadow, and our own creation, the legacy of our tinkering with being God.

PART II TREATMENT AND THE PHASES OF
           RECOVERY

My heart aches, and a drowsy numbness pains
My sense, as though of hemlock I had drunk,
Or emptied some dull opiate to the drains...
                                    Keats

Treatment needs to be focused on the
daily challenge of being drug free and
not drift prematurely into expansive
psychological, social service, and
family-related issues.
                            NADA

We shall not cease from exploration
And the end of all our exploring
Will be to arrive where we started
And know the place for the first time.
                            T.S.Eliot

A.A. is an utter simplicity which
encases a complete mystery.
                            Bill Wilson

Western chemical dependency treatment (as distinct from *recovery*) is an inherently paradoxical proposition because it developed, as a model, from the Western exclusionary templates of medicine, psychology, and religion, which are among the most crystallized manifestations of the problem it is trying to solve. Traditional Western drug treatment is grounded in the addictive paradigm. It has historically been a rather bleak landscape.

In the Introduction to this book, we said that a requirement for this work is "to speak two languages," and it is in the treatment arena where that demand is great. It is in the function of providing *effective* drug treatment that the addictive paradigm and the recovery paradigm must interface, and effective treatment must, in order to achieve its effectiveness, remain grounded and centered on the recovery side of things.

We have characterized the Alcoholics Anonymous Twelve Step program, which is the premier recovery paradigm, as a countercultural reaction to this failure of the dominant Western Rationalist systems of medicine, psychology, and religion, to provide effective alcoholism treatment. Most contemporary Western treatment, since the ascent of A.A., has the *pretense* of being grounded in recovery. It has, in general, co-opted, tacked on, or adapted the *exterior trappings* of the Twelve Step programs. But it hasn't, unfortunately, ventured to take any of the Twelve Steps itself!

Recovery, as a system, has gotten the reputation of being exclusionary, which is a characteristic we have been ascribing to the addictive system as well. There is a tendency, born of survival, for people trying to remain centered in recovery to *insulate* themselves from the addictive system. This "cloistering impulse" is as understandable as people not wanting to go outside during a hurricane (as understandable, indeed, as a health professional choosing to deal with chemical dependency from the comfort and security of the private practice). Consequently, recovery from the isolating malaise of addiction often results in more isolation. Ideally, as the center grows stronger, there is a sort of spiraling movement in and out of the two systems. But the fact is, since isolation itself is an addictive syndrome, there is no escaping the mouth of the tiger of addiction.[129]

The addiction treatment field is about the art of interfacing on multiple levels with the addictive system while at the same time remaining centered in the system of recovery. The most acute faces of the addictive system which manifest in the treatment arena include, of course, the *clients* themselves. Also included, however, are the *treatment funding community*, the *treatment administration and regulation establishment*, and, not the least important, *one's own unresolved personal addiction "trigger" issues.* The effective treatment program, based in recovery principles, is continually involved in the process of healing on all of these levels.

And so, in making the decision to accept the challenge of transforming drug and alcohol treatment through the development of acupuncture-based programs, we are compelled into the mouth of the tiger. This is a journey we must make. It will have its rewards.

One reward is that we will find increasing numbers of allies within these systems, people already in recovery who are trying to bring recovery principles to this work. We will need these people for support. They will become as our extended family, a network of people whom we need not *like*, but whom we need to *love*! Like an extended family, these are people who, "when you need to go there, they have to take you in." Among others we will find in this work are those who are experiencing sufficient desperation that they are open to the new perspectives of recovery. These are our clients, earnest in discovering the tools of recovery, and our teachers as well, reminding us of where we ourselves came.

Just as the chemically dependent person begins the recovery journey with a redefinition and transformation of his/her relationship with the "drug of choice," so we begin our journey into the acupuncture-based chemical dependency treatment field in Chapters Four and Five with a description of some clinical realities concerning detoxification from drugs, and with an examination of psychoactive drugs themselves. We, too, seek to redefine and transform our relationship with these substances. In the looking glass of modern American culture, few phenomena are as emotionally charged as are our attitudes about drugs and our stereotypes about those who use them addictively. Most of us have grown up learning about these substances in a Western context with a Western moral frame of awareness, profoundly influenced by the institutions of education, government, church, and the media, for whom these substances have been invested with great and morally connotative power. These drugs, so we have been told, threaten the very fabric of our civilization.

Yes, they have harmful effects (ironically, more so by far the licit than the illicit ones). There is indeed pathology here, and lesion. In some drug categories, extended chronic use - and, in some cases, abrupt *abstinence* from extended chronic use - is life-threatening. However, from a treatment (and "prevention") perspective, using these facts to justify a moralizing posture helps not one iota. Health and recovery do not come from proselytizing. And thus, it is our goal to come to an understanding of these substances as indeed potent, but also as *morally neutral*.

In Chapter Six of this section, we will describe the "mouth of the tiger," examining the Western models of treatment. Acupuncture can be effectively integrated into any of these models and can help to transform them toward recovery. Also, we will find elements of these models that indeed have efficacy of their own: counseling, residential treatment, urine testing, and even drug therapies. We will also discover structures of great value which cut across and transcend all treatment modalities, such as the group process and intervention. Acupuncture is among these transcendent systems.

Treatment is a *gateway* to recovery. It is never a replacement for recovery (though that is what most clients often will be seeking, what A.A. calls an "easier, softer way.") Finding one's *center* in recovery is a life-long process. Chapter Seven describes the various phases of this process and provides a more thorough analysis of the Twelve Step recovery programs, activities that complement them, some of their alternatives, and some of their more subtle resonances with the principles of Chinese medicine and acupuncture.

It could be said that little of what we have discussed so far has specific relevance to the day-to-day realities of the clinic where professional meets client. The moment we are in the clinic, our focus of attention is captured by the acute and chronic effects of the drugs our clients have used. The specific drugs and their effects, in other words, appear to be the most important issue in this work. Vomiting, diarrhea, the shakes, high blood pressure, fainting, seizure: these are what command our attention. It is, therefore, easy for us to become fixated upon pharmacology. One can even imagine our becoming as obsessed with drugs as our clients are!

The effects of drugs and the presenting symptoms are, of course, what has brought the client to us, and what has brought acupuncture to this difficult work. These acute drug effects, in one sense, are the most important issue. However, none of us will be very effective unless we have found a place to stand within ourselves to do this work. The manner in which we posture ourselves in the clinic, and the manner in which the clinic postures itself in relation to other components in the treatment program, will determine our degree of ultimate success. Therefore, before we begin a discussion of specific drugs and their actions, a few words are in order about the tenor of the clinic, and about the basic clinic posturing of the acupuncturist and other front line staff.

The information that has been discussed so far in this book, and some of what will follow, is presented in the hopes of providing a context for understanding, developing, and maintaining empathy for the clients we will meet. We will quickly discover within ourselves, when we begin interacting with clients every day, the sources of the moralizing and judgmental posture that society at large has historically taken concerning drugs and intoxication. These clients will, as the psychotherapists say, "push all of our buttons." They will exasperate, frustrate, confound, and disappoint us endlessly. We will need all the help we can get to remain centered, day to day, and the acupuncture service our program provides will need all of the help it can get from other components of the treatment program. Many of us will have hopes that acupuncture itself is all that our clients need. Our clients themselves will be hoping that this is the case, for they are addicts, searching for the magic fix! The demands for humility will be great indeed. We will discover, with the successful client, that here is something I cannot do alone. I need help. Therefore, the overarching daily clinical concerns are finding and maintaining our own center, taking care of ourselves, finding harmony and support in the adjunctive services our program offers, and avoiding the codependent pitfalls of becoming seduced by the addictive issues our clients present to us. In this sense, addressing the acute and chronic effects of the drugs our clients are using is the easy part.

From the acupuncturist's point of view, it would not be as easy if our clinical challenge was to diagnose, in the traditional manner of Chinese medicine, each individual client.[130] The pathologies seen in the drug treatment setting are complex indeed. They include the acute withdrawal symptoms of a myriad of psychoactive substances (often in a single client), and also the subclinical chronic effects of these drugs, such as liver, pancreatic, and lung disorders. Also presented can be a cacophony of accompanying issues ranging from malnutrition, acute stress, trauma, mental disorders, fatigue, and all of the infectious diseases that plague these communities, such as acquired immune deficiency syndrome (AIDS), tuberculosis, hepatitis, and sexually transmitted diseases (STDs).

Individual diagnosis would challenge everything that we know about Chinese medicine and Western medicine. It would consume all of our resources as well, for in the typical successful acupuncture group clinic in a drug treatment setting, an average treatment case load of twenty clients per hour is not unusual. This provides a treatment opportunity of three minutes per client! Naturally, this prospect may seem overwhelming and even frightening for the acupuncturist accustomed to the private practice setting. How, indeed, can we have any success at all in such a seemingly impossible situation?

Our potential for success begins with a simple and essential premise, a premise that the individual addict must finally come to as well if he or she is to survive: absolutely none of these attending symptoms will ever get better until the individual stops chronic drug use. We must, as in the clichés of Alcoholics Anonymous, adopt the position of "first things first," and "keep it simple! " The client's inability to accept this premise is a premier barrier to recovery. The client will be as concerned as we are apt to be with all of the attending symptoms. The client will bring to us, as part of his or her denial system, a hundred issues, real and imagined, and a great deal of concern about these symptoms, when in fact the only single concern ought to be getting clean and sober. "You will lose anything you put before your sobriety," is an old recovery adage. We must support that adage. Since the client is unable to put "first things first," we must employ a treatment approach that provides that message and that helps the client to establish this priority. This is an essential part of the wisdom we will find in the treatment protocol developed by the National Acupuncture Detoxification Association (NADA).[131]

The acupuncture needle points on the ear that have been identified in the NADA protocol are "sympathetic," "*shen-men*," "kidney," "liver," and "lung." The needles are inserted in these points in that particular order. Sympathetic and *shen-men* are always used; of the kidney, liver, and lung points, at least two are chosen by the acupuncturist depending upon sensing active points, and upon observation of the patient's symptoms.[132]

This protocol is recommended for all clients who come to us during the acute withdrawal phase. We will use the same treatment regardless of the particular drug of abuse. This treatment is repeated daily, and is not varied in the early phase. It therefore becomes predictable and reliable for the client.

Our treatment goal here is a simple and realistic one. We want to make the client feel better. The goal is not to make the client well. "Well" is not a realistic treatment goal in this phase.

"Better" is a realistic treatment goal. The client comes the first day, and receives a simple treatment, and feels a little better. Some of these clients will find their way back the next day, and the same thing will happen again. The client's symptoms will likely have changed by the second day because they may be 24 or 48 hours in withdrawal. He or she may be more depressed than they were the day before, or more anxious. But the treatment is the same, and the client will again feel a little better. They may complain of this or that symptom, and that's to be expected. However, the treatment remains consistent. The treatment, the client learns, is as reliable as their drug of choice was, and their drug of choice has been the only consistent, reliable thing in their lives for a long time. So, this is a good thing. This is progress. It's not perfect, but the client, having found something besides chemicals that will help them feel a little better in the present moment, will be motivated to come back again.

The foremost and obvious goal of all drug treatment programs is client retention,[133] a goal which follows our premise of setting priorities. If clients continue their chronic drug use, nothing else is ever going to improve in their lives. To stop their chronic drug use, they need to come to treatment. The reason they come to treatment is that they feel a little better without using drugs. This is a principle mechanism of Twelve Step programs as well. The Twelve Step meeting has a parallel consistency, because the basic structure is repetitive. It makes people feel a little better, and it addresses their recovery needs regardless of what stage in recovery they happen to be in. It is a structure that is horizontally flexible. People can take from the meeting what they need. It is a safe place, and uniquely nurturing. Our daily acupuncture protocol offers a similar systemic advantage. The treatment does not vary with the changes the client is going through.

Another central and unique feature of the acupuncture treatment protocol is that it is non-verbal. This does not mean that we don't talk to clients. It does mean, however, that the client's ability to provide accurate and truthful information about their condition is not a requirement for achieving benefit from program participation. The importance of this cannot be overemphasized. Western conventional treatment alone, which must rely upon pharmaceutical interventions and talk therapy, cannot provide this benefit. In order to make the client feel better consistently, every day, during the acute withdrawal phase, the conventional treatment provider has to use other drugs. Talk therapy cannot provide this, no matter how skilled the counselor is, because there will be days during which the client may not feel capable of talking with a counselor, so the client won't come. Since the majority of clients are in denial about their drug use, they will not generally be honest with the counselor. Therefore, the verbal information upon which diagnosis is made will not be accurate. If the client relapses, he or she usually won't come to treatment for fear of disappointing the counselor. Even if the client has an especially productive counseling session on one day, he or she may not come the next day for fear that the counselor will expect them to be able to function at that level again. Due to transference and other related issues, clients generally fear failure in the eyes of the therapist, so treatment that is based upon performance can intrinsically generate treatment drop-out.

Besides, from a cost standpoint, daily individual counseling is not generally a realistic goal in a public treatment setting. Group counseling is more manageable in terms of cost, and group counseling can indeed be an effective modality in early recovery. However, chemically dependent clients are usually resistant to groups, for fear of being exposed, or for fear of failing to perform adequately. The group acupuncture setting, in which there are no verbal expectations placed upon the client, offers a safe and comfortable prelude to a more interactive group process when the client is ready.

There is another profound benefit in non-verbal therapy. Perhaps what clients take exception to the most about conventional drug treatment, besides abstinence, is health lectures. Clients have already given themselves a thousand health lectures about how they should stop using drugs. Most addicts do that at least once a day. And because there are so many people in their past who told them the same thing, the addict actually has a "committee" in their head giving them lectures all the time about a whole host of things they should be doing with their lives: see a doctor, get a job, eat decently and take vitamins, go back to school, get this and that together. Adding another voice to the current bombardment will not be productive. Clients won't come to a treatment program if they expect to get another health lecture.

But here, in our simple acupuncture protocol, is something new: a reliable, consistent, empowering, accessible,[134] non-judg-mental, non-verbal, nurturing something that they do every day, one day at a time, that makes them feel a little bit better each time. Drug addicts and alcoholics are excessively conscious of product quality, and they recognize a very good deal here! Most acupunc-turists who work with this basic protocol on a daily basis also come to find that it is surprisingly potent, that it is sound and effi-cacious for a great number of issues presented by this population.

The benefits we describe are very important issues in determin-ing treatment program design. They are benefits which inform the manner in which the acupuncture interfaces with other components of the treatment program. These other components are essential to program success. Acupuncture alone will help, but it won't result in long term positive outcomes unless we have group and individ-ual counseling, case management, education, and other adjunctive services. But it is important, in overall program design, to distin-guish between simply having an acupuncture component "tacked on" to these other services, and having an acupuncture-based pro-gram. An acupuncture-based program means that the client can come to the program site and get all of the benefits that the acu-puncture program can offer without having to be screened, without having to talk to a counselor, without having to say when they last used, and without having to participate in any of the other services. While the other services are accessible, they are choices the client can make once they have stabilized.[135]

Acupuncturists, meanwhile, putting four or five needles in people's ears day after day, will be struggling mightily to hold back on their great arsenal of clinical knowledge which they are convinced would help all of the attending disharmonies that this individual is presenting. What do we do if the person has chronic back pain too? As Lincoln Hospital's Michael Smith has said, if you have an alcoholic with a bad back, what you want is a sober alcoholic with a bad back. We know that, in Chinese medicine, we have things that we can offer to provide relief for this disharmony. Our goal, however, is that this individual will remain in treatment long enough to achieve abstinence, that they will stabilize to a degree that they will be able to take advantage of all of these things we have to offer. We know that if they continue chronic drinking, this will not be an option. We realize that there may even be cases in which shifting our focus to attending, underlying, unmasked symptoms - symptoms which may in fact be precipitative factors in the drug use - could enable the client to continue chronic drug use by protecting them from the consequences of the drug use that are primary motivators for getting sober.

And so, we adhere to our premise of "keep it simple." Our greatest clinical concern is that we avoid the premature expansion of the treatment protocol. The moment we expand the protocol, we have begun individual diagnosis, which depends upon conversation with the client. We no longer have a non-verbal treatment program. For an expansion of the basic protocol to happen, we are going to have to become verbally engaged with the client, and the consistency will be lost. We will have acquiesced to changing the subject. The subject is no longer the cessation of chronic drug use; the subject is now bad backs. The focus has shifted.

These are the clinical costs of expanding our treatment beyond the basic protocol, and they are important costs, so they must be carefully weighed.

This basic NADA protocol is the clinical baseline. It is the treatment to which the client may return at any time, especially following a relapse, and still find all of the benefits that have been discussed. We can begin to see that expanded protocols using traditional Chinese medicine ideally will occupy a similar position in clinical design to all of the other treatment components such as case management and counseling. It will, in the ideal, be something that is available once the client has achieved a degree of stability. Perhaps one can see how programs have been able to operate with "detox specialists," non-acupuncturists who are trained in the basic ear protocol and who administer the protocol under the supervision of a licensed acupuncturist,[136] and how a program component designed in this way can be compatible with an adjunctive Chinese medical clinic. An acupuncture-based program with a Chinese medical component is the natural growth of our detox programs, whether or not they have detox specialists.

We will discuss the stages of recovery at some length in subsequent Chapters, but for our present purposes, it is important to see this distinction between the baseline protocol, with all of its advantages, and an expanded protocol based upon diagnosis. Individual clients will vary greatly in terms of specific time frames in which transition is appropriate from the generic to expanded protocols. An individual who has been sober for two weeks, coming every day, who has begun to attend Twelve Step meetings, and who has persistent insomnia or headache or diarrhea, is a candidate for a gradual expansion beyond the baseline to address the persisting symptom. For some individuals, earlier expanded intervention may be indicated. For others, we may want to wait. Over time, the practitioner will come to appreciate the wisdom in our earlier diagnostic restraint, finding that many of the disturbing symptoms the client presented the first hours and days of abstinence have disappeared "all by themselves." We will gain, through experience, a sense of what symptoms are to be expected in the acute withdrawal phase as distinct from subclinical symptoms that lie beneath acute withdrawal.

In spite of the generic clinical protocol we have recommended, which will apply to anyone regardless of whether they are an alcoholic, heroin addict, or cocaine addict, it is natural and helpful for practitioners to develop a somewhat detailed knowledge about both acute and chronic drug actions. We will present a classification of these common symptoms for each of the major drug categories. This information will be more than adequate to the needs of someone beginning work in this field. We have also provided, in Appendix II, an extensive list of references for those interested in additional information. Since traditional Chinese medical textbooks do not address chronic drug use, the issue of expanded treatment in this setting represents a significant frontier of its own. This is an exciting and challenging clinical dialogue that has begun among acupuncture practitioners in the chemical dependency field.

We will begin our discussion with a brief summary of the site of action of all psychoactive drugs.

Neuronal Pathways - The "Site of Action"

Psychoactive drugs are called "psychoactive" because they act on the central nervous system (CNS), particularly the brain. It is not generally easy for drugs to gain access to the brain. The brain, in fact, as one might suspect, works very hard to keep foreign substances out. It is protected by the *blood-brain barrier* (BBB). The anatomical basis of the BBB is believed to be the structure of the walls of the blood vessels supplying the brain. In addition, neurons in the CNS are densely surrounded by specialized cells called *glial* cells (*glia* from the Greek meaning glue). Extensions from the glial cells cover most of the surface of the blood capillaries in the brain.

Neuronal Action

The *neuron* and its branches (*dendrites*) are the basic cell unit of the CNS. The function of neurons is to communicate with each other and with glands and muscles. The basis on which all psychoactive drugs work is that they either alter the chemicals neurons receive or interfere with conduction. Most of the drugs that work on neurons don't need to actually penetrate the neuron, working "on" rather than "in" the cell.

Neurons, which vary greatly in size, are comprised of the *soma* (body), which contains the nucleus; dendrites, varying from one to many, which receive and carry information into the soma; the *axon*, which carries information out of the soma; the *axon hillock*, an intermediate area where electrical changes begin, and the *axon terminal*, a button, covered with *telodendria*, which sit above and nestle into (without touching) the dendrite spine of the neighboring neuron.

The space between the telodendria of the sending neuron and the dendrite of the neighboring neuron is called the *synaptic cleft*. The sending neuron is called the *presynaptic* cell; the receiving (receptor) neuron is called the *postsynaptic* cell.

Inside the axon terminal button of the presynaptic cell is the *cisternae*. It builds spherical balls filled with chemicals and sends them to the membrane wall. These balls are called *synaptic vesicles* (little bladders). When the neuron is activated, these vesicles go to the wall of the membrane of the presynaptic cell and release chemicals into the cleft. These chemicals are collectively called *neurotransmitters* or, more recently "information molecules." They are all synthesized in the CNS from various amino acid precursors, and collectively form the basis of the brain's information processing system.

Once released into the synaptic cleft, these chemicals float across and bind to *receptors* located on the dendrite of the postsynaptic cell. Receptors are built and recycled inside the neuron. Like sugar molecule receptors in the tongue, these are specific receptors, not general ones. They have shapes that are complementary with the neurotransmitter molecule, like a lock and key. Foreign chemicals from neighboring cells won't fit.

The postsynaptic membrane is riddled with openings which are plugged with proteins. They open only when the transmitter binds to the locking mechanism. The protein shape changes and moves and the gate opens and then the inside of the cell becomes accessible to *ions*. The ions pour in (the gate is open 1/2000th of a second), and travel down the dendrite of the postsynaptic cell to the soma. This triggers the release of neurotransmitters in the axon of the postsynaptic cell and the transmission process begins again, like links in a chain.

After the neurotransmitter has bound, it is either degraded enzymatically and eliminated, or otherwise inactivated. Or, through a process called *terminal reuptake*, it is drawn back into the originating neuron.

Most psychoactive drugs swamp most of these systems. Some drugs, such as nicotine and morphine, mimic certain neurotransmitter molecules, fooling the receptors so that they open the gate. These are called *agonists*; drugs that are similar enough to bind but not to complete the task, such as naloxone, are called *antagonists*; they tie up the channels but don't open them, and in the process block anything else from binding. Still others, such as cocaine, block terminal reuptake, causing a sustained proliferation of neurotransmitter molecules in the cleft, binding again and again to the post-synaptic cell.

Neurotransmitters

Following is a discussion of some of the neurotransmitters that are important in psychoactive drug mechanisms. Note that acupuncture has been shown to have an effect on the production of most of these chemicals.[137]

Norepinephrine (NE) - also called noradrenaline - is one of three *catecholamine*[138] neurotransmitters. It is found largely in the pons, where the peripheral autonomic nervous system modulates heartbeat, contractility, blood glucose, and pulorection sweating. Since these are functions of the so-called "fight or flight" reflex, it is postulated that NE is involved in the modulation of global alertness and vigilance, and is associated with arousal reactions and moods. It appears to play a central role in opiate and alcohol addiction and withdrawal.

Epinephrine (adrenaline) is also a catecholamine. Like NE, it is a hormone involved with the "fight or flight" reflex. It is the most potent stimulant (sympathomimetic) of alpha- and beta-adrenergic receptors, causing increased heart rate, vasoconstriction or vasodilation, relaxation of bronchiolar and intestinal smooth muscle, glycogenolysis, lipolysis, and other metabolic effects associated with quick mobilization in an emergency.

Dopamine (DA), is the third catecholamine neurotransmitter. Also called *3-Hydroxytyramine (3-HT)*, it is an intermediary in tyrosine metabolism, and the precursor of NE and epinephrine. Localized in the basal ganglia, it is associated with body movement. The dopaminergic system is thought to be a primary basis for cocaine actions, and dopamine deficiencies have been shown to be related to the neurological disorder Parkinson's Disease. Alcohol induces dopamine release when administered on an acute basis, but chronic consumption leads to a decrease in dopamine in striatal tissue.[139]

Acetylcholine *(ACh)* is released both inside and outside the CNS. It is produced at the ends of cholinergic nerve fibers and at the motor end plates in skeletal muscle. It is an acetyl ester of choline.[140] ACh is an excitatory chemical, triggering nerve impulse. Its release is particularly prompted by nerve injuries. Its function is not known, but there is a research hypothesis that it may have to do with creativity and short term memory. It is significant in most psychoactive drug actions, particularly nicotine and other stimulants.

Serotonin *(5-HT* - shorthand for *5-Hydroxytryptamine)* is present in the CNS and in many peripheral tissues and cells, including some carcinoid tumors. The 5-HT system appears more thickly interwoven and intricate than other neurotransmitter systems, and there are what appear to be at least a half dozen different types of 5-HT receptors.[141] Serotonin, along with NE and DA, is a *monoamine*,[142] and it inhibits gastric secretion and stimulates smooth muscle. It is also associated with the regulation of sensory perception and pain transmission, sleep, sexual behavior, and body temperature, and with a wide range of psychiatric disorders and with hallucinations in ways that are not understood. Early research showed 5-HT to have some similarity to LSD. It is highly concentrated in the limbic region of the brain, where emotions are regulated, and some researchers believe that it is the primary mood-modifying system. Animal studies show that 5-HT synthesis increases with chronic alcohol consumption, and falls in withdrawal. Its normal generation seems to be directly related to blood platelet levels.[143] Its levels are increased by alcohol, and by cocaine, which blocks its reuptake.

Gamma-aminobutyric acid (GABA) is an inhibitory neurotransmitter, blocking the transfer of a nerve impulse to an adjoining neuron. When its normal functioning is disrupted, convulsions result. It is affected by the sedative hypnotics and the minor tranquilizers. Its levels are increased by alcohol.

Tryptophan (*TRP*) is an essential amino acid[144] associated with sleep. It is also a metabolic precursor of 5-HT.

Enkephalin (from the Greek "in the head") is a pentapeptide (a combination of amino acids) associated with perception, emotions, and behavior. It is found in the pituitary gland and many parts of the brain, and binds to some opiate receptors possibly related to pain.

Endorphins, 40 times more powerful than enkephalins and 100 times more powerful than morphine, is the term collectively used to describe any natural, internal body substance with morphine-like activity. There are a variety of subtypes of endorphin: *mu, kappa, sigma, beta,* etc. It is a peptide and an analgesic. Rats become addicted to human endorphins. Endorphins play significantly in hallucinations and schizophrenia, and possibly in learning and memory. They also have a relationship with sexual activity - the higher the levels, the less the sexual activity.

Theoretically, endorphins act as hormones in a negative feedback relationship with the pituitary gland. The function of morphine itself (called an "exogenous opiate") is that it effectively ties up the receptor site and fools the natural feedback system.[145]

An important anomaly in terms of mind/body dualism has been the discovery that while it was originally assumed that endorphins were a function of the CNS only, both endorphin and endorphin receptor site activity have been discovered in the gastrointestinal, reproductive, and immune systems as well. Therefore, when we say that psychoactive drugs effect the "mind," we speak indeed in Western Rationalist metaphor.[146]

Using this model, we have two theories of opiate addiction which may be applied to other drugs as well. First is the *Receptor Supersensitivity Theory*. This theory has it that addiction is the body's compensation for the chronic presence of the drug. This compensation is tolerance. With chronic opiate use, the receptor cell produces more post synaptic receptors, so the receptor becomes super-sensitive. This is called *upregulation*. The drug's effectiveness is equal to the number of receptors bound, so the net effectiveness decreases with use. The brain is trying to maintain a homeostatic balance in the presence of the drug, so euphoria requires a greater and greater dose. Whatever was produced by the drug, the opposite will be produced by withdrawal; therefore, the effect of a huge number of receptor sites and no more drug to attach is dysphoria and pain. In the neuropharmacology of addiction, the search is for these calibrating mechanism of the brain.

The second addiction theory is the *Enzyme Induction Theory*. Morphine, this theory assumes, interferes with the amount of endorphin being produced, and, as a result, the smaller endorphin effect on receptors restricts enzyme production. Early research, however, indicating that endorphin production was abated during chronic opiate use has recently been challenged,[147] thus challenging in turn our own assumptions about the role that acupuncture plays in withdrawal. Since we know that acupuncture stimulates the production of endorphin levels in animals, and since we assumed that opiate addicts in withdrawal were suffering from an endorphin deficiency, our treatment made logical sense. But the recent research indicating that endorphin production may *not* be curtailed during chronic use has caused us to rethink this area of efficacy.

One conclusion we may draw from this is that the neurotransmission process is far more complicated than we have described here, and clearly more complicated than the current research has been able to explain. There are many steps in the process of neuronal conduction in the neurotransmitter chain: *production, storage, release, membrane penetration, binding, and reuptake*; all of these processes, and a variety of correlative factors could be discretely altered by ingestion of an exogenous psychoactive chemical, as could the receptor sites themselves. For we now know that these receptor cells are in a constant state of transformation from energy to particle and back again, much like the behavior of sub-atomic particles.[148]

And if, indeed, all of our discoveries about this intricate system have taken us to the door step of *intelligence* itself, then it is clear that a phase of the process is missing: the *transformation phases of energy into information in a patterned way*. This is something that we may not come to understand adequately using the conventional model of Western science. The implied hypothesis is that there is another discrete and as yet undiscovered system underlying or interfacing with the neuronal conduction system. From the Chinese point of view, we have then perhaps arrived at the doorstep of *qi*, the life force which lies hidden behind and flows through all living processes.[149]

Psychoactive Drug Categories

Psychoactive drugs have been classified in different ways. Any attempt to classify them thoroughly and accurately produces anomalies. For our purposes, we will classify them as follows:

1. Depressants
   a. Sedative hypnotics
   b. Minor Tranquilizers
2. Mood Modifiers
   a . Major tranquilizers
   b . Anti-depressants
3. Narcotics
   a. Natural Opiates
   b. Synthetic Opiates
4. Stimulants
5. Hallucinogens (Psychotomimetics)

Depressants

Depressants act to depress or inhibit the activity of the CNS. The sub-category of <u>sedative</u> <u>hypnotics</u> includes the beverage alcohol, chloral hydrate (a sleeping medication), and the barbiturates, which include phenobarbital, tulinol, and seconal. The Barbiturates are used for sleep. They are old drugs, fairly effective, with no serious side effects, but with dangerous alcohol potentiation actions and overdose potential. Their use has declined largely because the drug industry is geared to new drugs with new patents since that is where the big profits are. The barbiturates behave similarly to alcohol, can be lethal when mixed with alcohol or with minor tranquilizers, and, as with alcohol, can produce a fatal withdrawal due to seizure.

The most popular <u>minor</u> <u>tranquilizer</u> is the benzodiazapine *diazepam* (Valium). Structurally similar to a metabolite of *chlordiazepoxide* (Librium), it was marketed by Roche Laboratories in 1959 as a benign, non-addictive tranquilizer. We have since learned that it is among the most addictive drugs we see in our clinics. Librium, another minor tranquilizer, is an "anxiolitic" drug, a reducer of anxiety. Like Valium, it is frequently used in the Western medical setting to treat alcohol withdrawal because it acts on the same receptor sites.

Other minor tranquilizers are *flurazepam* (Dalmane), Vistaril (a drug of choice in treatment of irritability in early stage alcohol withdrawal), and Xanax, which has been marketed as a non addictive replacement for Valium; it is, however, similar to Valium, and just as addictive.

The benzodiazapines, especially Valium, were originally designed to replace another group of minor tranquilizers called the *meprobomates*, which include Equinil and Milltown, that were popular in the 1940s and 50s.

Alcohol
    <u>Psychoactive Mechanisms:</u>

A primary neuronal mechanism of action of alcohol is the GABA receptor. GABA, as we have discussed, is an inhibitory neurotransmitter, and alcohol is thought to facilitate this inhibition. The benzodiazapines Valium and Librium also inhibit the GABA receptors, and so are often used to treat acute withdrawal because they work partially on the same neurotransmitter system. Because the alcohol molecule is so small, and because alcohol is an astringent, a further mechanism of action is that it leaks in and out of the neuronal membranes and slows the signals. This process affects not only the GABA receptor neurons but every nerve cell in the body. A 5 to 10% concentration of alcohol shuts down the system. Besides the GABA neurotransmitter, alcohol affects tryptophan, dopamine, norepinephrine, and serotonin; the affects on these neurotransmitters may be of the acetaldehyde or other metabolites rather than of alcohol itself.

Acute Effects:

Acute effects are those immediately following the absorption phase. In the CNS, alcohol, in low doses, actually increases reflexes due to lower CNS inhibition (which gives the subjective perception that alcohol is a stimulant). The smallest amount of alcohol increases the workload of the heart and raises blood pressure. In moderate to high doses, reflexes - as well as memory, coordination, judgment, and concentration - decrease, therefore, alcohol probably works from the higher centers and moves down to basal functions. It is a mild hypnotic in low doses, and suppresses stage five (REM) sleep in medium doses (which yields, in withdrawal, REM rebound, resulting in very vivid, coarse dreams and poor quality sleep; the benzodiazepines suppress stage four sleep, but help restore stage five sleep.

Chronic Effects:

CNS: Chronic use of alcohol causes vitamin deficiency in compounds that affect memory, and both remote and recent memory function can be permanently impaired.

Circulatory System: The heart muscle damage from long term drinking causes atrial fibrillation by decreasing the ability of cells to oxygenate, though precisely how is not known. Alcohol drops body temperature, bringing blood from the periphery, and causing, with chronic use, high blood thermia.

Liver: Chronic alcohol use affects the liver in a number of ways. An indirect effect is that it penetrates and sedates the bone marrow, which is responsible for the production of red blood cells essential to the body's normal detoxification process. It also overworks the liver, competing for detoxification with the liver's normal processes, and it adds fat and clogs the liver, causing the cirrhotic condition; blood backs up and the esophagus bursts. As the cirrhosis builds up, NA_3 (ammonia) increases, causing dementia. In Western medicine, dementia (wet brain) is treated with diet and with the drugs lactulose (which produces a bacteria that absorbs ammonia), and with neomycin (which kills the bacteria).

Gastrointestinal Tract: In the gastrointestinal tract, chronic alcohol use causes hydrochloric acid excretion, which produces gastric ulcers. (The reason alcohol stimulates the appetite in low doses is because of the release of gastric enzymes.) Alcohol, in any amount, decreases nutrient absorption, especially the B vitamins which are co-factors in the enzymes that break down alcohol.

Other Chronic Effects: Chronic alcohol use:

- increases phosphate zinc and causes magnesium depletion in the kidneys;
- causes sexual dysfunction and loss of erection. Since a normal function of the liver is to break down the female hormone in men and the male hormone in women, and since alcohol interferes with this function, there are sex hormone imbalances which may have secondary effects relating to sexual dysfunction;
- suppresses normal adrenaline production;
- clogs the pancreas. Digestive enzymes can't get out, so the pancreas begins digesting itself;
- flushes calcium out of the bone.

Alcohol Withdrawal Reactions:

Acute alcohol withdrawal is typically from seven to 14 days. Binge alcohol withdrawal is often worse than chronic.

The first signs are minor, occurring six to 12 hours following the last drink, and include:

- irregular pulse;
- rising blood pressure.

These are key symptoms to be aware of in the detox clinic setting. The primary concern in acute alcohol withdrawal is seizure, and seizure will be preceded by alarmingly high blood pressure. In the general population, over 140/90, is thought of as high. 150/80 in alcohol withdrawal is not unusual. 120/ for young people and 160/ for older people is normal. The 180/ - 200/ range is cause for alarm, suggesting arterial cirrhosis. /90 is on the border, and /95+ is alarming. 190/95 is very subjective; the likelihood of seizure depends further upon pulse rate and shallow breathing. Symptoms further include:

- irritability;
- restlessness;
- tremors (shaking);
- sweating;
- loss of appetite;
- insomnia;
- tachycardia;
- hypertension;
- anxiety.

In the period of 24 hours to ten days, add to these:

- auditory, tactile, and olfactory hallucinations;
- cravings;
- disorientation;
- complaints of paralysis and numbness;
- hyperthermia;
- delirium tremens.

Delirium tremens (DTs) more typically have a two to three days onset, but can be as long as ten days if other drugs are involved. Because chronic alcohol use suppresses normal adrenaline production, there will be abnormally high levels of adrenaline during withdrawal. This was initially thought to be a precipitative factor in DTs, which are now thought to be more a function of neurotransmitters. The mortality rate from DTs, which forebode seizure, is estimated as high as 20% (without the use of acupuncture). Other estimates used are that five to 10% of chronic alcoholics in acute withdrawal will experience DTs; five to 10% of those will seize, and 5% of those seizing will die or suffer permanent mental damage, but there are in fact no good studies.

Seizures are of two types: *petit mal* or grand mal; the onset is typically 12 to 48 hours with up to five days known. Petit mal seizures are either *simple a.*, - a brief clouding of consciousness - or *complex a.*, involving a sharp spasm or convulsion (paroxysm) accompanied by atonia or twitching, coughing, or sneezing. Grand mal seizures involve extensive muscle contractions (convulsions) and respiratory arrest (jerkiness and irregular breathing). In the Western medical treatment setting, Valium is the drug of choice, placating DTs and seizure because it also works on the GABA mechanisms. It is administered orally or by IV injection, early, and aggressively: 50 to 100 mg's, depending on the size of the person and the chances of seizure, and then 50 mg's every one to two hours as needed for agitation. In 24 hours the dosage is cut in half again or stopped as necessary.

Seizure disappears nearly but not completely in the acupuncture treatment setting, even without medical intervention.[150] However, because this is a potentially life-threatening withdrawal syndrome, vigilance on the acupuncturist's part is required. Close attention must be paid to **client history of seizure**, and to any **changes in respiration, blood pressure, and pulse** before and during treatment.

Latent withdrawal symptoms (those that occur beyond the acute withdrawal phase) for virtually all psychoactive drugs are subtle symptoms compared with blood pressure, pulse rate, and are a difficult treatment challenge in the Western clinical setting. They include a cycle of craving, depression, and anxiety. Irritability is also common, frequently accompanied by sleep disturbances including "drug dreams" and insomnia.

One of the earliest researchers on latent withdrawal[151] was Jerome Jaffe. He suggested that latent withdrawal symptoms persisted in general for three months, but that it was individual-specific and could last from six to 12 months. He hypothesized that the length of time was related to drug's half-life.

Latent withdrawal was originally termed "protracted abstinence syndrome" or "post-addictive syndrome" by the Addiction Research center in Lexington, which suggested that a hyper-responsivity to stressful stimuli was the physiological substrate of the anxiety/depression/craving cycle. It is theoretically caused by chemical activity and inactivity. The length of time predicted for the latent withdrawal period has grown longer the longer that the research has been going on, expanding from 30 days to one to five years. Some researchers believe that the receptors probably never come back to normal. Western medicine has little to offer anxiety, depression, and craving besides talk therapy and other psychoactive drugs, so acupuncture is singularly effective in the treatment of post-acute withdrawal.

Alcohol-Drug Interactions:

Lethal with alcohol are the barbiturates ((phenobarbital and tulinol) and the benzodiazapines (Valium, Librium, and Xanax).

The Benzodiazapines

The benzodiazapines are classified as minor tranquilizers, and include diazepam (Valium), chlordiazepoxide (Librium), flurazepam (Dalmane), and the highly soluble Ativan. The minor tranquilizers are mildly sedative. With increasing dosage they are also hypnotic. They have all been widely used for anxiety, tension, behavior excitement, insomnia, lower back pain, convulsive disorders, and withdrawal from alcohol and opiate-narcotic dependence.

Psychoactive Mechanisms:

Specific drug receptors have been found for Valium and other minor tranquilizers even though no similar chemicals have been discovered to be produced by the body. None of the known neurotransmitters combine with these receptors, though GABA binding is suspected. What seems likely is that we generate our own "minor tranquilizers," but these have yet to be isolated.

Valium and other benzodiazepines potentiate the effects of the neurotransmitter GABA, which is believed to act as an inhibitor for certain parts of the brain and to be responsible for some of the symptoms of anxiety. An increase in GABA may lower the amount of norepinephrine and serotonin in the brain.

<u>Acute Effects:</u>

Minor tranquilizers produce drowsiness, lethargy, nausea, diminished libido, blood cell abnormalities, and increased sensitivity to alcohol. In high doses they can depress respiration, induce coma, and cause death.

<u>Chronic Effects:</u>

Aside from their addictive potential, here is no clear evidence of permanent, irreversible damage to neurological or other physiological processes, even with long term use of benzodiazapines. Skin rashes and irregularities in menstrual cycle are not infrequent.

<u>Withdrawal Reactions:</u>

Both barbiturate and benzodiazapine withdrawal are nearly identical with alcohol (see pp. 101-103). *Acute* withdrawal includes severe depression, hypotension, anxiety, headaches, tremors, tachycardia, and possible grand mal seizure and psychotic reaction. Prolonged use of hypnotic doses may cause rebound increases in REM sleep and insomnia.

Due in part perhaps to the long half-life of the benzodiazapines, the acute withdrawal is extremely protracted. It is also dramatic, and acupuncture is not adequate to ameliorate these acute symptoms following prolonged use; therefore, clients need to taper down gradually from their dose over time. A 30 mg-per-day addiction may require as long as six weeks or more, with a five mg decrease in dosage per week. Individual clients will need to find their own way, and, if the drug is being procured by prescription, the cooperation of the prescribing physician is, of course, essential.

For general support in these issues, acupuncturists are encouraged to contact their local affiliate of the American Society for Addiction Medicine or of the National Council on Alcoholism and Drug Dependence for a list of physicians in the local area who are sensitive to addiction and recovery issues (see Appendix IV, Section A).

Latent benzodiazapine withdrawal, like the acute phase, is keen and protracted. The classic anxiety/depression/craving cycle, with attending insomnia and other disturbed sleep, can persist for months, depending upon the duration of use.

Benzodiazapine-Drug Interactions:

Valium action is potentiated when used with Phenothiazines (Thorazine, Mellaril, and Compazine). There is also a potentiation of CNS depressant effect when combined with alcohol (also true of Librium, chlorpromazine, and Compazine). LSD and mescaline intoxication can be alleviated with a dose of chlorpromazine (Thorazine, a "major" tranquilizer) and to a lesser degree with Valium.

Mood Modifiers

We place the so-called mood modifiers in a class of their own. They have a low abuse potential, and are used largely in the treatment of psychiatric illness. They include the major tranquilizers Haldol, a dopamine antagonist generally used for treating schizophrenia; Thorazine, used for maintenance in the treatment of schizophrenia and acute LSD reaction; Stelazine, and Lithium, both used in the treatment of bi-polar disorder.

The anti-depressant Prozac is among the newer mood-modifiers. Drugs like Prozac have a low abuse potential because they are very slow-acting, requiring ten days to two weeks for effect. Prozac blocks the reuptake of serotonin on the theory that chronic depression results from a serotonin depletion.[152] Newer mood modifiers based upon the serotonin deficiency theory are Zoloft and Paxil.

Narcotics

Pharmacologically, narcotics are analgesics of the opiate family. (The legal definition of narcotics is different, referring to any illicit drug). *Natural opiates* include opium itself, which is usually smoked, and its naturally existing ingredient codeine. Morphine (from the Greek *Morpheus*, God of Dreams) is the primary psychoactive ingredient in opium. Diacetylmorphine (heroin), and hydromorphone (Dilaudid), are sometimes classified as *semi-synthetic* opiates. Dilaudid is shorter acting and two to eight times more potent than morphine.

The *synthetic* (man-made) opiates, sometimes called *opioids*, include methadone, which is the most refined and potent opioid form. It is a highly controversial drug, popular with law enforcement and the medical community in maintaining opiate addicts in a state of heroin abstinence by preventing the cardiovascular "rush" of intravenous (IV) injection. The synthetic opiate propoxyphene (Darvon) is a close relative of methadone, and more than 30 million prescriptions per year are currently sold for pain. It is less effective as an analgesic and less dependency-producing than natural opiates, and it has dangerous abuse potential because it is commonly used to potentiate other drugs. Other synthetic opiates are Percodan and Demerol.

The leading medical function of the opiates is in their analgesic properties. These drugs are thought to act by reducing both the sensory signals of pain and the affective properties of pain ("It still hurts but it doesn't bother me."). They are the drugs of choice for post-surgical pain, and they are sometimes used as anesthetics during heart surgery because, unlike other anesthetics, they have no depressant action on the cardiovascular system. The opiates are also antitussive. Codeine is a common ingredient in cough suppressants. And they also have peristaltic effects, so are used in the treatment of dysentery and diarrhea. Food moves through the intestines in a wave, and opiates slow the wave, causing constipation.

Oral administration of opiates results in a slow, continuous absorption, with little euphoria since euphoria is related to the steepness of the absorption curve. Intramuscular administration is popular for pain management in hospitals because it also steadies absorption. Subcutaneous administration ((skin popping) is popular with early stage heroin users, but the most popular route of administration for addicts is intravenous injection ("main line"), which makes the dose more potent for a shorter time.

Psychoactive Mechanisms:

For a discussion of the psychoactive mechanisms of opiates, see pages 93 - 95.

Acute Effects:

Tolerance and physical dependence develop rapidly with opiate use. There is typically depressed sex drive, appetite, and activity in general. The first three to six hours following use, there is drowsiness, stupor, and daydreams. The "rush" is cardiovascular warmth, which is not a central effect of the drug. The rising curve resulting from rapid absorption is where the hedonia is, producing a mild euphoria, a tingling sensation resembling sexual orgasm, flushing, and a sense of well-being. Unlike other CNS depressants, there is usually no loss of motor control or consciousness, nor slurring of speech, although there is a clouding of mental function in very large doses. There can be mental distress, fear, and nervousness, but these symptoms are not typical. More common is a constriction of pupils, constipation, and respiratory depression producing irregular breathing. Less common symptoms are nausea, vomiting, dizziness, and shortness of breath.

The symptoms of overdose are a stuporous condition, and a deep sleep from which arousal is difficult but very important since this can forebode death from overdose. Dangerous signs of this include low respiration, slow or shallow breathing and/or blueness of lips and skin, and pinpoint pupils. There are far more methadone overdoses than heroin overdoses. Methadone is the most refined opiate we have; anything over 100 mg. per day is a toxic dose, and 100 mg. is enough to maintain abstinence without withdrawal for a four gram-per-day heroin user. The danger of overdose from methadone is amplified by its failure to produce euphoria and by the use of illicit (street) methadone which may contain impurities and for which the precise dose is not known.

Chronic Effects:

The primary chronic effect of opiate use is the fear of running out! Opiates, including heroin, are far less harmful to the body than most other drugs, such as alcohol, if the product is clean and is used cleanly. The myths around the dangers of heroin likely have to do with severity of withdrawal. There has been reported degenerative nerve damage, but measurable degenerative nerve damage is rare, and the changes are subtle. Most of the dangerous chronic effects are secondary, due to needle use or to a contaminated dose. These dangers include HIV infection, viral hepatitis (B and C), blood vessel inflammation, festering sores, heart valve infection, and malnutrition due to the lifestyle often associated with chronic use of the drug.

There are clear dangers to women during pregnancy. Reported complications of heroin use in pregnant women include infection of amniotic fluid, spontaneous abortions, breech deliveries, premature labor, premature rupture of membranes, placenta insufficiency, and toxemia.[153] It is standard Western medical protocol for physicians to place pregnant heroin-addicted women on methadone maintenance for the term of their pregnancy rather than risking detoxification of the fetus *inutero* where withdrawal symptoms cannot be monitored. Acupuncture has become the treatment of choice for heroin addicted pregnant women in many regions of the country (see pp. 300-302, 324-327, 396-396).

Withdrawal Reactions:

Acute withdrawal reactions from IV opiate addiction are severe, and their severity is increased by virtue of the fact that the chronic heroin user has a deficiency or imbalance in the natural pain-ameliorating mechanisms where morphine has its impact. Tolerance to pain or to any physical discomfort is exceptionally low among this population.

Acute withdrawal symptoms are usually as follows:

4 hours:
- anxiety
- craving

8 hours (add):
- yawning;
- teary eyes;
- perspiration;
- runny nose

12 hours, add:
- dilating pupils;
- chills and "goose bumps" (hence the phrase "cold turkey");
- twitches ("kicking");
- aching bones and muscles;
- hot and cold flashes;
- loss of appetite;

18 - 24 hours, add:
- increased intensity of the above;
- rise in blood pressure, pulse, and temperature;
- insomnia;
- nausea;

26 - 36 hours, add:
- vomiting;
- increased blood sugar;
- diarrhea and intestinal spasms;
- cramps.

All of these symptoms will peak at around 24 hours, and by 36 hours following the last dose, the symptoms will greatly reduce, followed generally at 48 to 72 hours by sleep.[154]

With methadone withdrawal following months of daily use at 50 mg or more, these symptoms will be greatly intensified and protracted, lasting from four to eight weeks or longer, depending upon the length of use and the dose. While twice-daily acupuncture can generally reduce heroin withdrawal symptoms to something resembling a mild case of the flu, it is unable to provide manageable withdrawal to methadone detoxification. So, as with the benzodiazapines, the client must reduce the dose gradually over time, titrating down typically in increments of five to 10 mg. per week until a daily dose of 25 mg. is reached, and then decreasing by three to five mg. per week or less, depending again upon the length of the dependency and the size of the original "maintenance" dose. It is important in these cases to let the client find his or her own way in the process. Opiate withdrawal is not fatal. The cliché is that they will *think* they are going to die, and then they will *wish* that they would, but they won't.

Latent opiate withdrawal, like the others we have discussed, is characterized by depression, irritability, cravings, anxiety, and (not universally) insomnia. The relapse rate for opiate addiction is extremely high, and treatment failure with heroin, even in the acupuncture treatment setting, is exceeded only by treatment failure with nicotine, where, as with heroin, the acute withdrawal is relatively brief, and yet relapse is the rule.

Opiate-Drug Interactions:

Opiate antagonists (which occupy the morphine receptor site but let nothing through) include naloxone, which is derived from thebaine, another component of opium. Thebaine is chemically similar to morphine and codeine, however, it has stimulant effects. Interestingly, naloxone has been shown to potentiate the euphoric effects of cocaine, and also inhibits some of the effects of acupuncture. Naltrexone, similar to naloxone, is commonly used in heroin treatment. If the patient uses heroin with naltrexone, the hedonic effects of the heroin are nullified.

Stimulants

Cocaine

As cocaine has driven American drug policy, pervasive stereotypes about cocaine users have driven social attitudes toward the drug: "yuppie" users in the early 1980s; inner city African

American "crack" addicts and their "crack babies" in the late 80s and early 90s, and the stereotype that cocaine-using are "loose," immoral, and wealthy.

Though the *DSMIII* (as opposed to the *DSMIII Revised*) and the World Health Organization (WHO) have minimized cocaine abuse because it produces no "physical" withdrawal syndrome, cocaine is, according to researchers Spitz and Rosecan, "deceptively and powerfully addictive over time in a manner that is unique among substances of abuse because of subtle imbalances in brain chemistry produced." [155]

Cocaine, as it is used addictively, is *cocaine hydrochloride*, a refined alkaloid derived from the South American coca plant, which is in itself more benign than caffeine. Cocaine and its base crystals, "crack," have driven and shaped the strategies of our recent National drug policy in terms of legal interdiction, research, and treatment.

Pharmacologically, cocaine is an anomaly. It is water soluble, yet gets to the brain because it is also soluble in oil. Its use seems to produce effects similar to chronic depression, although it is a CNS stimulant and is used for its euphoric effects. And, although the prevailing medical and psychiatric view through the 1980s was that cocaine is relatively harmless, more recent laboratory research has proven it to be the most addictive of all psychoactive drugs.[156] There may be discreet genetic parallels between cocaine addiction, alcoholism, and mental illness. As many as 75% of cocaine addicts have an alcoholic parent, and as many as 50% have predisposing or attending affective disorders such as chronic depression and mood disorders.

Cocaine use tends to be intermittent rather than continuous, with typical concentrated "binges" interrupted by periods of abstinence. This pattern is typical of laboratory animals such as rats and monkeys as well, for whom cocaine is the most addictive of drugs, with unparalleled rewarding potency. Given a choice of food, water, or cocaine, animals will consistently self-administer cocaine without eating or sleeping during an uninterrupted five to 12 day binge. For these animals, a period of abstinence begins with exhaustion or seizures. If the cocaine is taken away, they will quickly return to a normal healthy state. But in some studies, if it isn't taken away, all animals will be dead in 30 days, some in less than five days.

Cocaine is a local anesthetic, interfering with exteroceptor neuronal conduction. It also produces vasoconstriction in mucous membranes, which reduces bleeding during surgery. In general, its medical uses have been superseded by synthetic drugs. Street cocaine sometimes contains as little as 10% cocaine, having generally been diluted by mixing or "cutting" with other substances. Oral administration produces a greatly diminished high due to the effective "first pass effect" in the liver (see p. 53), in which the drug is efficiently metabolized before reaching the bloodstream. Intranasal administration (snorting), is most popular for cocaine hydrochloride, resulting in rapid absorption and peak euphoria in 15 to 30 minutes. Intravenous administration results in a short-lived but intense high followed by an extreme dysphoria (crash) and intense craving 40 to 50 minutes after injection.

Crack - cocaine base crystals, vaporized when heated - and "freebase" - a cocaine alkaloid paste - can also be used through IV injection, but smoking is the most popular route of administration for these forms in which the drug reaches the brain in about six seconds.

Psychoactive Mechanisms:

According to Spitz and Rosecan, cocaine abuse can be seen as a "natural experiment in affective illness" since the neurochemical changes resemble those seen in depression, cyclothymia, and behavioral disorders such as residual attention deficit disorder. The primary neurotransmitters involved in mood regulation and affective disorders are serotonin (5-HT), dopamine (DA), and norepinephrine (NE). Cocaine presumably potentiates transmission of these neurotransmitter chemicals, and then blocks their reuptake.[157] The result in a rapid accumulation of these substances in the synaptic cleft. Cocaine itself also binds to DA receptors closely related to the reuptake site, the significance of which is unknown. Cocaine also causes an increase in the density of the postsynaptic DA and NE receptors (upregulation), with the net result, with chronic use, of a DA and NE depletion. This combination of DA receptor supersensitivity and depletion is the theoretical substrate of the crash/craving syndrome. 5-HT is in the raphe regions of the pons and upper brain. Its "circuits" are not well understood. According to Spitz and Rosecan, early LSD studies indicate that LSD exerts its hallucinogenic psychotomimetic effects by interfering with the inhibitory effects of 5-HT. Later research, however, indicated that LSD effects are more obscure and complicated. The source of the toxic effects of cocaine in high doses are in this system. Cocaine's effects here are largely inhibitory, depleting the system, and inhibiting reuptake not only of 5-HT but also of its metabolic precursor tryptophan.

Other neuro-peptides that interact with cocaine include vasoppressin, which plays a role in learning and memory, and GABA. Cocaine increases GABA synthesis and turnover and decreases GABA binding in some brain areas and not others. And, cocaine is structurally similar to acetylcholine (ACh) antagonists such as atropine. It stimulates choline transport and acutely increases ACh levels.

Acute Effects:

Cocaine (like Valium) is described as a "state dependent" drug in that the effects felt depend upon the state of the subject, environment, etc.

Besides euphoria, a toxic dose produces:

- restlessness;
- tremors;
- diaphoresis;
- hypertension;
- cardiac arrhythmias;
- death.

Crack results from anesthetic effects on the heart.

Chronic Effects:

Many of the chronic effects of snorting cocaine are nasal, including rhinitis, mucosal erosion, nasal septum perforation, and sinusitis. Smoking or IV use also produces bronchitis, ventral fibrillation and arrest, and respiratory arrest, including cerebral hemorrhage and hyperpyreia seizures. IV cocaine use also produces the same secondary effects as IV heroin use.

Regardless of the route of administration, the following:

Physical chronic effects:

- weight loss (due to appetite suppression);
- malnutrition;
- insomnia;
- impotence;
- exhaustion;
- muscular twitches, tremors, and weakness.

Psychological chronic effects include:

- grandiosity;
- depression;
- anxiety;
- severe paranoia;
- hallucinations.

Additionally, crack cocaine destroys lung tissue. The high temperature does great damage. One "joint" per day equals the lung damage done by one pack of cigarettes.

Withdrawal Reactions:

Acute cocaine withdrawal reactions are, from a physical point of view, a little blip compared with opiate and alcohol and barbiturate withdrawal, a fact that led medical community to believe that cocaine was not addictive. Crack produces often severe depression or "dysphoria" 30 or 40 minutes after use, which is not universally true with other forms of cocaine. Withdrawal symptoms following a single dose (although research on dose response relationship is pretty thin) include oversleeping and lethargy, overeating, and craving for more. After a high dose, symptoms may include headache, fatigue, myocardial infarction, and anhedonia.

Latent withdrawal studies for cocaine are ten years old, so they say the period for latent withdrawal is ten years. With a typical 98% recidivism rate for cocaine in the Western treatment setting, there is little good research on latent withdrawal. Clinically and anecdotally, cocaine addicts experience a "honeymoon" period lasting from 60 to 90 days following cessation of use, and then "hit the wall" with severe depression, anxiety, and a return of keen craving. Recurring cocaine cravings months following use seem more associated with external "triggers" and association or suggestion than do the protracted cravings associated with other drugs. One of the greatest areas of efficacy of acupuncture is in its application to both acute and latent cocaine withdrawal.

Amphetamines

The amphetamines are also CNS stimulants with actions and effects similar to cocaine. Sometimes generically referred to as "speed," amphetamines are also called "crystal" when injected, "crank" when ground up and snorted, and "ice" when smoked. They were widely used prior to regulation in 1980 as an appetite suppressant. Their popularity in urban areas has waned since the ascent of crack, but crank in particular is popular in rural areas. Crystal (or crystal meth) is melted and put in syringe. Both crystal and ice are highly debilitating, producing a rapid, intense, and short high and crash, with dramatic tolerance (like crack, it develops a progressively lower high and lower crash with each use, so people tend to keep increasing the dose). As with cocaine, patterns of use are generally binge/collapse.

Psychoactive Mechanisms:

Psychoactive mechanisms of amphetamines are similar to those of cocaine. Both noradrenergic and dopaminergic actions include enhanced release of the neurotransmitters, blockade of presynaptic reuptake, and inhibition of the enzyme monoamine oxidase. Amphetamines also enhance the release of serotonin.

Acute Effects:

Acute effects of amphetamines include mood elevation (euphoria), increased psychomotor stimulation, enhanced alertness and increased attention (it has been used in the treatment of Childhood Attention Deficit Disorder), and diminished appetite (anorexia). Physiological effects also include sympathomimetic actions, increased systolic and diastolic blood pressure, bronchiodilation and increased oxygen consumption, elevated respiratory rate and depth, increased urinary retention, hyperglycemia, lipolysis (elevated plasma-free fatty acids), increased metabolic rate (in large doses), and mydriasis (pupil dilation).

Chronic Effects:

Toxic chronic "psychological" effects include anxiety reactions, sleep disturbances, paranoid schizophrenic symptomatology, rebound depression, and, particularly with ice, acute psychotic reaction. Physiological effects include cardiac arrhythmia, angina pectoris, hypo or hypertension, circulatory collapse, cerebral hemorrhaging, and brain electroencephalographic seizure activity.

Withdrawal Reaction:

There is little abstinence syndrome or withdrawal except for irritability, depression, and anger, so motivation for seeking treatment is low. As with cocaine, these withdrawal syndromes generally respond very well to acupuncture.

Hallucinogens

The hallucinogens, sometimes called *psychedelics*, or *psychotomimetics* (in that some of them are known to mimic the symptoms of various forms of psychosis), are perhaps the least understood class of psychoactive drugs. Depending upon the individual and the circumstances of use, they sometimes act as stimulants and at other times as depressants. The most common is the natural hallucinogen cannabis (marijuana), which is sometimes considered in a pharmacological class by itself since it displays both hallucinogenic and depressant properties. Mescaline, also a naturally occurring hallucinogen, is the psychoactive ingredient in the peyote mushroom.

Perhaps the most famous synthetic hallucinogen is lycergic acid diethylamide (LSD). Because it produces some of the same symptoms as schizophrenia, a great deal of research was done on its actions in the 1960s and 70s, but laws prohibiting further research were enacted in the 1970s. Other synthetic hallucinogens include methylenedioxyamphetamine (MDMA), also called "ecstasy" and sometimes classified as a stimulant. It was used in veterinary medicine around the turn of the century, but no other medical use has been found. Phencyclidine or phencyclohexyl piperdine (PCP) is another synthetic hallucinogen with a high "abuse" potential, though its popularity has been largely replaced by crack cocaine. It is used by the National Park Service to immobilize grizzly bears. It is perhaps the most socially dangerous of all the hallucinogens because of the severe psychological disorientation it produces - feelings of unreality, separation from the environment, restlessness and panic, and paranoia.

Hallucinogens are not generally thought of as addicting because they produce neither tolerance nor classic withdrawal (although the protracted withdrawal from chronic marijuana use produces a low-level anxiety and sleep disturbance which contributes to a high rate of relapse).

As we have noted, daily acupuncture treatments will make all of the symptoms of acute and post acute withdrawal manageable in the vast majority of cases, even in cases of polydrug in which more than one drug as been used chronically. The exceptions to these cases, however, require constant vigilance. Acupuncturists, especially in the beginning, will want to use blood pressure and pulse diagnosis for acute alcohol, barbiturate, and benzodiazapine withdrawal where seizure is a risk. Inservice trainings with public health officials is desirable at program start-up so that the symptoms that forebode serious withdrawal complications, such as seizure and dehydration, as well as toxic drug reactions, may be recognized. The program staff is also urged to consult with NADA veterans concerning special individual cases, particularly regarding detoxification from methadone and the benzodiazapines from which gradual cessation of chronic use is recommended.

Chapter Six   **Western Treatment Models and the**
                         Acupuncture Interface

In general, treatment modalities follow funding, and funding, in turn, determines what goes on clinically. To be eligible for certain types of funding, treatment programs must adhere to certain licensing and/or certification requirements, which dictate clinical protocols. The *medical/pharmacological* treatment programs, therefore, are creatures of either the public or private insurance industries. State supported Medicaid Drug and Alcohol programs,[158] for example, whether outpatient, or the more recent designation "day treatment," must have Western medical supervision. The medical supervisor may or may not be a psychiatrist, and may or may not actually be on the program staff; he/she may be a physician employed by the local county to provide clinical oversight, signing treatment plans for clients he/she may never meet, and providing for physical examinations, or, more frequently, signing with a rubber stamp "Physical Exam Waivers" based upon a medical history taken by a counselor at the admission site. Drugs to treat withdrawal may or may not be prescribed, but all of these bureaucratic and medical services must be provided for in the budget and in the clinical protocols.

These state Medicaid-billable cases require meticulous paper documentation of clinical treatment plans and progress notes and must come under the scrutiny of periodic state "Site Visits" and of monthly "Utilization Review Committee" (URC) meetings or their equivalent. The URC is usually made up of staff members under the supervision of the URC-approved Clinical Supervisor or, again, more often than not, his/her designee. This administrative, control- and-accountability-based paper trail may or may not reflect what really goes on in the program.

Acupuncture is, as of this writing, not a billable treatment event in these programs. However, there are no restrictions that prevent an acupuncture component from being a part of these programs, and certainly no restriction prohibiting acupuncturists from being designated as program *counselors* if they meet other counselor requirements of the Program, as determined by the county or state funding agency. Billable treatment events include individual and group counseling/education, urine testing, drug administration sessions, and other specially defined "treatment episodes." In Medicaid-certified day treatment facilities, the "billable event" is a unit of time - either a day, or a minimum number of hours in a day - in which a minimum number of treatment activities such as those listed above take place, and these activities may include acupuncture.

Private treatment programs that bill third party payees (private insurance companies) must also operate under Western medical oversight. Such programs, whether residential or outpatient, are often operated adjunctive to a general hospital. The conventional private inpatient programs, whose popularity is waning (see p. 29), are typically 28 days long and cost from $15,000 to $35,000. They operate medical detoxification services on the front end, usually the first seven to ten days, and outpatient aftercare, usually individual and group counseling, following discharge. The balance of the inpatient program is devoted to individual, group, and family psychotherapy and/or counseling; education on drug and alcohol issues and on dysfunctional family systems; generally some kind of physical therapy, and attendance at Twelve Step meetings either inside or outside the facility. These Twelve Step meetings are often supplemented with "step-study" activities or discussion groups. Some of these programs may also have innovative adjuncts such as art therapy, nutrition lectures, or "trust-building" nature outings. Patients are kept busy, and there is often limited contact with the "outside world." [159]

Private medical/pharmacological-based *outpatient* programs are also often operated adjunctively to a hospital, or perhaps to an inpatient program, and usually cost around $3500 for an intensive (six weeks or so) evening and weekend program. Due to decreasing popularity with the insurance companies that support all of these medical/pharmacological programs, these hospital-based programs are currently in the process of diversifying, and many now include programs for eating or sexual disorders or other private insurance billable psychiatric illnesses.

The potential for acupuncture to become a part of these private programs depends upon having a respected physician advocate who has influence with the Board of Directors and/or the Clinical Review Board of the hospital of which the treatment program is a part to advocate such treatment.

The drug therapies in these medical/pharmacological programs are used to control the patient and make him or her more comfortable during acute withdrawal. Common drugs used include Valium in the inpatient setting and, in the outpatient program, Valrelease (timed release Valium) or "kickpacks" of Librium or Clonidine (a fairly benign blood pressure medication often prescribed in patch form that is helpful for withdrawal from opiates and nicotine). Haldol, sometimes used for amphetamine withdrawal, is a major tranquilizer used for psychotic episodes that helps with extreme anger, mood swings. Other frequent pharmacological interventions used include antabuse for alcohol and naltrexone for heroin.

Methadone treatment for opiate addiction is in a class of its own. It is generally available only in a state licensed outpatient setting, and dispensation of the drug must comply with federal regulations that include urine testing. There are some self-referred clients in methadone programs, but many others arrive as a condition of county, state, or federal probation or parole, or of local child protective services. These "mandated" clients are usually recently released from prison or county jail, often having violated parole or probation with a positive urine test. Some parolees viewed as high risk for relapse may be summarily referred upon release from custody by an understandably nervous parole or probation officer whose task, after all, is not to effect recovery of individuals but to prevent the resumption of criminal behavior.

Methadone clients either have to pay for the treatment themselves, usually around $200 per month, or apply for a publicly funded "free" slot, for which there are usually long waiting lists. The methadone is administered daily on site in an oral liquid dose.

Illicit methadone is also widely available on the street, and is often used to supplement the prescribed dose, or to self-medicate heroin withdrawal. Methadone clinics themselves are generally private entities operated for profit.

Methadone programs usually have two protocols: *detoxification* and *maintenance.* Detoxification is a 21-day program with a daily dose tapering down from 40 or 50 mg. Maintenance is a daily dose ranging from 40 to 100 mg. depending upon the length and severity of the opiate dependency. Some methadone programs have begun a 120-day protocol that includes both a detoxification and a brief maintenance phase. Some of these programs are supported by ancillary counseling, education, and/or Twelve Step services. Methadone maintenance is currently increasing in popularity, and recommended maintenance doses are rising, as a result of increased evidence of the risk of spreading the HIV virus through shared needle use. At the same time, there is a trend away from public funding for unlimited maintenance services. Some California counties have recently placed a two year limit on publicly funded maintenance slots, and a recent Oregon law requires that individuals try acupuncture detoxification before receiving publicly funded methadone services.

There are places in the country, such as Lincoln Hospital in New York, Bayview Hunters Point in San Francisco, and programs in Texas, where acupuncture has been successfully integrated either on site or in close proximity to methadone programs. "Twenty-one day" opiate detoxifications using methadone are far more successful when accompanied by acupuncture.[160] People who have been on methadone maintenance for a period of time find that the withdrawal from methadone itself is exceedingly protracted and difficult. This withdrawal is so severe that people should not be encouraged to quit "cold turkey," but should instead taper off the methadone gradually on an individually developed schedule. The Bayview Hunter's Point Clinic has found that Chinese medicine and full body acupuncture has been helpful for individuals on methadone maintenance in making a decision to attempt withdrawal.

Aversion therapy is another medical/pharmacological-based treatment approach that is quite controversial. This intrusive therapy is, not surprisingly, the forerunner of modern medical treatment. Drugs that are either enzyme antagonists for the target drug or nausea-producing drugs are administered prior to ingestion of the target drug so that a violent toxic reaction to one's "drug of choice" is elicited. This procedure is often combined with "negative feedback" audio or video tapes. Mild electric shock is also sometimes used, especially to accompany cigarette smoking.

Drug-free treatment programs that depend for therapy upon the social interaction of clients are sometimes called *Social Model* programs. Other drug-free treatment programs use cognitive oriented treatment such as case management, counseling, or psychotherapy. The Rational Emotive Therapy (RET) of Albert Ellis has gained some recent popularity. These latter approaches are rationally oriented, focused on changing thinking patterns and one's life through cognitive, rational means; the former, Social Model programs, have roots in "religious therapy" (such as Salvation Army or Rescue Mission type programs), and also in the Twelve Step programs.

In the earliest days of A.A., sober members and their families often took alcoholics into their homes to provide a safe and sober living environment during the transition period. The sole therapy provided was lots of A.A. meetings and A.A. sponsorship. This form of recovery-based "treatment" survives in residential "clean and sober living environments," usually gender-based and operated by private nonprofit corporations on a self-supporting basis, with the residents working outside, paying room and board, and sharing in housekeeping chores. Similar programs are operated by churches or other religious organizations where the therapy, either in addition to or in place of the Twelve Step programs, includes religious services, Bible study, and "work therapy."

Unfortunately, while these are prime settings for on-site daily acupuncture treatment, and are in fact often solvent enough to afford it, any sort of organized treatment on site is generally prohibited by lack of licensure of these programs. Under the legal designation of "Clean and Sober Living" environments in California, these programs are currently able to avoid the regulation and scrutiny of the State Department of Alcohol and Drugs; understandably, they cling aggressively to this status.

Some residential programs, based on the social model, have crossed the line into "treatment" and have become licensed as *Therapeutic Communities* or *Residential Recovery Homes*. Therapeutic Communities began with the Esalen Institute, founded in Big Sur, California, in the 1960s as a "Growth Resort." They became part of the pop culture and experienced growth and popularity through the 1970s, using a blend of ideas ranging from cooperative living and group encounter therapy to Zen and "Dale Carnegie." There is currently renewed interest in the general concept, especially among law enforcement and advocates of the "Cocaine Camp" alternative to incarceration for drug offenders.

Long term (90 days or longer) Residential Treatment programs usually add to the Twelve Step-based template such activities as group and individual counseling and education. Some of these provide social model (non-medical) detoxification while others require that people detox prior to admission. Some homes are co-ed, but most are gender-specific. Some derive funding from public sources administered by the state, county, or city (see Chapter Eight). Others may be operated by, or under contract with, the State Department of Corrections. Still others, often funded by county probation departments, target specific populations, such as adolescents, or pre- and postpartum women, a few of which have been funded by the Federal Center for Substance Abuse Prevention (CSAP). All of these are excellent target programs for on-site acupuncture. For an acupuncture component to do well in such facilities in which clients are mandated, however, the support of the non-acupuncture program staff is essential. If the acupuncture is scheduled as optional in a "free time" slot, when other activities are mandated, client participation can be problematic, requiring intensive staff support for the acupuncture component and assertive education concerning acupuncture and Chinese medicine for both staff and clients.[161] In residential settings, where people have already detoxed and where relapse generally results in program expulsion, we need not adhere as strictly to the five-point auricular protocol, although it is still important to keep the substance abuse-specific protocol as a basic template from which to expand to other Chinese medical protocols.

Outpatient drug-free programs, both public and private, proliferate the drug treatment arena. They include drop-in center type services, staffed by volunteers, which offer crisis and referral counseling and education; day treatment or outpatient group and individual counseling programs; protective payee case management for alcoholic or drug dependent SSI recipients;[162] private counseling or psychotherapy by a licensed Marriage, Family, and Child Counselor (MFCC) or Therapist (MFCT), licensed Clinical Social Worker (LCSW), or psychologist, and specialty treatment such as massage, bio-feedback, hypnotherapy, behavior modification, and, of course, acupuncture and Chinese medicine.

By far the largest alcohol outpatient case loads in most communities are in "Drinking Driver" programs. Anyone convicted of driving under the influence (DUI) of alcohol in many states is required to enroll in a First Offender DUI program and attend classes. Subsequent convictions require completion of a Multiple Offender DUI program in order for driving privileges to be restored by the state's Department of Motor Vehicles. Multiple Offender programs typically involve individual and group counseling/education sessions. Clients must pay for these programs themselves, and the program protocols generally require strict approval and oversight by the State Department of Alcohol, and any treatment outside of these protocols is prohibited. There is little substantial measurable impact of these programs on the drinking driver population (the rule of thumb in the Multiple Offender programs is that the more offenses a client has, the deeper the denial and the more resistance to counseling and education!). As the number of DUI arrests escalates (and law enforcement reports that only a small percentage of offenders are caught), and as the political pressure of groups like Mothers Against Drunk Driving (MADD) and state police organizations increases, there is a grow-

ing level of desperation on the part of the planners of these programs, making them a fertile target indeed for acupuncture programs.

Some therapeutic processes transcend all treatment protocols
and modalities. Acupuncture is among these, and as we describe
these transcendent processes, we will begin to gain a better clinical
understanding of the role of acupuncture as a complement to them.

One of these transcendent therapeutic processes is the dynamic
of *groups*. Whether the group is a Twelve Step meeting, or a room
full of people receiving acupuncture treatment, or a counsel-
ing/education session, group dynamics are a salient therapeutic
mechanism in recovery, establishing a ground for healing relationship. Herbert Gravitz (see *n.* #10) has said that alcoholics and
addicts were wounded in relationship, and they must ultimately be
healed in relationship. So, group acupuncture, Twelve Step
meetings, and perhaps a gender-based support group would, taken
together, form a very potent program of early recovery apart from
whatever content was being addressed in each group. Not
surprisingly, the individual addict or alcoholic will generally and
impulsively resist group participation or activity, preferring the
relative but dubious comfort of isolation where there are no cognitive expectations nor opportunities for social failure. A fundamental aspect of our success with acupuncture is that it takes place in a
group setting. Here, people have an opportunity to be involved in
a group process, but without any expectations being placed upon
them. It is a safe group, which, for the practicing addict, is a contradiction in terms! This is a nice paradox with which to introduce
an individual to recovery.

Another therapeutic process that cuts across all treatment lines
is the process of *intervention*. Most private medical treatment programs such as those we have described also offer intervention
services. The intervention concept was developed in Minnesota in
the 1970s, and involves the alcoholic's or addict's "significant others" - family members, friends, employer, minister, etc. - in a
carefully planned and orchestrated confrontation with the
"identified patient," a confrontation in which admission to the trea-

tment facility is made an ultimatum. The concept of intervention is a major treatment breakthrough. It acknowledges the *addictive family system* as an essential aspect of the alcoholic's or addict's disease, and a skilled intervention counselor will use the intervention as an opportunity to heal the system itself; in this regard, there is no such thing as a failed intervention, because even if the identified patient declines treatment and chooses the pre-orchestrated consequences of continued drinking or drug use, the codependent circle of family and friends will come to see their own part in the addictive system in which they have been functioning. Recent alcohol and drug prevention efforts, including the Robert Wood Johnson Foundation's "Fighting Back" grants, and CSAP's "Community Partnership" grants, have an opportunity to apply the dynamics of family systems intervention on a *community systems level*.

This is an important concept in our work, for it provides a way of understanding the role of acupuncture in treatment. Intervention is based upon the valid premise that the most endemic feature of the addictive system is *denial*; denial is, in fact, the foundation symptom of alcoholism/addiction. Denial does not necessarily or even typically refer to use of the drug. Most chronic alcoholics/addicts will admit that they drink or use drugs a lot. Clinical denial refers instead to the *consequences* of the addictive use.

In the original philosophy of Alcoholics Anonymous, it was assumed that an alcoholic had to "hit bottom" before he/she would be ready to accept recovery. What "hitting bottom" means is that the *consequences* of the chronic use of the drug have become sufficiently felt so that a *conscious connection* is made between *use* and *consequences* of use; hence, denial is broken. The alcoholic/addictive "bottom" takes many forms. It may be financial (destitution, loss of job, or the threat of same), social, marital, or familial (divorce, abandonment, or threat of same), moral (shame at actions while under the influence), legal (incarceration, drunk driving arrest, etc.), or physical (medical consequences). Unfortunately, most addicts and alcoholics die before they reach a bottom sufficient to develop the conscious willingness to seek help. So, the notion of intervention is to "raise the bottom," to bring the consequences to consciousness. The well-rehearsed intervention session says to the identified patient, "here are the specific consequences of your alcoholism/addiction, and this is specifically what is going to happen if you continue this way." Period.

Intervention only works when the underground currents of motivation are heading or tending in the same direction as the intervention. In our view of recovery, we always assume that this motivation is present. No matter how keen the denial, how deep the identification with the addictive behavior, or how fearful the identified patient is of letting go of the addictive ground, there is always a deeper, wiser part of the person to whom the intervention speaks. If clients could just stop using drugs, they would just stop using drugs! Every addict wants freedom from the addiction, if they only knew *how* to *do* it. This, we assume. Those of us with an appreciation of the principles of Chinese medicine are fortunate to be justified in embracing such optimism, for we are able to view the organism as a *balance-seeking* system with the intrinsic capacity to heal. And we understand acupuncture to be a method of bringing support to this agenda of balance. Acupuncture as intervention - or, perhaps more appropriately, *innervention* - invites the individual's attention toward the inner resources of healing.

In a way, as we have suggested earlier, *physical* denial is the most pervasive and certainly the most personal form that denial takes. We can even go so far as to say that physical denial is the *original* form of denial in the addictive state, for the ascent, crystallization, and dominance of ego (mind) in the Rationalist system involves a splitting off of consciousness of body. This sense of separation and isolation from body can be seen, therefore, as the fundamental addictive template.

Recovery manifests as assuming responsibility for one's life, and, in a sense, one's mortal life begins (and ends) with one's organism. The organism, and not the abstract mind, is the true seat of consciousness, of emotions, of wisdom, and of healing. While the essence of addiction is turning off and distorting internal messages, the essence of *recovery* is having the inner channels open: being accepting of, in touch with, and responsive to the internal processes of balance, healing, and life.

We can see acupuncture, then, as a *physical intervention* on a level that addresses the *core issue* of the disease of addiction even beyond the clinical efficacy of particular point location. Chronic drug use not only produces denial as a symptom; it in fact *requires* denial for its continued survival. It is virtually impossible to be accepting of, in touch with, and responsive to one's body *and* chronically use psychoactive drugs at the same time, because *the agenda of the body is always balance*, and if one *feels* oneself to be one *with* one's body, then acceptance of life, and, by implication, the state of recovery, follows. As with most fundamental truths, Alcoholics Anonymous has a pithy aphorism to describe this: it is the alcoholic's psychic pain of sitting in a bar "with a belly full of booze and a head full of A.A.." This is not, homeostatically, a comfortable state!

And there is more here to lead us to an understanding of the efficacy of acupuncture in dealing with addictive systems, because the original dualism, the original denial of self, as we have suggested earlier, is projected outward from mind/body to self/other. Addiction is sometimes called, as we have also suggested earlier, a disease of isolation. Just as chronic addictive use requires denial of the inward, physical consequences of use, it also requires denial of, through isolation from, the external consequences of addictive use.[163]

This is the operating dynamic of addictive institutions as well, and the source of their dysfunction. As Anne Wilson Schaef has pointed out, these institutions are like classic dysfunctional families, often with a practicing addict (identified patient) in a position of authority, who may be an alcoholic, a workaholic, a rageaholic, a sex addict, etc., whom everyone moves to protect and cover for. Everyones agenda is to take the focus away from themselves. So, the system is characterized by - indeed *thrives* on - control, manipulation, scarcity, dehumanization, and crisis. It is a closed system. If one of the actors leaves for some reason, someone else moves in to take their place and play the role in the addictive drama. Everyone knows their parts, because they learned them in their own historical family of origin.[164]

Traditional Chinese medicine, practiced as it normally is in the West in private treatment rooms and in response to uniquely reported and diagnosed symptoms, may function to address the original inward denial we have described; but acupuncture as it has evolved in the public group treatment setting with NADA protocols has the added potential of opening up the addictive system of isolation from external energy. The *qi* flows *outward*, *yin* energy is nourished and is manifest in the room, and, for the moment, the focus shifts, and there is the possibility of the *consciousness* of unspoken connectedness and participation. Just as the addict cannot be accepting of, in touch with, and responsive to his/her body *and* chronically use psychoactive drugs at the same time, neither can he or she sustain the external consequences of the addictive behavior while being in a state of participatory consciousness.

The frontier of Western treatment (and a current "buzzword" as well) is *relapse prevention*.[165] This concept has been born, in part, of the failure of treatment whose focus has been on detoxification and the first thirty days of recovery. Clients will often negotiate this phase successfully, only to resume drug use upon release from the program or shortly thereafter. This reality is notoriously typical of nicotine and cocaine, and common as well with alcohol, the opiates, and other psychoactive drugs. Relapse prevention as a focus has also been borne of the increasingly sophisticated research on the persistence, into abstinence, of the discreet alterations of neurotransmitting mechanisms that result from the drug use. And, its focus has also been influenced by general clinical and recovery experience that indeed alcoholism/drug addiction is, as the American Medical Association has described, a disease *characterized by relapse.*

Before discussing "relapse prevention" specifically, it will perhaps be helpful to be aware of the notion of different *phases* of recovery. These phases have been extensively broken down and analyzed in the literature of relapse prevention, but, for our purposes, we will simplify them, and suggest three general phases: *transition, stabilization*, and *empowerment*. The more we understand about the dynamics of these phases of recovery, the better understanding we will have of how acupuncture can be integrated with traditional treatment to enhance recovery at each phase.

It might be assumed that the transition phase of recovery begins with abstinence. Indeed, it is traditional for recovering members of Alcoholics Anonymous, Narcotics Anonymous, and Cocaine Anonymous to count their "time in recovery" from their first day of abstinence, even celebrating "birthdays" with token "sobriety chips" and birthday cakes.

But our experience in the acupuncture clinic, as well as our image of a new world view emerging from recovery, warrants a less "use-specific" definition, one that tends less to define recovery as commencing with a static event, such as abstinence, and instead one that emphasizes the notion of *recovery as process*. We will suggest that *the transition phase begins with the consciousness of the consequences of addictive drug use* and extends for weeks, months, or even years in a manner that is unique to each individual.

The transition phase is a scenario of the balancing of physical and emotional extremes; it is the period of time required for the addict to become relatively comfortable with the idea of abstention. It is a period characterized by "slips and starts."

One subset of the transition phase is detoxification, or acute withdrawal, a period lasting from three to fifteen days following abstention.[166] We can describe this state as Michael Smith has, as a "crisis in elimination,"[167] or as the body's homeostatic efforts to achieve balance in the sudden absence of the chemical, or as a subclinical period in which attending pathologies are still masked by the toxic effects of the drug. The recommended treatment for this detoxification period, as we have noted, is daily auricular acupuncture according to the NADA protocol (see p. 85).

A client may go through detoxification several times during the transition phase, moving from Bateson's rigidity to collapse again and again (see p. 58). The transition phase is the period of radical center-seeking described in Chapter Three. It is a weaving in and out of many different kinds of energy, from romantic "honeymoon glows" to periods of brooding, deep depression, anxiety, grieving, and fear. It is a period of wide swings from "white-knuckle sobriety" to "this is the greatest thing that has ever happened to me." It is a period of great emotional vulnerability, a time of "easy does it," when major life decisions are best avoided. It is a time of being patient with and learning to honor and trust the process of one's own healing. And it is often a time of the emergence of secondary or accompanying addictions.

In "Twelve Step time," it is the period of taking the first three steps, the period of ego dissolution, of dethroning the king and discovering the meaning of the words powerlessness, humility, surrender, and gratitude. And, it is a period of self-forgiveness.

We emphasize that this period is not a static event but a dynamic process. It requires a transformation of one's relationship with the drug, and a transformation of one's basic identity as a person who *uses* drugs. There is also generally crisis in one's identity with friends, family, and vocation. It is a period of coming to terms with difficulties one has never imagined, and of bitter disappointment that God has not chosen to reward abstinence with "instant wellness! "

We can say that, in a typical successful recovery scenario, this period lasts about eighteen months following abstinence.[168] But one of the more harmful things we can do is to make an inflexible blueprint of this period. The challenge is to give people "markers," assure them that they are "right on schedule," that it will get better if they don't drink or use. But making an issue out of these time zones and "phases" is dangerous because of countertransference, a projecting of our own hopes, fears, and expectations upon the client who will then think they are doing something wrong because they think that, "by now, they *should* be feeling thus and so."

To be efficacious as a gateway to recovery, treatment will honor and support this recovery process on every level. The way that this support is offered is through *validation of experience.* We suggested in Chapter Two that a central dynamic precursor to addiction is unvalidated trauma, the psychic splitting off because of shame, and the crystallization of the fundamental dualism. This denial of experience and of sensation has become the central problem of existence in the transition phase of recovery. Validation (like the drug-induced state of intoxication) speaks "yes." But while drug use speaks "yes" by turning off the parental messages of authority, guilt, and shame, and blurring external negative feedback, *genuine* validation says, *yes*, you are experiencing these things; *yes*, this is very difficult and painful; *yes*, you are healing, and you have the inherent ability and right to heal; you have suffered grievous losses, and, *yes*, the consequences of your drug use are real.

Pragmatically, the primary disease concept is of great value in this phase, because it allows the essential process of self-forgiveness to begin. "We are not bad people trying to become good; we are sick people trying to become well." The survival frame is alternately useful: we are not victims of addiction, but survivors of our life experiences.

It is, as we have suggested, in its ability to offer a fundamental validation of experience, and of the possibility of healing, that acupuncture fills the experience-based gaps that exist in traditional Western treatment. It is a physically supportive, predictable, non-judgmental, and validating experience that the client can access on his or her own emotional schedule. One of the reasons that the acupuncture treatment needs to be available daily, consistently, on demand, throughout the transition phase, is so that the client may come into the clinic for treatment regardless of how they feel that day, without the fear of being judged, or of being asked to become cognitively engaged in a conversation about how they are doing. Again, this is what we mean by "barrier free" treatment.

Following the detoxification phase, the acupuncturist, at the client's request, may begin to provide more expansive treatment beyond the NADA protocol, treating attending or unmasked symptoms that are presented. But, again, it is essential that the basic treatment continue to be available daily on demand so that the program can become malleable to the client's unique and changing needs, rather than coming to depend upon diagnosis for its success. In this way, our treatment mode becomes empowering in its form, validating the client's personal process of recovery and placing the responsibility for recovery not with the clinic but with the client. This is a new experience for the client, and for the drug treatment establishment in charge of program evaluation. It is not new to the Twelve Step group, which says to the newcomer, "it works if you work it! "

Ideally, crisis, referral, or group counseling is also available "on demand" at or nearby the acupuncture clinic site. And, ideally, the counseling will mimic the acupuncture, also being supportive, non-judgmental, and validating of experience. It will remain focused on the consequences of the drug use, rather than expanding prematurely into other emotional, social, and psychological issues. The counseling posture will usually be most supportive if it is done with a strong Twelve Step orientation in combination with Rogerian, "client-centered" organizing principles.[169] This means that the counselor will be speaking the language of the Twelve Step paradigm, even though the client may not as yet have embraced the Twelve Step program, and that counseling sessions will be ethically guided by the Rogerian principles of genuineness, spontaneity, non-judgmental acceptance, honesty, and accurate empathy. We recommend that group counseling sessions be gender specific, since fundamental issues of sexual identity are an essential part of recovery. Mixed gender groups may be available in later stages of recovery.

There will come in this process a weaning from the treatment program as the client becomes more and more centered in the Twelve Step recovery program. The treatment program is never a replacement for recovery, even though it is potentially addictive; clients (and staff!) can get hooked on the client's remaining in treatment. It is an essential part of program planning and design to look for structures that will serve as supportive "bridges" *out* of the treatment program and back into the client's community.[170]

The *stabilization phase* of recovery commences with the onset of longer and longer moments of time in which the individual is at last comfortable inside his or her skin with the idea of non-use of psychoactive drugs. This period often begins with the client's taking the 4th and 5th of the Twelve Steps,[171] and extends for three to five years into recovery. Primary identification has shifted from chemical use to non-use. There has been a surrender. One has turned from the old drug-centered acquaintances and the old haunts. Recovery has been embraced as a "lifestyle." New friends are clean and sober, and the new haunts are usually Twelve Step meeting halls. The client may sporadically return to the acupuncture clinic for "tune-ups," or perhaps to begin the transition phase of nicotine recovery. Secondary or "unmasked" symptoms and conditions will begin to be addressed, and there will likely be major career and relationship decisions made. There will be a sense of commitment to sobriety, and a sense of confidence that one is at last "out of the woods." However, the fact is, the risk of relapse is high during this period. Many return to use of the "cunning, baffling, powerful" (and patient) drug of choice. But we realize that it is not in reality the *drug* that warrants this description. It is the addictive culture, manifest in the need to "get it right," in the need to control, to be what and who one is *supposed to be* instead of realizing that *who one is* is enough.

This is the phase in which unmasked issues are addressed. Acupuncture continues to have a vital role, and we will have moved beyond the basic NADA protocol to more expansive diagnoses and treatment, including traditional Chinese medicine. The private practitioner plays a significant role, not only the acupuncturist, but other professionals, particularly those involved with body work. Nutritional needs will begin to be addressed. Secondary addictions will become primary - nicotine, eating disorders, sex addiction, or relationship addiction. Other Twelve Step groups may be sought out to address these other addictions. Psychotherapy may begin to play a role as the client becomes ready to begin to address family of origin issues in the new awareness that his or her affliction has a systemic origin and nature.

One's family may also become involved in treatment. Incest issues or other historical issues of violence and unresolved trauma will surface and, untreated, may precipitate relapse.

In this phase, gender, racial, and ethnic identity issues play a central role. Women, supported by recovering women, will become aware of the internalized oppression of the patriarchy which has been an underpinning of their addictive behavior. They will find from other recovering women *validation as women* and support for coming to trust their feelings. They may experience the spiritual crisis of coming to question the God of their understanding to whom they have surrendered "their will and their lives" in Step 3, and begin to find a new and stronger identification with female archetypes as they move away from the subjugation and internalized oppression of the patriarchy in their movement toward empowerment.[172] People of color, supported by others of their race or ethnicity who are in recovery, will experience the psychic pain of their woundedness without the mask of anesthetizing drugs to defend them from memories of oppression, rage, and abandonment. They too will gain a consciousness of how the historical oppression in their lives became internalized, and self-imposed limitations will be uncovered and faced. New and deeper sources of racial and ethnic pride will be discovered and transcended as they move toward individual empowerment. Men will become conscious of the repressed feminine both outside and inside, and will move through the pain and guilt of their participation, however tacit, in the system of oppression which they too have internalized as their addictive legacy. New, healthy masculine archetypes will provide touchstones for balance and completeness as human beings.

All of these paths are fraught with difficulties, and most travelers will shift addictions along the way to political, spiritual, or gender movements - a new "fix" "out there." Those well enough supported to return again and again to their own center may learn the way to true empowerment, the discovery and expression of who they are as individual people living one among many. They will come to appreciate the paradox that "the path of excess leads to the palace of wisdom." With the Buddhists, they will learn to "chop wood and carry water" in a state of serenity, a state of "peace that passeth understanding."

The third phase we have called empowerment, and there are many "stuck points" in negotiating the transition from stabilization to empowerment. The empowerment phase is the ascendancy of the "newly constituted self" to the relinquished throne. It is the acceptance of ourselves for just exactly who we are. This is a difficult phase because every message from every institution in which we function in our society - as well as an active "committee" of parental and other historical messages in our heads - is saying the opposite, that we need to perform better, act better, accomplish more, acquire more, control more resources and energy, look better, get our lives together, set goals, lose weight, and aspire to *be* somebody at last. These are all *things* for which all referents are *outside*.

Recovery doesn't work in a vacuum. It works "where the rubber meets the road," in the daily and moment-to-moment interface with the addictive systems in which we must function. We are vulnerable to being seduced back into our addiction on a thousand levels - in every relationship, in every new memory of earlier pain, in every enterprise, in every unmet childhood desire, in every sexual impulse, in every wish for intimacy, in every setback, in every achievement, and in every transition that constitutes our daily lives. It is not enough simply to be attending meetings, getting acupuncture, having a sponsor, and abstaining from psychoactive drugs. We must live *in* our recovery, in our growth, in our own spirituality, *in the process of our lives* in order to realize empowerment. The old dethroned king awaits in the shadows; his admonishments are: *How could you be so stupid? I told you the world was really f---ed. I told you this wasn't worth it. I told you you would never amount to anything. If this is what sobriety is, you might as well be drunk,* and so forth.

This relapse process has been analyzed from the Western treatment perspective by Terence Gorski and others. In a 1973 study of 118 patients by Gorski and Alcoholism Systems Associates, he identified 37 common progressive symptoms preceding alcoholic relapse.[173] It may be fruitful to examine them:

1. Apprehension about Well-Being.

This is the initiatory step in relapse, regardless of the phase of recovery. It is a sense that something is wrong with who one most deeply is. It is Alice starting to change size again. This is a generalized rather than a specific apprehension, a nameless and shadowy fear, as awaking from a terrible but unremembered dream. We would argue that a generalized apprehension about well-being is a perfectly normal response to the "vale of tears" we call life, but this apprehension may be especially true of life on the planet in the late 20th century. It is something beyond specific concerns about population, abortion, the rain forests, global warming, liability insurance, race relations, economic imperialism, and on and on. It is a toxic accumulation of bad news. In this scenario, however, the recovering person doesn't see the malaise as having an external locus. Instead, the apprehension is perceived as a *personal failure to "measure up"* under the circumstances. It is a self-centered inward blaming for not having done whatever is necessary to feel good at the moment. It is the sense that somehow, for reasons unknown, one is no longer "on schedule."

This is also a repetition of the drama of unvalidated trauma in the dysfunctional family, where things were perceived and sensed as being not quite right, but, since the system denied that anything was wrong, the observer child assumed that there was something wrong with *him/her* at having sensed the disharmony to begin with.

2. Denial (reactivation).

And the systemic denial is now *internalized*. Instead of sharing with someone else, like a Twelve Step sponsor, friend, or counselor, the apprehension that one feels, and instead of owning, acknowledging, and honoring one's senses, one moves in the other direction away from the center and assumes the facade that there is, indeed, "nothing wrong here! "

3. Adamant commitment to sobriety.

The generalized apprehension becomes focused on the fear of what is seen as the ultimate moral failure: resumption of drug use. Since one has by now made an identity investment in being a non-user, the resumption of use is a primary threat. So, the fortress is shored up: "Well, at least I'll never drink again." Thus the first half of Step One - "admitted we were powerless over alcohol/drugs" - is undone, and the idea of the chemical substance as a moral agent returns to the landscape.

4. Compulsive attempts to impose sobriety on others.

This is the basic human defense of *projection.*

5. Defensiveness.

The old ego has returned to the throne and is digging in. This is perceived by friends in recovery, pointed out, and yet denied.

6. Compulsive behavior.

Like projection, compulsive behavior is always a defense of something, a shift in emphasis from inner to outer conditions, a search for the "fix." Each compulsive behavior goes with a feeling one wants to repress.

7. Impulsive behavior.

The central craving for oneness has returned. Impulsive behavior is a disregard for consequences, a necessary precursor to relapse.

8. Tendencies toward loneliness.

With the impulsive behavior usually comes a distancing of one's self from others. The original addictive state of isolation and self/other dualism becomes crystallized again.

9. Tunnel vision.

More disregard for consequences.

10. Minor depression.

Now the serotonin is acting up, too. Little wonder!

11. Loss of constructive planning.

DuWors says that there are two primary paths to relapse. One ends with the expletive, "f--- it," and the other with the technically true but history-denying statement that "one won't hurt." [174] A loss of constructive planning is a set up for the former.

12. Plans begin to fail.

The evidence mounts that sobriety isn't worth it. Room is now created either for self pity and an ultimate blaming of God for one's failures, or for the more generic, "f--- it." One has moved back into the director's chair of the drama. Things *ought* to be thus and so because this is the way I *planned* them and this is the way I *want* them. Thus is undone the *second* half of Step One- "(admitted) that our lives had become unmanageable."

13. Idle daydreaming and wishful thinking.

The gap between acceptance of the reality of one's life and the fantasy of what one would wish it to be widens and deepens.

14. Feelings that nothing can be solved.

Notice the movement in the opposite direction from empowerment. We again quote *Alcoholics Anonymous* that the dilemma for the alcoholic is not alcohol. The "dilemma (of the alcoholic) is "power." [175]

15. Immature wish to be happy.

This implies the state of the pre-rational child, but in anger, not innocence.

16. Periods of confusion.

Disorientation is always present in any paradigm shift, and we are in fact describing here a *regressive* paradigm shift.

17. Irritation with friends.

More justification for isolation.

18. Easily angered.

19. Irregular eating habits.

20. Listlessness.

21. Irregular sleeping habits.

This cluster of symptoms signals a return to the early transition phase of sobriety which was characterized by the imbalance of emotional and physical extremes.

22. Progressive loss of daily structure.

We are back on the original battleground on which early sobriety was first won. The polemic of rigidity/collapse returns, and the contest of mind over body has been rejoined. The re-seated ego, now perceived as the shadow self, has returned with a vengeance, and there is a great deal of sabotage manifested. The ground is now established for a return to drug use with the following array of symptoms:

23. Periods of deep depression.

24. Irregular attendance at treatment or Twelve Step meetings.

25. Development of an "I don't care" attitude.

26. Open rejection of help.

Though in fact, intervention is at least theoretically possible at any stage of this process.

27. Dissatisfaction with life.

28. Feelings of powerlessness and helplessness.

29. Self-pity.

30. Thoughts of social drinking. ("One won't hurt.")

31. Conscious lying.

32. Complete loss of self-confidence.

33. Unreasonable resentments.

34. Discontinuance of all treatment/recovery activities.

35. Overwhelming loneliness, frustration, anger, and tension.

36. Beginning of "controlled drinking" episodes.

37. Loss of control. ("F--- it.")

Relapse, in any phase, is viewed by the client and often by the treatment program as catastrophic. In the Western treatment setting, it generally equates with treatment drop-out, and hence a treatment failure. In the acupuncture based program, however, particularly with daily urine testing as an adjunct to acupuncture (see p. 291), it can be viewed not as treatment failure but as treatment *opportunity*. It is an opportunity for the client, particularly in the transition phase, to examine the dynamics of his or her use and to become aware of the cyclic patterns underlying that use. Since the acupuncture-based program is barrier free, where abstinence is not a condition of coming for treatment (as is generally the case in the Western setting), the clinical opportunity is present to adhere to the fundamental clinical ethic of validating the client's experience. And, as we have seen, it is the *in*ability to validate one's experience that is the core precipitative issue in the relapse process.

The early transition phase is an opportunity for the client to practice sobriety. An oft-quoted example is that of a female cocaine addict at Lincoln Hospital's acupuncture program who had over 280 dirty urines in a row, and then got sober! Western treatment generally views relapse, as it views recovery, as use-specific. That is, the moment of relapse is the moment of returning to use of one's drug of choice. But again, relapse is not a static event but a dynamic process of being drawn back into the addictive system. Relapse is about patterns, a process or cycle in which substance use is simply the culminating event/symptom. Obsession with abstinence is yet another imbalance, and can itself become another addiction.

The clinical posture toward relapse should be led by our desire to place drug use in a position of moral neutrality, to move the focus away from the event of drug use (the external fix), and toward the process of self-forgiveness and of validation of the client's experience and of the possibility of healing from within. When acupuncture becomes the foundation for the treatment setting, this clinical posture becomes possible, and it becomes the clinic's central organizing principle.

Anne Wilson Schaef has said that Twelve Step recovery is the most important spiritual movement in the history of the world. She believes that the really significant question is, are we willing to accept the fact that we are going to be led into the new paradigm of the 21st century by a bunch of drunks and drug addicts? [176]

Schaef was a feminist and a psychotherapist in private practice and a feminist in the early 1980s when she wrote her first book, *Women's Reality*.[177] In that book, she developed the theory that there were three systems functioning in modern society. The first was the "Dominant (White) Male System," which she defined as the Newtonian, Cartesian world view in which the universe is a machine, in which truth lies in non participatory, linear, reductionist, scientific objectivity, and in which the mind is eminently supreme over the body. This system, as Ernest Kurtz pointed out, thinks it's God.[178] It is what Robert Bly called the "Old Position." [179] It is what we have been calling the Theology of Exclusionary Rationalism.

The second she defined as the "Reactive Female System," feminine energy that had been thwarted, convoluted, and seduced into a position of service and support for the Dominant Male system.[180]

The third she defined as the "Emerging Female System," which she saw as feminism, with dimensions in the ecology, peace, and Civil Rights movements.

Then, in her private practice, Schaef began to see more and more addicts and codependents as clients, and she began to recognize codependence in herself, and became involved in her own recovery from codependence, or what she would ultimately come to define as "relationship addiction." [181] As she became involved more and more in this process of recovery and of working with addicts, she noticed that the addictive system closely resembled the Dominant Male system; the codependent system resembled the

Reactive Female system, and the recovery system resembled the Emerging Female system.[182]

Then she took the next rather quantum step: these systems didn't just *resemble* one another; *they were in fact the same systems.* Her awareness that codependence is actually an addiction in its own right resulted in a simplification of her original theoretical model from three systems to two: the *addictive system* and the *recovery system.* It is important to realize that she is not suggesting addiction as metaphor, but as *reality.* In contemporary society, *one is either in the addictive system or the recovery system.*[183]

No third choice.

This is a fairly hard-line position. One may question such a radical posture. What about those of us who are "well," who aren't addicts? And, does this mean that everyone who is an addict has to go to a Twelve Step program? Is A.A. the answer and the *only* answer for every alcoholic? - Narcotics Anonymous for every drug addict, and so forth? Aren't there individuals who aren't suited for the Twelve Step program format? Shouldn't people be free to choose an alternative?

In Schaef's unequivocal view, everyone who grew up in the West in the last three or four centuries *is* an addict. People who do not *appear* to be addicts are simply people who are able to function very well in the addictive system. They are similar to early stage alcoholics who use their substantial tolerance for alcohol as evidence that they don't really have a problem, when in fact tolerance is a *primary indicator* for alcoholism. Mindy Fullilove, previously quoted from a talk she gave at a recent NADA conference, has said, "those who view themselves as non-addictive are the greatest culprits." And, if you're an addict, you can go to, or do, anything you wish in order to stop drinking, or using, or practicing your addiction of choice, but if it isn't a Twelve Step program, it better *look* a lot like a Twelve Step program if *recovery* rather than simple abstinence is sought. For our purposes, we are not interested in abstinence, but in recovery. We are interested in a "gestalt switch in perception," a "turning in the deep seat of consciousness," a transformation in one's view of the world. We are looking for the witch's broomstick, for true empowerment, for a new pair of looking glasses. We want to get the message to Alice that there is nothing wrong with *her*. It is Wonderland that is nuts. And the solution is not in the banning of mushrooms from the kingdom! As healers, our attention is on Alice, the "identified patient," but we are also interested in the healing of the Mad Hatter, in getting acupuncture needles into the ears of the Caterpillar, in helping the poor Queen down from the position of arbitrary power she has fraudulently assumed out of her own addiction to power.

And here is the test of our own "codependence" - our "neurotic need to help others." We wish to help, yes, but we need to help *in order to heal ourselves*. The moment we shift the focus from our *own* addictive woundedness, we are in our collective disease, assuming that "oh, yes, *they* need help, but not *me*! "

This awareness is the core of the radical center of recovery. So many strong and vital healing movements have been occluded by the addictive system in the past: Civil rights, feminism,[184] the peace movement, ecology, public health, and earlier counterparts that we have discussed such as Romanticism and Populism. The salient aspects of these movements continue to be re-seeded because the healing needs are so glaring. But they are co-opted and transformed again and again, becoming themselves addictive substances upon which people get hooked in their own urgent desire to feel good about themselves, and in their denial that in the looking glass is a reflection of themselves. People get seduced and hooked on the rush and drama of the movement, and so the focus, the radical center, is lost. The end result is not the intended empowerment, but its opposite - the *dis*empowerment that comes from losing one's center for the sake of a "cause." This is the Great Compromise. This is Romance Addiction.[185]

Political and social movements are goal-oriented, and goals are antithetical to recovery. With goals and planning, the emphasis is on outcome rather than process, the future rather than the present moment, and we are back in Exclusionary Rationalism, assuming control (the *illusion* of power), and centered in (future) results. The focus is on external agendas rather than internal growth. And there is nothing, absolutely nothing we can do to get the outside to straighten up and turn out right until the inside is honored because healing always manifests from the inside out. We may wish to reform systems because that is where the glaring symptoms are, but any efforts to do so will be ineffective until our own house is in order. Alice has to *get it* that *she is okay* before Wonderland will transform. When, in the awaking from her dream, she at last becomes her "right size," the beheading Queen and all of her cohorts turn into nothing but a pack of cards. In a parallel manner, while Dorothy seeks the broomstick "out there," attaining that which it represents comes from her acceptance *within* of the courage, wisdom, and compassion necessary for its acquisition. Once these are realized, the externalized evil Witch melts away at nothing more than a simple pail of water.

Traditional Chinese medicine is at risk of being included in this list of potentially addictive movements as it strives to gain a foothold within the dominant Western medical system. Because it is so much needed in the current crisis in health care delivery, because it is resisted, and precisely because of its intrinsic wisdom about the internal sources of healing, advocates can find themselves drawn into a polemic in which they become co-opted by the system they are trying to change. NADA is also at risk for this as it gains increasing success as an organization and becomes tempted to place money, status, and prestige above principles. This is, above all, the most essential aspect of our work, remaining centered in a new and transforming paradigm. As we have suggested, Western history is against us in this, and our own denial of our own part in the addictive system is how the center can be lost.

An examination of the historical influences and the systemic qualities of Twelve Step programs provides insight into the processes of the transformations required for recovery from addiction. There were a variety of historical strands that influenced the development of Alcoholics Anonymous, the first Twelve Step program. The influence of Eastern philosophy was present, but the substantive influences were endogenous to Western Culture. Paradoxically, in fact, the very institutions of Western medicine, psychology, and religion - against which A.A. was a counter-cultural movement - themselves provided much of the essential wisdom.

This is an extremely important point for two reasons. First, it illustrates what we have said earlier that systemic Exclusionary Rationalism, at whose feet we lay the blame for our inherently addictive society, is not itself inherently malignant. Its basic fault is not in its fundamental tenets of Rationalist philosophy, dualism, reductionism, and "scientific objectivity." Rather, its fault is in its insistence that these tenets are *factual and exclusive reality* rather than simply *one way of looking at things*. Its error is one of mistaking the map for the territory, the looking glass for that which is perceived when peering through it.

It is not wise to "throw out the baby with the bath water." The solution to the *mechanisticism*, for example, of Rationalism, is not to destroy all of our mechanical devices! Because, while it is true that the universe is not a machine, *looked* at a certain way, it *appears* as a machine, and such a view can provide productive insights. This view has given us the conceptual basis for inventing clocks, indoor heating, bicycles, and much more besides. And, while the whole is always greater than the sum of its parts, breaking things down into their elements (as we are currently attempting to do with Alcoholics Anonymous), can often be helpful in providing understanding. And, while the mind as we think of it in the West is not preeminent over, nor in fact separate from, the totality of one's organism, its activities (as well as its temple, the brain) are absolutely essential in navigating through our lives. Our purpose, therefore, is healing, not further separation.

One of the revealing chapters in the book *Alcoholics Anonymous* is entitled "We Agnostics." [186] In conceiving of this chapter, the assumption was made that chronic alcoholics were, practically by definition, going to be resistant to A.A. because of what were perceived as its "religious overtones" - references to God, prayer, and spiritual experiences. It was understood that agnosticism - which, like Rationalism, is a *philosophy of doubt* - was part and parcel of the pathology of late-stage chronic alcoholism.

In "We Agnostics" we find the philosophy of doubt challenged (and the underpinning theology of Alcoholics Anonymous stated), as follows: "...we had to fearlessly face the proposition that either God is everything or else He is nothing." [187]

What is apparent here is that one's belief about the nature of God defines the way in which one relates to self and others. For example, E. A. Burt's previously quoted reflection in 1932 that "the 17th century, which began with the search for God in the Universe, ended by squeezing Him out of it altogether," applies as well to the development of Western individual consciousness. An individual tends to identify with the God of his or her understanding. If one's God, for example, is seen as immanent within creation, then one generally tends to feel themselves at home in the same creation. If, as is more generally the case in our addictive culture, one's God is experienced as an outsider, one feels oneself as having the same estranged standing. If, as Shakespeare said, "all the world's a stage," then the alcoholic/addict is watching the drama from the wings, and A.A.'s central theological challenge is either to walk on stage - which is to embrace participatory consciousness - or quit the theater!

The chapter, "We Agnostics," takes a curious tact. Rather than bolstering frontal arguments about why the alcoholic should embrace a spiritual orientation to life, Bill Wilson presents Western science and technology *as theology*, things which are, after all, taken on *faith*. "Without knowing it," he asks, "had we not been brought to where we stood by a certain kind of faith? " He argues that *where we stood* has been with *abject faith* in a "God of Reason." [188] This God of Reason, of course, is the estranged God of Descartes, and the "abject faith" has been in the absolutism that is the chink in the armor of Exclusionary Rationalism.

And yet A.A. is not anti-science, nor anti-reason. In drawing its wisdom, as we shall see, from essentially Western ideas, it contains within its tapestry the seeds of redemption of the system against which it was a reaction, the system which spawned the alcoholic for whom the book was written. While modernity is characterized by a theology of exclusion, A.A. is fundamentally a theology of *inclusion*, spacious and roomy enough for all who suffer. Even God.

A second reason for the importance of the fact that A.A. drew much of its central wisdom from the dominant Western systems of the day has to do with the endogenous versus exogenous sources of recovery in general. The psychologist Rollo May has pointed out that much of the current renewed interest in mythology in our culture is in fact an interest in *non-Western* mythology.[189] While May believes that the revitalization of myth is essential to the survival of Western culture, he believes that we will not be well served by stepping outside of Western consciousness to bring mythic significance to our lives. We can walk to the garden gate and peer in and enjoy the beauty and elegance of myths from other cultures, but for our salvation we must find the roots of meaning in our own cultural consciousness.[190] This is also the message of *The Wonderful Wizard of Oz*. The witch's broomstick, which symbolizes empowerment for Dorothy, is not outside the kingdom of Oz (Dorothy's dreamscape of consciousness) but within it.[191]

The relevance for acupuncture is clear. It is not Chinese *philosophy* that we overtly bring to our work with the Western crisis of consciousness that we call addiction. This would not be successful, and in fact we can see the failure of countless Eastern movements to take root in American culture in the past decades. The transformation of recovery is a mythic journey, and it requires Western referents. To step outside of endogenous Western culture for the "fix" would become just that: another fix. We can learn from the Chinese experience of successfully integrating Western medicine into their culture. The turbulent period for Chinese medicine from 1917 to 1945 notwithstanding, it has been in fact Western medicine and not the *theology* of Western medicine but rather its *tools* that have been integrated in China.

We draw a rather sharp distinction, then, between transplanting exogenous theology *en masse* and integrating the salient *wisdom* of those theologies. This distinction is born out by the fact that acupuncture has been most dramatically accepted by Western institutions when presented simply as a "tool that we don't understand very well" and not as a system involving the *yin* and *yang* of *zhen-jiu*, wormwood, mugwort, impulse points, meridians, and so on. It is still true that "a rose by any other name is still a rose," and the fact is that the salient elements of acupuncture are of course universal,[192] but we are transitional figures on a transitional landscape, and we are well advised to adapt the very Western philosophy of pragmatism in our work.

The single greatest influence on Alcoholics Anonymous, according to co-founder Bill Wilson, was the Western physician and psychotherapist Carl Jung.[193] In 1931, a wealthy industrialist from the Northeast by the name of Rowland H. went to Dr. Jung in Zurich for treatment of alcoholism. He remained in psychotherapy with Jung for a year, completed treatment feeling he was cured, but in a short time had returned to alcoholic drinking. He came back to Jung a second time, desperate, but Jung had bad news for Rowland: he told him that his case was hopeless, that there was nothing that psychiatric treatment could offer that would alleviate his condition. Jung told Rowland that he had, however, heard of a few cases in which alcoholism that had progressed to the degree that it had with Rowland had in fact been arrested. These alcoholics had had, Jung said (as paraphrased by Bill Wilson),[194] "vital spiritual experiences." Jung said that Rowland's own religious convictions, however, would not suffice. He would need to seek out some sort of *spiritual* movement that he found palatable, and then *pray*. The alternative was alcoholic death. No third choice.

Rowland followed the advice and became involved with the Oxford Group, a non-denominational fellowship which had begun in 1908 as "The First Century Christian Fellowship." Their gatherings involved inspirational readings and sharing of experiences; their theology involved confession, absolute honesty, restitution for past transgressions, and doing the "will of God" through unselfish service to others. Through the Oxford Group, Rowland was able to remain sober long enough to "carry the message" to another alcoholic by the name of "Ebby T.," who in turn carried the news of his conversion to his old drinking friend Bill Wilson. The fate of Rowland is not recorded. Ebby would die an alcoholic death, and The Oxford Group would disappear into the Moral Re-Armament movement in the 1940s, but in these events were sown the seeds of the formation of Alcoholics Anonymous in 1935.

Bill Wilson had been under the care of Dr. William D. Silkworth at Town's Hospital in New York. Silkworth had shared with Wilson his theory that alcoholism was a disease comprised of an "allergic reaction" to alcohol coupled with an "obsession of the mind." [195] By embracing this notion, and with support from the spiritual fellowship of the Oxford Group, and - pursuing Oxford theology - his own act of surrender to "God's will," Bill Wilson was able to achieve abstinence. His wife Lois provided the final piece of Bill's "program of recovery." He had been bringing to their home numbers of chronic alcoholics in order to "convert them" to sobriety. This had dismally failed, and at length, Bill complained to Lois that he hadn't gotten one single alcoholic sober.

"But," she pointed out, *"you* have stayed sober! "

It was this insight that Bill Wilson brought with him to his first meeting in Akron, Ohio, in 1935, with another "hopeless case" - and another Western physician - Bob Smith. Bill had found himself in Akron on an ill-fated business trip, alone and depressed and fearful of returning to drink. He realized that his only hope was in finding another alcoholic to talk to. A church directory in the lobby of his hotel led him to the physician's home, and the two spent the night exchanging stories about *what it was like*. Instead of preaching to or trying to "convert" Dr. Bob, Bill simply shared his own experience. This was the first A.A. meeting.

There are three conspicuous elements of Carl Jung's final session with Rowland that form the foundation of A.A.'s "theology." First was the message of the *hopelessness* of Rowland's malady. When Jung told Rowland that his condition was beyond the help of medicine, psychiatry, or religion, Rowland's "abject faith" in these systems was taken to the wall. He had to "give up" seeking the answer "out there."

The second related message was the disarming news that the alcoholism was beyond Jung's ability to treat because it was *not a symptom of an underlying psychological state.* It was a *primary condition.*

Jung's diagnosis warrants exploration. We have described the beginning of recovery as the conscious awareness of *consequences* of (in the case of the alcoholic) drinking. The *pre*-recovery state of denial operates through a curious *inversion* of the phenomenon of consequence. Instead of attributing one's problems to alcoholic drinking, one attributes the alcoholic drinking to one's problems. *Life* is the problem; the substance (alcohol) is the nurturing and necessary *solution.* Alcoholics (and other drug addicts) seek other solutions at this stage, as did Rowland in seeking out Jung. Though this is a spiritual quest, a search for wholeness, a tacit goal of this search is always to achieve, by addressing these "life problems," *control* of their drinking/using.

Here, then, is another fundamental paradox in treatment and recovery. While it is clear from virtually any vantage point that alcoholism or other drug addiction, genetic markers notwithstanding, arises from a deeper psycho-cultural malaise and is itself not the primary problem, unless it is *treated* as the primary problem, the condition is in fact hopeless. As we have said, the kindling of recovery requires as its centerpiece *relationship with the substance,* and the maintenance of recovery requires as its centerpiece *sobriety.* The folk wisdom of A.A. has produced the following slogan: *I will lose anything I place before my sobriety.* Sobriety, therefore, must supersede relationship, vocation, economic standing, gender, race, and any and all personal historical factors.

This apparent paradox, like our other radical "no third choice" propositions, suspiciously resembles the either/or thinking that is characteristic of the addictive system itself. It seems a violation of the natural homeostatic state. It is unacceptable to the alcoholic who has for so long been driven by the desire to *minimize* drinking/using, and for whom control has been the burning agenda; it seems an anathema to the fundamental creed of health, that *balance* in all things is desirable, and it flies in the face of reason to relegate cause to symptom.

Alcoholics Anonymous settles the problem in the way that the First Step is grammatically structured: *"(we) admitted we were powerless over alcohol - that our lives had become unmanageable."* Any cause and effect relationship between the two conditions is canceled by the use of the hyphen which separates them. Condition, symptom, and cause are rendered linked as separate but equal.

So, is alcoholism/addiction *root* or *branch*? - *cause* or *effect*? - *primary disease* or *symptom*? We have come to the nub of resistance to recovery, and perhaps its most fundamental paradox as well. This is not just a double bind from the standpoint of intellectual theorizing; it is the central existential dilemma for the chronic alcoholic/addict, a dilemma that constitutes the major barrier to treatment and recovery. It is the staging ground for denial, but it goes beyond denial to the heart of the Rationalist's quandary about existence. It is the central clinical issue in transitional recovery, and, it is the pivotal point in the paradigm shift we have been discussing.

What is the essential nature of this paradox? Is the paradox intrinsic to the field we are observing, or is this, like the Batesonian box we considered in Chapter Three, another case of "what we are looking at, we are looking with? "

In the case of the box...

> All Statements within this frame
> are untrue.

...we discovered that the statement was in fact true, and the statement was in fact false, and the reason that our rational intellect rebels at that proposition is because, while what is contrived here appears to be a *closed system* with no external referents, we realize that this is not the case. The locus of the paradox is in something we bring to the configuration - namely, the violation of a tacit and arbitrary rule of rational logic: "A class cannot be a member of itself." This is a rule that resides in the paradigm we bring to the configuration, and not in the configuration itself.

Similarly, the apparent paradox in the problem of whether alcoholism is root or branch lies not in the proposition itself but in the linear, effect-follows-cause logic we *invest* in the problem. The answer again is, "yes, to both questions," but the salient point is that the field we are observing draws its meaning from a *larger system* of which it is itself only one aspect.

This thinking is reminiscent of the adolescent riddle of "which came first, the chicken or the egg? " The answer to the riddle, as the solution to Bateson's box, lies in transcendence of the polemic that is posed. "Egg" is not a *thing* but a *process* that holds within its essence *chickenness*. Chickenness *is* eggchickening. We can imagine that the chicken-or-egg dilemma is one shared not only by children on the eve of their indoctrination into the dominant paradigm, but, if we may indulge for a moment an anthropomorphic metaphor, by the embryonic chicken living *inside* the egg as well! From his or her "rational" point of view, there comes a time when the dilemma takes on existential proportions. When the sole alternatives of *hatch* or *die* of suffocation become manifest, the embryonic chicken must surrender on faith to a larger reality than that of the perceived polemic. By surrendering to this larger process (which might well seem to the chicken in the egg as the end of the world!), the polemic is transcended and his or her destiny is realized.

A.A.'s Second Step, *"Came to believe that a power greater than ourselves could restore us to sanity,"* presents the same solution to the perceived polemic. It invites transcendence, pointing to the possibility that the existential dilemma is not a static state of hopelessness, but simply one aspect of a larger process. The word sanity comes from the Latin root *sanus* which means *whole*, and so, hope of resolution of the central addictive state of unconnectedness, within and without, is provided. Step Two proposes *belief* in a process beyond self, and Step Three asks for *surrender* to that process: "Made a decision to turn our will and our lives over to the care of God *as we understood Him*." And so, Jung's third essential message to Rowland was that recovery from alcoholism was going to be essentially a *spiritual* (and hence non-rational) proposition.

We can see that these first three steps of Alcoholics Anonymous, often called the "foundation" steps, are framed in the language of traditional religion with a masculine deity. This is understandable in that the steps were written by and for White male alcoholics with a Christian background suffering from the grandiosity peculiar to White male egos living in the patriarchal system of post-17th-century Rationalism. The original draft of Step Three, as a matter of fact, was: "Made a decision to turn our will and our lives over to the care of God" period. An atheistic member of the original fellowship insisted that the phrase *"as we understood Him"* not only be added, but underlined for emphasis as well!

Some contemporary Twelve Step groups, with a consciousness that such a frame promulgates the myth of the patriarchy, have further modified the Step to read,"...God as we understood *God.*" - deleting any gender references from the reading of the steps. Charlotte Kasl[196] has been a pioneer in advocating alternative language for women and people of color for whom "God," in the traditional patriarchal consciousness of Western culture, is the disempowering image of White masculine authority to which far too much surrender has already been made. The Twelve Steps, she feels, in using language inherent to the patriarchy, fail to adequately "unmask" the Wizard. She argues eloquently for alternatives to A.A., especially for women and people of color, and recommends for those for whom A.A. does not "work," more secular versions, such as Secular Organization for Sobriety (SOS), Women for Sobriety, Rational Recovery,[197] and her own essentially Rationalist "sixteen step" model of recovery.

Kasl suggests that the "grandiosity of ego" suffered by the A.A. founders, who were, indeed, primarily White male businessmen, is quite a different dilemma than that of women or people of color who suffer alcoholism and drug addiction. She suggests that addiction, most fundamentally, is *internalized oppression*. This internalized oppression is the operational dynamic of what we have been calling the ascent of Exclusionary Rationalism, the autocratic shutting off/down of feelings, intuitions, and the natural balancing and healing mechanisms of the body. But is it, in fact, a different dilemma for people of different classes, gender, or race? Our search in recovery, as Kasl's, is for a deeper center of wisdom and action, the true source of power. Is the estrangement from this sense of self that is suffered by white, male, middle and upper class alcoholics and addicts functionally different than the estrangement felt by *any* individual for whom systemic dysfunction in family, community, and culture has produced a psychic splitting off of consciousness from these inner sources of power? Is not addiction a universal syndrome for those who have invested the crystallized center of conscious attention and volition with the exclusionary, God-like, illusion of the power of *control* of the people, places, and things around them? Do exterior conditions of poverty, oppression, and discrimination alter this basic dynamic, or do they simply act to reinforce it?

As Schaef implies, the Twelve Steps of Alcoholics Anonymous represent an *intrinsically feminine system.* Recovery is living in the process of one's life, finding a nurturing center in *interior* rather than *exterior* reality. It fosters and nurtures *yin* energy. The theology of A.A. is not static, and neither is *it* God. The challenge is to move through the external trappings to a fundamental, radical (root) wisdom that will address the crystallization of Exclusionary Rationalism *on a systemic level.* Nothing less than this will provide a way of linking the global crises of ecology, economics, and consciousness with the human problems of gender, racial, and ethnic oppression, whether internalized or overt. Any attempts to seriously address these vital social concerns using the framework of the old addictive paradigm will be (like treating psychoactive drug addiction with psychoactive drugs) little more than mowing down the weeds. [198]   The issue is not A.A., but the process of recovery to which the Twelve Steps lead. The process of Rationalism, like the process of addiction, is cunning, baffling, and powerful, and will argue for more "reasonable" alternatives to such folly as a "turning in the deep seat of consciousness." It will argue for an easier softer way.

And, it is appropriate again to point out that Rationalism is not the locus of evil. The problem lies in the use to which it has been put, the pedestal upon which it has been placed, and the theological reverence with which it has been promulgated through the veil of family, church, school, medicine, psychology, government, and so on. Just as, when Alice becomes her proper size at the end of her dream, the Queen and her Court become nothing but a pack of cards, so will the false-tyranny of external gods fall in the awaking from the dream of addiction. The limitations "out there" will be seen as reflections of the limitations we have imposed "in here," a monster created by the collective unconscious of separation of self from self, self from other.

On the other hand, the *external trappings* of internalized oppression that we find inherent in the *language* of early A.A., still, not surprisingly, survive and permeate A.A. *groups.* All of the "sins of the fathers" survive and are manifest in these meetings which are, after all, organized, run, and attended by sick alcoholics and addicts! In this sense, Kasl's argument for finding any road possible to begin the journey is a valid one. If we hold with her that the journey itself is one journey, but that there are a variety of roads, then what is required as the crucial elements that these paths must have?

They must, like the Twelve Steps. be intrinsically *yin*, or feminine. They must direct the conscious attention of the recoverer, in other words, inward to intuitive and healing resources, a movement toward *acceptance of feelings*. They must provide a forum by which the individual is obliged to address the core issue of his or her relationship with the addictive "substance of choice." The tacit agenda of *controlled use of the substance* must be dismantled. And, they must provide the opportunity for fundamental *validation of experience*, validation of the original trauma, and of the pain of early recovery. They must involve some mechanism by which shame and self-loathing can be addressed so that *self-forgiveness* can begin. And, all this needs to happen *in the process of relationship*; it cannot happen at home alone listening to tapes or plugged in to an electrical stimulator, or in a one-on-one, non-equal, or "one-up", or romantic relationship in which the other party is assumed to have "the answer" or is expected to provide through physical intimacy the longed-for connectedness and gender validation.

These are the primary requirements for the transition phase, the developmental phase of early sobriety. Many people, not ready for this experience, will indeed choose other options, and this needs to be honored as part of their journey. People are and need to be ultimately free to travel any path they choose.

The second phase of recovery, which we have called the *stabilization phase*, can be seen, as suggested earlier, as beginning with the Fourth Step: *"Made a searching and fearless moral inventory of ourselves."* This step is best followed immediately by Step Five: *"Admitted to God, to ourselves, and to another human being the exact nature of our wrongs."*

These two steps might be thought of as a combining of the maxim of Aristotle, the grandfather of Rationalism, that "the unexamined life is not worth living," with the significance of the Catholic confessional. They do indeed include both of these Rationalist and religious elements, but there is a synergy operating as well, and the process suggested here is more than either a linear historical examination or a confession. As we described in Chapter Three, the center now expands from the relationship with the addictive substance or activity, and the relationship with self, to the relationship between self/other. One begins to see one's disease in the context of historical and current primary relationships. The primary relationships addressed are those involving trauma-producing guilt, shame, and resentments. For many alcoholics or addicts, going into this trauma can precipitate relapse if attempted too soon following abstinence. Many Twelve Step sponsors recommend that people wait until they have been sober for a year before beginning Step Four.[199]

The language of Steps Four and Five seem harsh to the degree that the onus or responsibility for one's life issues are directed to one's self. There is understandable resistance here, especially when we remember that this entire movement is toward empowerment. Given what we have uncovered about the root of addiction, it seems more rational to seek restitution for the moral harm that *others* have done to *us* than to focus on our own "wrongs! " But, from a homeostatic view, we can see that the energy spent in blaming others for our problems from the posture of victim, even though the blame may be entirely justified, must ultimately be dismantled and transformed if we are to be truly empowered, and Steps Four and Five represent the difficult beginning of this movement. The sensation is one of fleeing a burning building only to stop, turn, and walk back into the flames!

To blame others is to remain in the wings, off stage. The clusters of unvalidated trauma of our lives that caused the psychic splitting off of self are what has made us non-participants in our lives and driven "God" from our universe. We must now return to this emotional stage as participants in the pain. It is a descent to the pre-rational stage as well, the original traumatic ascent from which was born of emotional survival. We are, in effect, going to the castle of our dreamscape to throw a pail of water on the Witch so that she won't bother us any more. It's a dangerous and scary journey!

It is important that this is not to be undertaken alone. Immediately following the inventory step, we involve another person to share in our trauma, which provides the essential and heretofore missing human validation of the experiences. But we also enlist the support of God. The Twelve Steps are not written in random order; in Steps Two and Three, a bid has been made to establish a personal relationship with a power that is capable of restoring us to wholeness, a power beyond the God of Mind has been invited back into the landscape of our lives, and we have made a surrender to that power. Step Four is begun from this new consciousness, as an act not of our own will but of God's. We can of course, with Morris Berman, view this God as the unconscious, the deeper emerging self. [200] When Dorothy enlisted the assistance of her companions in her journey to the Witch's castle, she was enlisting her own inner - though as yet unintegrated - resources of wisdom, courage, and compassion. This was an act of faith.

As we have suggested, perhaps the most fundamental and human psychological defense is projection, and Step Four is designed from a psychological point of view to carry us to the genesis of our emotional disempowerment. An example of this dynamic can be seen in the nature of the perpetration of sexual abuse. A vast majority of sexual abusers were themselves sexually abused as children, so they are both perpetrators and victims. We can recognize that laying all of the blame for acts committed by the perpetrator on the original perpetrator leads to a process of endless rationalization that has no potential of breaking the cycle. It can be seen, in Chinese medical terms, as *yang* excess heaped upon *yang* excess. We can see that a continuum of complete healing will require going to the root, but how does one enter the cycle? Beginning with the "sins of the fathers" may be soothing, but it doesn't contain the emotional power required to break the cycle. Steps Four and Five take the most difficult emotional tack. The individual's acts as perpetrator are where the projected emotional energy is crystallized. It is where the original pain can be accessed.

The Step Four inventory is done in writing, and it covers areas of emotional, sexual, financial, and relationship history. It should contain the deepest secrets (one A.A. cliché is "we're as sick as our secrets! "). It is generally quickly followed by Step Five, and the role of the person with whom Step Five is taken is, of course, critical. A.A. recommends that this step be taken with a sponsor, a priest, or someone who will listen without judgment. This is, as we have said, the essential process of human validation. The difference between Step Five and the Catholic confession is that the person receiving the testimony is not vested with the power of absolution. Something subtle and very significant begins to manifest in the precise wording of the steps. It is the awareness that atonement is not a function of forgiveness, but lies instead in the process of disclosure itself. We are not approaching the "other human being" in Step Five for penance. This is not a sacrament whose implication is judgment on the part of the Creator, or penitence for our "sins."

This is affirmed in the next two steps: (Six) "Were entirely ready to have God remove all these defects of character," and (Seven) "Humbly asked Him to remove our shortcomings." [201] These two steps are not about penance but about surrender. We aren't even asked to "perform surgery" upon ourselves or "undo" or "work on" our own defects or shortcomings. To attempt to do so would be tantamount to reclaiming rational *control* over our lives. These steps, instead of leading us back into the precarious landscape of fixing ourselves, are a movement toward increasing surrender of control. This surrender may seem, especially to the Rationalist, a further moral abrogation of responsibility. To the practitioner of Chinese medicine, however, it is the revelation of the simple truth that healing of the body is not under the sole direction of the brain!

And yet, the Sixth and Seventh Steps are not without cost. What is asked is the willingness to change and to heal. This is a difficult thing, particularly given the strains of self-destruction and self-loathing that characterize living in the addictive system. More relapses are promoted by an unwillingness to accept the grace of healing than by any other single factor. Acupuncture can be a very supportive part of this difficult process of acceptance of the sources, possibility, and validity of healing.

Another important aspect of these two steps to notice is that the recoverer does not get to decide which things are defects and which are not! Due to the self-loathing mentioned above, addicts and alcoholics are notoriously judgmental and harsh on themselves. Practicing Steps Six and Seven teach the recoverer much about patience, because, generally, many of the things about one's self that are perceived as shortcomings or defects, instead of being removed, will ultimately be found to be strengths! Rather than becoming "fixed" as a result of taking these two steps, one discovers the truth revealed in *The Wizard of Oz*, that what we were looking for, we were looking with. One's self-perceived "weaknesses" are often in fact one's strengths turned inside out. This is because the primary experience of the addict in life has been attempting to do and be and say and perform "right" against society's perceived standards, and falling short every time, which gives one a terribly convoluted sense of one's actual strengths and shortcomings. One may perceive one's self, for example, to be too sensitive, too soft, too critical, too talkative, and learn through the process of recovery that these are one's greatest attributes: being able to feel deeply, to care, to perceive, and to express. Such indeed are the lessons of a wounded artist!

Probably the most feared Steps are Eight: "Made a list of all persons we had harmed, and became willing to make amends to them all," and Nine: "Made direct amends to such people wherever possible, except when to do so would injure them or others." [202] Here, the movement is again away from self and toward human relationship - relationship and forgiveness. R. D. Laing wrote, as we quoted earlier, that "True sanity entails in one way or another a dissolution of the normal ego, that false self completely adjusted to our alienated social reality; the emergence of the 'inner' archetypal mediators of divine power, and through the death a rebirth, and the eventual re-establishment of a new kind of ego-functioning, the ego now being the servant of the divine, no longer its betrayer." [203] The ego is seen here as *the feeling of conscious separation from*: from others, from God, from the universe, from one's own being. Newcomers at recovery ask: "Does one *really* have to completely lose one's ego? " "No," said one A.A. old timer. "But you better lose it long enough to take the first nine steps! "

In fact, the first nine steps are a frontal assault on the ego. They are the process by which crystallized consciousness becomes dismantled, by which surrender is negotiated to a power beyond self. They are the means by which the seeds of humility are sewn.

The last three of the Twelve Steps are often termed the "maintenance steps:"

(10) Continued to take personal inventory and when we were wrong promptly admitted it.

(11) Sought through prayer and meditation to improve our conscious contact with God as we understood Him,

praying only for knowledge of His will for us and the power to carry that out.

(12) Having had a spiritual awakening as the result of these steps, we tried to carry this message to alcoholics, and to practice these principles in all our affairs.[204]

While the first nine steps were about the sewing and cultivation of surrender, humility, acceptance, and relationship, the last three are about the *practice* of these qualities, with the final charge being one of service to others.

These steps, developed by Alcoholics Anonymous in 1935, are clearly not about alcohol. They are, as we have said, about the *dilemma of power*, which is the core issue in alcoholism and addiction. In the addictive system, as the rational ego ascends to the position of "God," genuine power is surrendered, and the subsequent need for control emerges.

Let's spend a moment tracing the dynamic of how this happens. Exclusionary Rationalism, like any theology, holds its power through ritual and other means by which the sanctity of its tenets are affirmed. In order to prevent heresy among the rank and file, the system invokes guilt or shame-based compliance with its rules, both overt and tacit, through the use of certain "theologically charged" code words and concepts. In the theology of Exclusionary Rationalism, examples of these code words and concepts include *mind, reason, control, responsibility, goals, structure*, and so on. Mind - which is of course the conceptual *raison d'etre* of the theology itself - is the initiatory shame-invoking concept used on children to take them out of their senses and into the adult theology. Perhaps the most common invocation is *"you mind me! "* This phrase, or course, makes no sense whatever to the child when first heard, so it needs to be demonstrated, usually through physical coercion, that what is expected when this phrase is used is acceptance of the imposition of arbitrary (exogenous) will and volition.

The emotionally charged early experiences of this are the first lessons in internalized oppression, the internalization of the will of another, and here begins the process of the splitting off of mind from body, the ascent of the false god to his throne. We use the pronoun *his* deliberately, because what is cut off can be seen as the feminine, internal, non-linear sources of information and wisdom.

"Mind me! " shifts developmentally to such commands as *"Think! "* and *"Use your head!"* There is an apparent shift of power here from oppressor to victim, (adult to child), but this is not what is intended. These are simply variations on "mind me." To "Think" means to "think like me," or to "think as I have taught you to think." Similarly, "Use your head" translates: "follow the rules I have told you to follow." These commands evolve later into the seductive and similar exorcisms, *"Be reasonable! " "Get control of yourself! " "You have to take responsibility for your actions." "You have to have goals (a goal) in life." "People need structure,"* and so on. The sexist forms are the familiar *"Why don't you act like a lady? "* and *"Nice girls don't behave that way! "* The gender inversions are *"Big boys don't behave that way,"* etc.

Such phrases are emotionally charged and admonish us to comply with the dominant theology, to divorce ourselves from our inner wisdom and succumb to the imposed canons of intellectual and moral authority. By the time we are "grown up" addicts, of course, we no longer need a "real" parent figure in our lives to carry on the internalized oppression; we are perfectly capable of doing the deed ourselves, through self-talk.[205]

One can see that especially these initiatory invocations are sometimes survival-based. "Mind me" is not always born of the parents insecure need to manipulate and control the child. One can, for example, imagine being raised in a loving home in which one's introduction to "Mind me" was associated with hot stoves, light sockets, matches, crossing the street alone, and so forth. But the error, of course, is in excluding from the learning process development of, or, more important, faith in, the child's internal sources of wisdom. When these inherent sources of information are denied, survival in a hazardous world becomes a rote enterprise depending upon the following of imposed rules rather than upon judgment. One ends up looking in both directions before crossing the street because that is what was taught, *not* to avoid getting hit by a car!

Understanding this distinction we can see how genuine power has been relinquished in the addictive system. This surrender to external referents and arbitrary "rote" authority is most keenly experienced among racial and ethnic minorities and women, but the dynamic is systemic and therefore universal in the addictive culture of modernity, so that even White males, who invented the system historically, are its "victims" as well.

The great lesson of recovery, again, is that *truth lies in paradox*, and here, in the Twelve Steps, is a demonstration of what appears to be an unthinkable thing for the alcoholic or addict: *the surrender of power*! That, one feels, is the *problem*, not the *solution*!

And yet, it is through the dissolution and giving up of the old guard, the old seat of internalized oppression and defense, that the original self may emerge in legitimate power and strength. This process of *empowerment*, the final phase of recovery, is where the recovery journey truly begins.

PART III ACUPUNCTURE-BASED PROGRAM FUNDING AND DESIGN

Remember, your program is always
sicker than your sickest client.

Michael Smith, M.D.

In this section, our book becomes something of a manual. It includes information on getting a program started, about how public and private funding for drug and alcohol treatment works and is accessed, and about the process of education of communities about the efficacy of acupuncture. It is also about the process of acupuncture program planning, design, proposal, and implementation, whether the program is to be developed as a free-standing program or adjunctive with other services. If you, the reader, are an outsider to drug and alcohol treatment, this section of the book will offer strategies on how to get in. If you are already experienced in public funding of chemical dependency treatment, this section will help with such matters as budget design, proposal writing, and other organizational considerations specific to acupuncture, including a vision of the future of acupuncture-based program design.

As of this writing, public funding for all areas of public services is uncertain at the federal level, and in serious decline at the level of most states, counties, and cities. We have suggested that all addicts eventually hit "bottom." That bottom may be physical, moral, familial, and so on. One can certainly speculate that, if, as Anne Wilson Schaef claims, *society* is an addict, its potential bottom will be *financial* in nature, for the crisis of public funding of all treatment, prevention, social, criminal justice, and health permeates all governmental levels and departments in our society, reaching its apex of course with the problem of national public indebtedness. Fittingly, what is sometimes termed the "Black Belt" of Twelve Step programs, or the "last stop on the Twelve Step track," is *Debtors Anonymous*!

This crisis in funding for social and health, chemical dependency, and criminal justice services makes acupuncture program start-up prospects seem bleak; paradoxically, however, these drastic funding shortages are bringing into sharp focus the fact that society can no longer afford the luxury of paying for the terribly expensive *consequences* of alcoholism and drug addiction, such as those that are born by the law and justice, health care, and social services systems. The simple and emerging truth is that *untreated* alcoholics and drug addicts represent a far more expensive proposition for government than does the cost of effective treatment. This combination of emerging wisdom and desperation on the part of government makes the prospects for acupuncture in the next decade very good indeed, because acupuncture is portable, flexible, easy to administer, inexpensive, and effective. This does not make our job of program development *easy*, but it at least makes it *possible*.

The structure of public funding is different in different states. Some smaller states administer drug and alcohol program services directly, or contract them to private service providers. Larger states distribute funds and delegate responsibility for the administration of programs to counties or, less frequently, larger cities. Some local jurisdictions rely solely on state and federal funds for substance abuse and related issues, and others use local tax revenues to pay for such services, either by providing the services themselves as governmental entities, or by contracting with private agencies.

For purposes of explanation in this section of our book, we will use the fairly common structure of drug and alcohol treatment administration that is in place in California. It is important to note that *the process of accessing the system* is the same, regardless of the way in which the system may be organized in the reader's locale. That is to say that all expenditure by government of public funds requires some degree of public scrutiny and accountability. In California, for example, the mechanism for this is the County Drug and Alcohol Advisory Board. This mechanism may be different in different states, but the mechanism will be there in one form or another, and may be discovered by contacting the local or state agency responsible for administration of drug and alcohol treatment funds. We have provided in Appendix IV, Section B, contacts in each state for information about local funding mechanisms. Whatever form that mechanism takes in the reader's own region, the basic procedures outlined in this section can be applied.

In general, program funding is dictated by politics. Political issues whose recent popularity has influenced chemical dependency treatment funding include fear about the costs of caring for drug-exposed infants, and fear about the spread of HIV and AIDS through injecting needle use. Funding trends have consequently been moving toward treatment for pregnant and parenting women, and treatment for injecting drug users. Current political trends indicate that future funding patterns will have special emphasis upon chemical dependency clients who are members of ethnic and/or racial minorities, or who are homeless and/or dual diagnosed.

These funds will arrive in the local area through a variety of channels, and we now turn to a discussion of the mechanisms by which public funds are administered, and a recommended strategy for accessing these funds and gaining information about use of these funds for possible acupuncture treatment. We begin with the general area of drug and alcohol treatment, which remains the premier entry point for us into broader areas where our work will be of value.

Funding for drug and alcohol treatment in general is made available by every level of government: federal, state, county, and (depending upon the size) the city. The majority of funds come from the federal and state governments, and, in California and most other states, the *county* is the responsible agency by which these federal and state alcohol and other drug funds are administered. State law in California requires each *County Board of Supervisors* to create a position of *Drug and Alcohol Program Administrator*, and to appoint a *Drug and Alcohol Advisory Board* to represent citizens in each Supervisorial district to advise the Administrator on the administration of these funds. In larger counties, the Drug and Alcohol Programs may be administered separately, with two Advisory Boards and/or two administrators. In smaller counties, they are often combined.

Your county Drug and Alcohol Program may be under the administration of the County Health Department, Mental Health, or County Department of Human Services, or it may stand on its own, with the Program Administrator answering directly to the Board of Supervisors. Some counties may have two- or three-year funding cycles, but in general, all funding is awarded and administered on a fiscal calendar year (July 1 through June 30), because this is the calendar on which budgets are generally enacted at all levels of government.

The individual county itself may provide, from these state and federal funds that it receives, *direct treatment services* through Programs it has established, or it may *contract* these services to private *service providers*, usually agencies operated by private nonprofit corporations, or sometimes to other county departments such as mental health, county probation, or the county jail. Larger counties will do a combination of both. If the county administrator is aggressive and creative, the county may also receive and administer funds from private foundations, or be open to developing grant proposals to these foundations.

There is at each state level a *State Department of Alcohol and Drugs*, which is also generally served by citizens' Advisory Boards or their equivalent (see Appendix IV, Section B, for addresses of these departments). Most federal funds designated for drug and alcohol treatment arrive at the state as *block grants* that are designated either *discretionary* (funds that must be used for alcohol or other drug treatment or prevention, but in a manner that is at the discretion of the state), or *non-discretionary* - sometimes called *categorical* (funds that must be used in a prescribed way or to treat certain populations such as IV drug users, pregnant women, etc.). The State Department of Alcohol and Drugs in turn typically allocates these funds, as well as funds provided by the state legislature, to counties, again in discretionary and non-discretionary categories.

Overall, these funds are used not only for treatment services, but for drug and alcohol *prevention* and *intervention* services as well. By state law, First Offender and Multiple Offender Drinking

Driver Programs are usually also administered by the County Alcohol Program, even though these Programs are financed primarily by client fees. Treatment/education protocols for Drinking Driver Programs usually require approval of the State Department of Alcohol.

In addition to federal and state block funds, the county may administer public grant funds it has been awarded through competitive application to the state, or to federal agencies such as the Center for Substance Abuse Treatment (CSAT - formerly the Office of Treatment Improvement) or the Center for Substance Abuse Prevention (CSAP - formerly the Office of Substance Abuse Prevention). Sometimes, chemical dependence treatment funds are also allocated through the federal office of Housing and Urban Development (HUD) in which case they may arrive through the city or county housing authority.

Federal CSAT funds are formally awarded not to an individual or private agency, but to the state, who will in turn transfer the funds to the county where the grant originated. The county in turn may have designated a "lead agency" to manage the grant. New and different channels may be used by the current Federal Administration than have been used in the past, and current proposals of health care reform may fundamentally alter the manner in which these funds are administered. The reader can keep apprised of any changes in this regard by following the suggestions described in this chapter, and may have an opportunity to be involved in the origination of grant applications as a subcontractor of acupuncture services at the local level.

Federally funded drug or alcohol treatment *research* grants are awarded by the National Institute on Drug Abuse (NIDA), the National Institute on Alcoholism and Alcohol Abuse (NIAAA), which are both divisions of the National Institute of Health (NIH) (see Appendix IV, Section B), or by the National Institute of Justice (see Appendix V, Section A), and are generally awarded directly to public or private research institutions such as universities or research hospitals. Some treatment research also originates at the state level, and some is funded by private foundations (see Appendix IV, Section A).

While there may be other public or private funding mechanisms in the reader's particular locale, this is currently the *primary treatment delivery system*. In the fiscal crisis that states are experiencing as of this writing, there has not been a substantial decrease in funding for alcohol and other drug treatment programs because, as we have mentioned, there is a partial consciousness on the part of both state and federal legislators that alcohol and other drug problems, if ignored and untreated, will end up costing the government far more in medical, criminal justice, and social services expenditures than the cost of treatment. Increasing numbers of people in government agencies perceive that alcohol and other drug treatment is cheaper than paying for the negative consequences. It is essential to be aware that it is this fiscal (as opposed to humanitarian) concern that motivates funding sources. In this system, to advocate for treatment because it is the humane thing to do is often considered naive. In the "tough and tumble" bureaucratic and political world in which the tyranny of the budget reigns supreme, such a view is condescendingly referred to as the "social worker mentality." For this reason, all of our approaches to this system should keep in mind a bottom line of potential *savings to the system*. Acupuncture, in other words, is a desirable modality not because it helps more people and makes them feel better; it is desirable because it can reduce the fiscal impact of alcoholism and drug addiction on the health, mental health, criminal justice, and social service systems of government, the very services whose increasing cost is responsible for a very large measure of the current fiscal crisis. Not surprisingly, therefore, we find many advocates for our work among the most conservative communities. A recent jail program in Santa Barbara, for example, was funded by downtown merchants in order to reduce public inebriation in and around a new shopping mall, and new acupuncture-based outpatient programs were recently funded in New York City under the banner of a "tax-payer's revolt." These are the economic realities of our work; acupuncture makes strange bedfellows!

At this juncture, as we begin to discuss strategies for program development it is good to remember that we are dealing with the *addictive system* in all of its most glaring manifestations. As we proceed, we will be able to perceive the frustration and hopelessness of those well-intended and highly motivated public servants who have invested their energies into this process. As we begin to interface with this system, we will witness the institutional face of codependent enabling in its most highly evolved crystalline state. The bureaucratic mentality that has evolved as the *modus operandi* of this system, driven by control, is parallel to the arbitrary rules that govern the dysfunctional family system. The people we will meet have learned their roles well, for they have doubtless learned them in their own personal dysfunctional family systems.[206]

Remember too that this addictive system is not only cunning, baffling, and powerful, but seductive as well. If you begin becoming involved in these activities in your local area, you will have an opportunity to measure your own tolerance for the addictive system. Your own personal historical issues will be triggered, and you will be "invited in" - however tacitly - to play your own dysfunctional role. It is precisely here that one needs to remain centered. If you become angry, confused, frustrated, anxious, and depressed, don't forget that these are normal reactions to working in this system! The posture is to be as kind and supportive with the people you will meet in this arena as you would be with any addicted client. The overreactive danger is to become proselytizing and condescending. These postures, as well as confrontation, are generally as ineffective here as they are in the clinic setting.

To remain centered, it is good not to have to enter this arena alone. Seek out allies at every turn. Develop networks who understand what the realities are. The more broadly based the network is, the better. It may include acupuncturists. It may include professionals you have met at Twelve Step meetings such as CoDA, ACA, or Al-Anon. Be open to the cultivation of such allies at every step, choose them carefully, and use them to process the things you experience as you proceed. Our survival strategies as we move into the fray are to go to lots of Twelve Step meetings and get lots of acupuncture!

Where acupuncture has flourished in local regions, it has done so as a result of two factors. The first is through interest and support at the grass roots. The second factor is that a political leader of some influence has taken the initiative to advocate for acupuncture treatment. This individual may be a County Supervisor, a physician, a judge, a wealthy private benefactor, a police chief, etc. It is important to be open to the arrival of that individual in your community at every phase of this process!

Our ultimate goal is intervention, and interventions must be preceded by assessment. Assessment, therefore, is our first objective. The initial work is to learn the "ins and outs" of the primary funding systems in your own county.

The process recommended here for involvement at the County Drug and Alcohol treatment level may be repeated at any level or department in your area where funds are allocated for alcohol or other drug treatment.

1. Telephone your County Drug and Alcohol Program office and ask for the following:

a. the time and location of Drug and Alcohol Advisory Board meetings (or their equivalent[207]); ask to be placed on the Advisory Board(s) mailing list. These meetings are open to the public.

b. a list of all county treatment service providers, both public and private. *Ask also for the names of any programs or individuals currently providing any acupuncture services in the county.* If there are current providers, it is essential that you contact them before you begin. Meet with them and ask how you can help.

c. copies of any current *County Plan* or *Needs Assessments* that have been developed, and information concerning any current planning or needs assessment *activities* or *committees* that are open to private citizens.

2. The best vantage point from which to do the reconnaissance work of assessment, getting an overall view of funding in your county, is to begin attending the County Drug and Alcohol Advisory Board meetings. They are generally held monthly. Planning for the upcoming fiscal year - which is the time of reallocation of funds - usually begins in January. It will be good to be as educated as you can when this planning phase begins.

As you begin to attend these meetings, find out who the members are and what their special interests are. You will find that they usually represent law enforcement agencies, the clergy, the academic community, the business community, parents, and other concerned citizens. They will generally *exclude* representatives of agencies who are the recipients of county drug or alcohol funds. Such membership would constitute a conflict of interest; however, California allows that counties may have a certain number of program service providers on the Drug Board.

These boards are not vested with great power because they are *advisory* only, but individuals or funding committees may in fact have varied degrees of influence with the County Program Administrator, and they may have influence with the County Supervisor whose district they represent. It is the County Board of Supervisors who has ultimate authority over the administration of all discretionary funds in the county, even though this approval is often of the "rubber stamp" variety. Note that the funds that are being administered in this process are not funds that *originated* in your county, but rather at the federal and state levels; therefore, the Board of Supervisors is not necessarily going to have as keen a political interest in their expenditure as they are in local tax revenue expenditure.

3. Research your list of the county treatment service *providers* (contractors). As suggested above, the county will provide you with a list of all such providers. If you find that the Alcohol and Drug Program itself provides treatment services, find out the specific nature and extent of these services and who is in charge. Some services are likely contracted out. The agencies to whom county contracts have been awarded to provide treatment services

may be private agencies - generally nonprofit corporations - or public agencies such as the county probation department or the county jail. This represents an expenditure of your personal tax dollars and is public information.

You will perhaps find, as you attend the Advisory Board meetings, that these agencies have representatives in the audience. These people, too, are potential allies. Find out what type of treatment each agency provides based on the information in Chapter Six.

4. In this education process, review the *County Plan* and *Needs Assessment* documents you have received (item 1.c above). From them, gather statistics that are relevant to treatment. You may be overwhelmed by the volume of such information. These documents may or may not represent what is actually going on in the county, but their value is that they will reveal the overall needs, goals, and objectives that are currently supposed to guide all funding policy in the county. You will find statistics and language in these documents that may be helpful in supporting the proposals you will later draft.

5. As you go through these steps, become involved with any National Acupuncture Detoxification Association (NADA) members in your region (see Appendix III). If there is a state NADA chapter, join; if not, try to get one started. In any case, find out who else in your area is interested in this work, and network with them. Share strategies and information with others.

6. When you have a good general overview of funding in your county, it is time to meet with your own County Supervisor in the district where you reside or practice. The size of your county and district will determine how easy it is to get an appointment. It is likely that you will have to begin with a meeting with his or her assistant. At this meeting, you will have two objectives:

a. To provide information about the efficacy of acupuncture in treating chemical dependency.

Leave them a copy of a video (see p. 249). Perhaps leave a copy of the article "Acupuncture: New Perspectives on

Chemical Dependency Treatment" (Appendix VIII). Or write a short descriptive document using other Appendix resources. The document you present should be brief, and should include:

- a summary of acupuncture research in the treatment of chemical dependency.
- brief descriptions of the major successful programs in the country.
- a statement about the cost effectiveness of acupuncture compared with traditional treatment modalities.
- the importance of acupuncture as an *adjunct* to these other modalities.

If you are an acupuncturist, or can network with an acupuncturist who has learned about this work, it is very important to offer your audience a demonstration auricular treatment. Honor their decision if they decline. No one who is uninitiated likes being poked with needles! - but show them a sample of the ear needles that are used. Let them know about NADA, so that they are aware that this is not something you have come up with on your own, but that instead there is organization, substantial experience, and research behind these ideas.

The language you use to provide this information is very important. If you are an acupuncturist, even if you happen upon an individual who has been going to an acupuncturist regularly for years and has a high regard for Chinese Medicine, it is good to stay as far away from Chinese medical descriptive vocabulary as you can. If your audience perceives that you are there to ask them to take a *political position* as an *advocate for Chinese medicine*, they will probably not be receptive, even though they may be *personally* open to alternative medicine. You are there instead to provide helpful information on a "new" *tool* that has proven effective in the treatment of alcohol and other drugs in a variety of settings. You are not there to revolutionize what is going on in the county, but to provide information on a technique that will enhance what the county is already doing. You are not asking to *replace* but to *help* existing service providers. You are there not to tear down but to honor and support the efforts that are already in place. You are not there to tell them that current drug and alcohol treatment strategies have not been very effective; they *know* that. Nor are you there to educate them about "paradigm shifts" or "gestalt switches in perception." At least not overtly! This is a seed-planting time. We wish not to impose, not to offend, not to be invasive. The first rule of planting is to honor and understand the nature of the soil in which the seed is placed. Harvest comes later.

b) The second objective is to find out the specific goals and concerns this Supervisor has in the area of drugs and alcohol. What do they perceive as the priorities in the county, especially in the area of treatment? Tell them that you have been attending Advisory Board meetings, and that you are interested in helping in any way that you can with the county's drug and alcohol problems. Ask for suggestions about how to proceed that will help to address the priorities that are of importance and concern to the Supervisor. Take notes.

Then follow their advice! If they suggest that you talk to "so and so," ask if you may use their name by way of introduction. If they ask you to serve on the Advisory Board representing their district, agree.

Accept whatever miracles happen at this meeting, but don't expect any. Be humble. You are still in the learning and assessment phase. You may learn from this meeting that your Supervisor is going to be resistant. Or you may find here a potential ally for later.

7. Approach the Chair of the Advisory Board and ask if you may be placed on the agenda of a future meeting to make a presentation about acupuncture.

If you have been attending Advisory meetings, you will have seen other presentations made on a variety of topics. The organization for your presentation will be the same as Objective a) above for the Supervisor. Come prepared with a demonstration treatment on volunteers, and plan to show a brief video. The essential information you want to present (items 6.a.1 - 4. above) should be made before you begin the acupuncture demonstration, because once the treatment begins, the audience's attention will be on the treatment itself, and you can answer questions as they come up.

If you are turned down, or if their schedule prevents giving you space on their agenda within a reasonable period of time, ask if you can make a presentation to a *committee* of the Advisory Board.

8. Approach the County Drug or Alcohol Program Administrator(s). Tell them that you have agreed to make a presentation to the Advisory Board and suggest that you meet with them and their treatment people in advance of your presentation to the Advisory Board. This is a political courtesy, paying deference to the Administrator's desire to remain in control of the Advisory Board.

Your presentation should be the same as the presentation to the Supervisor (item 6 above).

9. Approach the Executive Directors of the agencies you have researched (item 3 above) and ask if you can make a presentation. These agencies are the likely sites for your ultimate acupuncture demonstration project, so this is a "good will tour." Again, follow the same basic presentation outline suggested, although here you may provide additional clinical information on exactly how the acupuncture part of their clinical program would operate. Ask if you may submit a proposal for their next funding cycle, and ask if you can make a presentation/demonstration to the agency's Board of Directors.

Even though these agencies receive county administered funds, it is likely that they are not *solely* funded by the county. They have other sources of revenue as well.

The funding track we have been describing in general is the primary drug and alcohol treatment funding mechanism in all counties in California, and is typical of other regions as well. As we have mentioned, the funds we have been describing do not originate *in* the county but are state and federal funds administered *by* the county. Depending upon the size of your area, there may be other funding tracks as well. Some counties may fund treatment from county general funds, or other local special revenue sources, through a variety of agencies. This information can be obtained from your County Administrative Office. The expenditure of all public money is the public's business, and you are the public! Therefore, be as assertive as you need to be to learn about what these other mechanisms are.

You may find that your county provides funds or accesses state and/or federal funds for alcohol and other drug treatment through any of the following county departments or agencies:

- A Human Services Commission;
- The Department of Social Services;
- The Department of Public Health;
- The Department of Mental Health;
- The Department of Probation;
- The Sheriffs Department;
- A Public Housing Authority.

Each of these agencies will have a more or less formal mechanism for involving the public in the expenditure of these funds. There may be Commissions or Advisory Boards similar in structure to the Alcohol/Drug Advisory Boards. If you learn that there is discretionary funding that is used for treatment available through these agencies, follow the same process that is recommended above for the County Department of Alcohol and Drugs.

Your city may or may not provide direct funding for alcohol and other drug treatment services. If it does, the political structure by which such funds are allocated will be parallel to that of the county. In this case, the City Council or its equivalent will be the ultimate authority, and funds may be administered through a city Human Services or Health Department that is advised by a Commission or Board designed to reflect public interest.

Multi-Government alliances may have been formed in your area to apply for special funding that may include treatment. There has been a recent trend in which regional or multi-county grant applications are viewed more favorably by funding agencies in order to avoid duplication of services across county lines.

Homelessness and HIV/AIDS

Programs targeting homelessness and HIV/AIDS are, as we have mentioned, other potential sources of funding. In most Counties, there will be a county (or perhaps a city) *Task Force* which has been established to address each of these issues. You can find out the schedule of the meetings of such task forces or commissions through the county Administrative Office. These bodies will function in a similar fashion to the advisory boards described above. They will likely not have any power themselves, but they will be attended by service providers and public officials in each area, and funding opportunities will be discussed. You will want to network with other individuals in attendance and be watchful for opportunities to make presentations and demonstrations and submit proposals to agencies or governmental departments who are the recipients of funds designated for these populations, including the County Public Health and Human Services departments.

As mentioned in the article in Appendix VIII, most promising is the use of acupuncture in homeless shelters, where alcohol and drug treatment often is resisted due to the unmanageability of withdrawal symptoms in such a setting, and where shelter client safety has become an increasing concern. Homeless shelter services are generally administered by either the City or County Department of Human Services, and our standard auricular protocol can be implemented on-site in shelters or in out-patient at ancillary service centers. The Santa Barbara program mentioned in Appendix VIII, operates an acute detoxification program with clients who are under the custodial care of a homeless shelter at night. Clients receive two acupuncture treatments daily, and the program has had a minimum of withdrawal-related medical emergencies, seizures, or social altercations. Shelter staff report that the program has had a positive effect on management of the facility in general. The program has a 90% program completion rate.

Our standard NADA auricular detox protocol is also an appropriate entry point for HIV or AIDS treatment because it conveys to the patient the message that the sources of healing are not *ingested* but come from within. This is essential information that AIDS patients need to receive if they are to survive with quality life. It is also, of course, essential information for people with HIV. Our protocol has further potential with these populations because there already exists a level of clinical acceptance of Chinese medicine and acupuncture in the treatment of AIDS.

Clients with a Dual Diagnosis

Dual diagnosis clients are generally trapped between the drug and alcohol services delivery system and the mental health system, and are generally not well served by either. Neither system knows what to do with these clients. The mental health services in your region are administered through structures similar to those described in the areas of drug and alcohol treatment, and mental health programs, like chemical dependency programs, are both residential and outpatient in design. The department of mental health in each region will have a chief administrator, generally advised by a Mental Health Advisory Board whose meetings are also open to the public. Acupuncture can be an important bridge between these two systems and can provide support to case workers and counselors who function in both. The perceived and real problems with dual diagnosis clients are:

- they abuse illicit drugs and alcohol, attempting to self-medicate their mental condition;
- they don't show up for appointments;
- they show up for mental health appointments too intoxicated to respond to counseling;
- they "fall through the cracks" of referral to necessary health and social services;
- they misuse and abuse their prescribed medications;
- they won't/can't stay clean and sober long enough to receive effective treatment for their mental health problems;

- the mental health problems that emerge when they detox from alcohol and illicit drugs and misused prescription medications are beyond the scope of the chemical dependency treatment program, so they relapse.

The best application of acupuncture and Chinese medicine for this population is to offer the standard outpatient NADA protocol in outpatient and residential mental health settings with the two objectives of (a) detoxification from illicit drugs and alcohol, and (b) stabilizing clients in their prescribed medications. Once people have detoxed and medications are stable, Chinese medical protocols can be added at the clinical discretion of the program to address the psychiatric diagnoses.[208]

In spite of successes, this all can be lonely and discouraging work because of the frontier position we occupy and the state of current funding. For moral and professional support, remain in contact with NADA members and programs in the state and elsewhere. Visit these programs if you can. You will find these people willing to lend support and ideas wherever they can. Your challenge in getting a program started, like that of the farmer, is to prepare the soil and plant, which involves (1) *doing the footwork* and (2) being patient! Build your grass roots network of people who express interest, and stay in touch with them. Keep abreast of new research and program developments in the field, and develop a mailing list of key people. Keep acupuncture in their consciousness. Send them copies of NADA newsletters and articles that you receive. Be prepared to submit proposals on request (see Chapter Nine and Appendix XI Section A). Follow all leads. Be open to creative and surprising avenues!

The Criminal Justice System

As we have mentioned earlier, a substantial degree of funding for acupuncture treatment in the United States comes not through traditional alcohol and other drug treatment sources but from the criminal justice system. This funding has been concentrated in the programs in Miami, Florida, and in Portland Oregon. But even programs that do not receive direct funding from the criminal justice system draw substantial numbers of clients from this system, and often find their most influential allies there as well.

When the consequences of alcoholism or drug addiction become *legal* consequences, a premier intervention opportunity presents itself. For many individual addicts and alcoholics, the criminal justice system - including incarceration - provides not just the *best* but sometimes the *only* opportunity for intervention,[209] regardless of one's philosophical views concerning the morality or efficacy of drug laws, enforcement, or justice administration. In fact, if the addictive system itself is our foremost client, no institution is more deserving of our services and of our attention than the institutions of law and justice, for here is where social energy is the most glaringly burdened, deficient, and stagnant. It is our great challenge to enter this system with vision, compassion, and healing.

The psycho-historical reality of course is that, in society's addictive desperation to "fix" a broken white male dominant culture, we have locked "Frankenstein's monster" away, and, in an act of repression as much as of oppression, have incarcerated our collective shadow, our "identified patient." As Kurt Vonnegut obliquely but bitingly reveals in his book *Hocus Pocus*, the social and moral reality is that we have become witness and perpetrator to what is perhaps the most scandalous and abominable chapter in the history of American ethnic and race relations: using drug laws to imprison the rich diversity in our culture in order to assuage our white historic guilt.

From a pragmatic political point of view, the burden, deficiency, and stagnation of the law and justice system translate directly into fiscal terms. And so, it turns out that the "bottom" for this particular addictive client is a particularly *economic* one. The former Governor of Texas, Clayton Williams, said that he would "spend the last dime Texas has building jails." He was subsequently and roundly defeated by Ann Richards, marking a change in consciousness in law enforcement. From this political and practical point of view, there is a growing necessity to get the alcoholics and drug addicts out of jail because there is no room there now for the real and dangerous criminals against whom society deserves genuine protection.   Leaders in the law and justice community who have spent their entire careers trying to figure out how to get people in jail are beginning to realize that they now have to turn their best energies to trying to figure out how to get them *out!* [210]   *Inmate reduction* has become a political banner in some county sheriff elections and indeed the formal order of some county Superior Courts.

The cost of incarceration of drug addicts and alcoholics is threatening the fiscal viability of many local jurisdictions in the United States, and, of course, of many states themselves.   The Drug Policy Foundation[211] has reported that in the United States, we incarcerate more people per capita than does any country on earth.   California leads the nation in this.   Typical counties in California spend more on incarceration and probation services than on any other single activity, including education, public works, or health care!   And it is only a matter of time before the people will demand - possibly, as has begun in New York, under the banner of a "tax-payers' revolt" - that we provide to addicts the tools of recovery so that they can become contributors to, rather than depletors of, the tax base.   This is not only the fiscally sound policy; it is also, of course, as Dade County's former "Drug Czar" Herbert Klein has said, "the right thing to do."   But even though the reasons of the system for embracing alcohol and other drug treatment, like some of the reasons addicts get sober, may not be the most noble ones, or the ones that we would choose, they will do!

It has become clear that no jurisdiction of society - city, county, state, or federal - is going to adjudicate its way out of the drug crisis in America.   It must turn to treatment if it is to survive. And the treatment must not be at the current token levels in which, out of an inmate population of 1000, 20 or 30 individuals are singled out for a treatment program; the dire need is for the means to reach hundreds and thousands of individuals on the criminal justice continuum.

Let's consider the fiscal arguments for treatment. In a representative county, using the most conservative estimates, 85% of the jail inmate population, 75% of filed criminal offenses, and 65% of welfare aid to families with dependent children are *directly related to alcohol or other drug dependence.* That's an average of 75%. In typical counties, the total of all local tax dollars used for law and justice, public assistance, and health care (the three areas where substance abuse has the greatest impact) amount to 65 to 70% of all local tax dollars used. If we assume that on average 75% of those costs are alcohol/drug related, then we can estimate that roughly *half of all local county revenues are being used to react to the negative symptoms of our growing drug and alcohol problem.* Of incalculable further cost are revenues lost that would be generated were these alcohol/drug dependent individuals productive, contributing, tax-paying members of our communities.[212]

Still, political and governmental officials are skeptical about treatment, and rightly so, because historically, drug and alcohol treatment has been relatively ineffective and very expensive to deliver on a cost-per-unit basis. Our challenge is to demonstrate, region by region, the efficacy of acupuncture as a means of bringing large-scale and cost-effective treatment to sizable numbers of addicts and alcoholics in the criminal justice system with success rates comparable to those of acupuncture programs that are currently operating.

Let's envision, for a moment, from a cost point of view, an ideal integration of acupuncture services in a hypothetical county or other jurisdiction. We will project figures per a population of 200,000. If we budget for the integration of acupuncture services at all of the jurisdiction's local corrections facilities, probation offices, public defenders' offices, community health clinics, mental health clinics, welfare and child protective services facilities, and other identified community-based locations where substance abuse interventions are appropriate, delivering a potential 2,000 treatments daily per 200,000 population, and if we estimate a realistic cost of $1.50 per treatment delivered,[213] these programs can be operated at a cost amounting to about 1.5% of the money that typical jurisdictions are spending *from local county tax dollars alone* on the *symptoms of alcohol and drug abuse.* Therefore, *a 1.5% treatment success rate would theoretically justify the expenditure*; a 20% success rate would save a typical county over eleven million per year per 200,000 population, and a more typical 50% success rate would amount to a veritable windfall.[214]   Again, in order to achieve such a dramatically successful outcome, political and administrative as well as financial support from the jurisdiction would be required - a willingness to provide a concerted and unified effort to generate support for this initiative on the part of all of the agencies listed above.

An argument can be made that simply because we typically have, in each county, a state and federally funded County Alcohol and Drug program, the county itself can no longer look exclusively to the state and federal governments for the wherewithal to address the drug crisis. The resources aren't there. Instead, the resources must be developed from within the local community, and from the law and justice system itself. This idea seems a fiscally sound and politically wise argument. Selling it to county departments of law and justice, social services, and public and mental health, however, is difficult because each of these departments is becoming increasingly protective of its own shrinking budget. Therefore, it is more likely that an infusion of funds to initiate these changes on a grand scale will have to come from outside the system.

In the meantime, the more realistic goal of beginning small programs, treating small numbers of people, and demonstrating success in each of our communities is essential to insure that acupuncture's efficacy is brought into the public consciousness now. Then, when the system reaches gridlock, as it had in Miami when the acupuncture-based Drug Court diversion program there began, local support will be in place.

When we speak of the "criminal justice system," we mean the entire continuum of law and justice services, from crime prevention through post-release services. It is a good strategy to initiate demonstration/presentations to all of the elements of this continuum, which include the following:

1. Prevention:

Private (or even public) *crime prevention alliances* have formed in many communities. These may be either:
   a. politically conservative groups with a vested economic interest in the prevention of criminal activity;
   b. formal or informal alliances that have formed to target neighborhood "gang" activity;
   c. neighborhood "watch groups" or citizens groups such as Mothers Against Drunk Driving (MADD);
   d. citizens' "task force" efforts directed against offensive police tactics.

These groups may have limited power and resources, but they may hold public hearings or meetings. These meetings are a potential target for an acupuncture presentation and demonstration. These are good seed-planting opportunities since such meetings are often attended by leaders in the law and justice or political communities, and by the press.

2. Arrest:

A major current fiscal concern of local city police departments and county sheriffs' departments is the problem of arrest and disposition priorities with alcohol and drug offenders. Due to declining funds, many departments have shifted priorities away from public inebriation and drug possession, directing their diminishing resources toward drug dealers. Disposition of the lesser offenders is a problem. Most officers wish there were a program (such as an outpatient acupuncture program) to whom they could "site release" these offenders. There is an increasing consciousness among some law enforcement officers that treatment is far more appropriate than incarceration, especially for their repeat offenders. The chief of police and county sheriff are therefore prime targets for outreach presentations/demonstrations. If you live in a fairly large community, your local police department likely has a division of community affairs, and this is also a good outreach focus.

3. Adjudication:

Judges at both the municipal and superior court levels are increasingly overwhelmed in their case loads by repeat alcohol and drug offenders. They are generally cynical about conventional alcohol and drug treatment, and are open to new diversion and/or referral ideas. New York City, Miami, Florida, Portland, Oregon, and Santa Maria, California are model acupuncture diversion programs, and have enjoyed significant judicial support. Municipal and superior Court judges are, therefore, also vital targets for making presentations and demonstrations, especially because of current publicity about "Drug Courts."

4. Incarceration:

Jails are operated by all levels of government: federal, state, county, and city (smaller cities may use county jail services rather than operate their own). The State Department of Corrections in Minnesota has become very supportive of acupuncture programs within the state prison system, and certain officials in the California State Department of Corrections are keenly aware of and interested in acupuncture treatment; however, county and city jails are the most accessible to us in terms of local program start-up. County jails are generally administered through the sheriff's department. Even though the sheriff is an elected official in most jurisdictions, the jail budget and operations is subject to oversight by the county's Board of Supervisors. County Superior Courts have interceded in jail operations in some jurisdictions due to jail overcrowding and the subsequent violation of state laws that govern incarceration.

Incarceration is the single most expensive service that most counties deliver, and there is increasing political interest in treatment in the incarcerated setting and in alternatives to incarceration. Special state and federal funds are also available in these two areas, and will often be administered and accessed through the county drug and alcohol programs.

Find out what treatment is currently being provided in your county's jail, and what agency is providing it. You may decide to make a presentation to this treatment provider, or to develop a proposal for a new and separate acupuncture program, or both. You may find financial support from a variety of sources for this, including private sources you are able to access through the prevention network (# 1 above). You may also ultimately find financial support for this directly from the Board of Supervisors.

5. Post-Release:

County offenders are generally released on *probation*. A probation department is likely operated by your county, and its director generally answers directly to the Board of Supervisors. State offenders are generally released on *parole*, and will be under the jurisdiction of the State Department of Corrections or Justice, which has a parole office in various regions of the state. State Departments of Corrections may also contract with private providers of halfway houses for state offenders who, prior to release, will sometimes be placed in such facilities to assist in vocational and social re-entry into the community.

All players in this process are targets for informational outreach presentations, and will be a major referral source for clients once your program is started.[215]

In the journal article appearing in Appendix VII, we cite a 1991 concept paper written by Paul S. Puccio, Director of Policy, Planning, and Research for the New York State Division of Substance Abuse Services.[216] This paper is important for two reasons: first, it has been rare as of this writing that a State Department of Alcohol and Drugs formally advocates acupuncture treatment. Second, it eloquently points out the most essential efficacy of acupuncture as it concerns criminal justice populations. Puccio describes acupuncture as a "threshold technology," most effective in "assisting cocaine and/or alcohol addicted clients who *resist initial treatment ... who may not be initially receptive to verbal, interpersonal intervention or counseling due to active drug use, the presence of withdrawal symptoms, or denial*" (emphasis mine). Acupuncture, according to the paper, "works in concert with traditional drug abuse treatment approaches [and] transcends the barriers to all treatment components."

The ability of acupuncture to overcome these treatment "barriers of resistance" is borne out by the Miami Drug Court re-arrest data, and by NIDA research findings in Miami. The first phase of the three-phase NIDA research grant, focused on IV needle users in Miami, has just been completed as of this writing, and the experimental group receiving acupuncture has demonstrated a faster rate of delivering clean urines than groups receiving counseling only. The most significant finding, however, is that, with acupuncture, *court referred* clients responded more favorably than *self-referred* clients compared with the controls.[217]

The Miami program, under the direction of the Metro/Dade Office of Rehabilitative Services, is on a continuum that begins with treatment in the Dade County Stockade and with a Drug Court diversion program for first and second cocaine offenders. The program was designed by Michael Smith of Lincoln Hospital and by Superior Court Judge Herbert Klein, who was then Dade County "Drug Czar." United States Attorney General Janet Reno, who was State's Attorney for Dade County at the time, was also involved in the planning of this program. Klein involved the Community College district in vocational rehabilitation for this very creative and intensive three-phase program which is considered the "showpiece" for acupuncture treatment.[218]

According to Metro/Dade Office of Rehabilitative Services, after two years of the Drug Court's operation, 4,296 felony drug possession arrestees had been diverted to the three-phase program, the first phase of which involved daily acupuncture and urine testing. Of the 4,296:

- 1,600 had graduated the program with a 3% re-arrest rate;
- 1,153 were still in the program with a 7% re-arrest rate;
- 500 had their charges dismissed after program entry;
- 1,043 failed to comply with the program.

Additionally:

- 90% of felony arrestees who were offered the program accepted the program (the other 10% were arraigned in regular Superior court);

- No screening for "treatment-readiness" was conducted; therefore, this is a non-selected, typical group of cocaine addicted offenders;
- 60% of the program graduates required at least a brief in-patient stay during their treatment;
- Most of the "failure to comply" drop-out group left the program in the first three weeks of participation;
- 30% of the drop-out group later returned to the program (either voluntarily, by summons, or by repeat minor arrest);
- Re-arrest rates were calculated for the year following graduation or time of participation; computerized finger-print checks were used to survey all Dade arrestees;
- Cost after two years of operation was given at $750 per client per year. Clients paid mandated fees, and the program was partially funded by a special fine levied on a certain class of traffic offense. When the program began, seized assets were used for part of program start-up costs. It should also be noted that the Drug Court is structured in such a way to preclude the need for probation officers; the judge acts as probation officer, with clients reappearing at intervals with computerized urine results and clinical records.

These outcomes and the success that they reflect are almost embarrassing in the success indicated. If we attempt to convince people of the efficacy of acupuncture based on these numbers alone, we will surely arouse suspicion as to our integrity. No treatment intervention could be this successful! Something must be wrong with either the numbers or the methods by which they were obtained.

The following qualifying comments should be made:

- The people diverted to this program were first and some-times second offender cocaine possession cases. People with multiple repeat offenses or additional felony charges were not diverted to this program;

- The incentive given defendants in the program was that their arrest record would be expunged if they completed the program, and these people were highly motivated to attain this result. People more recently diverted to this program have been more serious and chronic cocaine addicts, and the success rate has subsequently declined;
- The personalities involved in efforts such as these are often contributing factors to great success or failure. In this case, Judge Stanley Goldstein, who heard all the cases, brought a singular charisma, compassion, and presence to the process. He is an extremely caring individual, and is most supportive of defendants in their efforts to get clean;
- There was an amazing degree of cooperation in place in this program among the various elements of the criminal justice system (court, defense bar, jail, and prosecutor), *and* the treatment program. A treatment program counselor often sat in session with Judge Goldstein, providing in depth and current information on each client reappearing. Defendants were also transported to the treatment program immediately following their initial court hearing, so that there was a minimum of "falling through the cracks;"
- In addition, this program contained *all* elements of a successful treatment program, including vocational education and the cooperation of the community college, daily urine testing,[219] and a highly dedicated administrative, counseling and education staff.

This "Drug Court" was the first and only one of its kind in the Country, dealing exclusively with a certain class of drug offender, but many other jurisdictions have expressed an interest and some are starting Drug Court programs of their own as of this writing.

At present, over 120 inmates are treated daily in the Dade County Stockade, with no re-arrest data due to political problems with jail administration. Anecdotally, however, the program has had a positive impact on inmate management and reported productivity of counseling sessions. Unhappily, we have no good jail research to date. As reported in Appendix V, Section B, a preliminary study of Santa Barbara County Jail inmates indicated that those receiving 24 or more treatments during the last 30 days of their incarceration were two thirds less likely to be re-arrested in the two months following release than those receiving six or fewer treatments. Subsequent to that study, we examined re-incarceration rates of 29 Santa Barbara County Jail female inmates. Compared with an historical control group, the women receiving acupuncture had a 17% lower re-incarceration rate overall, and women in the control group were twice as likely to be re-incarcerated during the first 120 days of release than women in the acupuncture group. As in the earlier study, there appeared to be a relationship between incarceration rates and the number of treatments the experimental group received. Women receiving 32 or more treatments while in custody had an overall re-incarceration rate 26% lower than the controls, and 17% lower than those receiving fewer than 32 treatments.

Acupuncture programs have been in place in the Minnesota State Prison system for three years, and some research is currently going on, but no results have been released. Early indications, however, are that inmates receiving acupuncture make fewer requests for medical services and that there is also improvement in inmate management. In California, other jail programs have been started in San Luis Obispo, Santa Clara and Los Angeles County correctional facilities, again with no outcome studies as yet.

On the criminal justice continuum, we are currently burdened by the federal designation of acupuncture as an "experimental medical procedure," which prevents it from being a mandated part of sentencing, probation or parole. All programs, therefore, must be structured to allow the client to "volunteer" for acupuncture. It is our sense that when this barrier is lifted and prosecutors and public defenders and judges are brought into a treatment alliance, we will be able to see much more dramatic effects of acupuncture on the overburdened law and justice systems.

Hopefully, after you have made a presentation to one of the public or private agencies described in the preceding chapter, you will be asked to submit a proposal. The agency will likely require that the proposal include a budget, so we will open this discussion of program design with the bottom line: money. How much money should you ask for? How detailed should the proposal and budget be? How are you supposed to know what things to include in the budget and how much they cost? If you guess too high, there is a chance of being turned down; if you come in too low, the program, if funded, won't function well. This chapter will answer these concerns.

As we have said, acupuncture is an exceedingly fluid modality, and will fit nicely into any existing program. An outpatient acupuncture detox clinic can also flourish all by itself, without being contained by an existing agency or existing services. In the former case, you will be developing a proposal for an acupuncture *component* of an existing program. In the latter case, developing a program and budget for a complete and self-contained autonomous program, the budget demands, as you might expect, will be a little more complicated.

Let's assume, to begin with, that you are developing a program budget for an acupuncture component in an existing program. It really doesn't matter if the existing program is a neighborhood community health clinic, a social model outpatient counseling agency, a perinatal day-treatment program, or a residential facility. Your concerns will be essentially the same.

If you are an acupuncturist

If you are the acupuncturist who is planning to do the treatment in the program, the first considerations are to take care of yourself, to take care of your profession, and to take care that our work goes on under standards that will maximize chances for a successful outcome. These three things can be accomplished all together.

You cannot expect to be compensated for the time you spend developing the proposal and the budget, nor for the hours you spend getting to the point of being able to make the proposal. But once the program is established, your own compensation should be the first consideration. Assuming that you are going to be the acupuncturist, what should you charge? The best answer is probably "all that the traffic will bear." What that means is that you need to set your rate competitively. You don't want to ask too little, because you are apt to be locked into the fee you set initially, and it will be good for the profession if you can set a reasonably high standard in the fees acupuncturists should be getting. On the other hand, you don't want to set your fee so high that you might be easily outbid.

If you have done a good job in your approach to this agency, and studied this book well, then you have presented yourself as someone who is knowledgeable about chemical dependency, and you will have convinced them that it is essential that they use acupuncturists who are familiar with traditional chemical dependency treatment and with recovery issues. More than that, you will not have presented yourself as a "lone wolf." You will have told them about NADA, explaining that there is intelligence and planning and research behind the protocols you will be using in their program, and that NADA will be involved in program start-up and will be available for on-going consultant services, and that you yourself are (or soon will be) a NADA Certified acupuncturist.

But, when they read the budget section of your proposal, they will have forgotten about all of that. It is best to assume that the agency you are approaching, once they have your budget in hand, will look in the yellow pages of the phone book and call a few acupuncturists and ask what they would charge to do the work you are proposing. The people you have approached probably know nothing about acupuncture. They know nothing about NADA. If you have asked for $60 per hour, and a few phone calls on their part reveal that there are acupuncturists in your community willing to come in and needle people five mornings a week for $15 per hour, then you, of course, will probably be bypassed (even though they may keep your proposal!). This scenario is less than satisfactory; not only have you lost a personal professional opportunity, but the risk is that they will do their acupuncture trial using an acupuncturist unfamiliar with the protocol and design elements that will enhance success, creating a major setback for everyone involved. Therefore, it is essential that you have some sense of the financial status of acupuncturists practicing in your community. You may already know how well they are doing in private practices. If you ran an ad in the paper advertising for acupuncturists at $35 per hour, how many responses would you get? This is the sort of common sense you need to use in establishing your rate.

If you are not an acupuncturist

If you are not an acupuncturist, and are designing a program proposal, you will need to do the same kind of research described above, finding out how many acupuncturists there are in your area, and what a reasonable hourly rate is. You will not necessarily need to budget the per hourly rate at the same rate that the practitioner would charge privately because the work that will be available in your program is daily and on a regular schedule, unlike private practice clients. However, you also have an interest in protecting the integrity of the Chinese medical profession by helping to assure against exploitation. It will be well to educate yourself about licensure, certification, and educational requirements for acupuncturists in your area. It will also be helpful to discover if there are any acupuncturists in the area who are aware of and interested in this work. If so, involve them in your budget and program planning. You can also contact NADA (see Appendix III) and ask for the official NADA representative nearest you. Call them and tell them of your plans.

Hours of operation

Let's assume that you live in an area with many acupuncturists, and you have decided that $25 is a reasonable and competitive hourly rate for the acupuncturist's rate of pay. Of course, this is not likely to be $25 per hour for a forty hour week. And so, your next step is to determine the number of hours of operation of the acupuncture program.

We'll begin with the assumption that you will probably need to start small. It is likely that the agency you have approached is interested in exploring acupuncture on an experimental, demonstration, or trial basis, perhaps for six months. Despite the research you have shown them, they will want to see for themselves if it is going to help their program and their clients. Once the success has been demonstrated, expansion of hours will be possible, but to begin with, you will want to propose that the acupuncture be available one or two hours daily, depending upon the number of clients in their program. For example, if it is a day treatment perinatal program operating at a capacity of twelve client "slots," and since a treatment should last 45 minutes, one hour will be ample to treat everyone. On the other hand, if it is a residential program with 45 clients, two hours will be required. If it is to be a drop-in, outpatient setting, try to propose that the clinic be open for two hours, which allows a one hour and fifteen minute "window" during which people can arrive. In this setting, the acupuncturist can comfortably treat 20 clients per hour. Your ultimate goal is to have the clinic open an hour or two in the morning, and an hour or two in the evening seven days per week, but you may not be able to begin at that level with your demonstration. The importance of having the treatment available daily must be stressed, however. Treatments are offered in some residential settings only three times per week, and these can be helpful to clients, particularly if they are not in acute withdrawal, but you should establish five days per week as the minimum treatment availability in an outpatient setting where detoxification is a treatment goal.

For purposes of designing our first sample budget, let's assume that you are proposing a one year demonstration program that offers acupuncture for two hours each morning five days per week, and that you have established the pay for the acupuncturist at $25 per hour.

If the proposal is to a private, nonprofit agency, the next step in planning your budget is to add $5 per hour to that rate to cover the cost of malpractice or general liability insurance. Even though there has not, to our knowledge, ever been a liability suit filed against an acupuncturist working in a chemical dependency setting, the board of directors of the agency you have approached will likely insist upon it, and rightly so. As board members, they are legally and sometimes even personally responsible for any claims against their corporation. There are risks of infectious disease due to double-stick of needles, and HIV/AIDS and TB risk will be high among the clients you treat. Withdrawal from some drugs, as we have discussed, such as alcohol and barbiturates and minor tranquilizers, can be life-threatening. Hence, there are risks, both real and imagined, and they certainly *will* be imagined and anticipated by those who govern the agency that is considering your proposal. A surprising but obvious risk that some private agency boards have considered is that the treatment won't work; if it is presented to clients as something that will help them get sober, and a client continues to use drugs and causes an accident or dies, it is feared that the board will be liable.

The agency you are approaching may or may not have general professional liability insurance that covers acupuncture. If they are a medical agency, then it is probable that the acupuncture will be covered under their general medical liability policy. If they are a non-medical agency (and most of the more approachable agencies are), it is likely that they are not covered for acupuncture, especially for contract acupuncture services. In fact, acupuncture is specifically excluded in many general liability policies at that level. Even if acupuncture is covered, there may be an expectation that the acupuncturist will carry his or her own professional liability insurance.

Therefore, it may well be up to the acupuncturist to provide the coverage required, generally $1,000,000. In this case, the policy will be purchased to cover the individual acupuncturist, and will list the agency on the policy as additionally insured at an added rate. The premium for this will be around $1600 the first year ($500,000 coverage is available for around $1,200 per year), and will go up each year thereafter because extended coverage will need to be purchased each year for the previous year(s) at a level required by the agency. Some insurance providers offer financing for the premium so it doesn't have to be paid for all at once, and the $5 per hour added to the acupuncturist's hourly rate should cover the annual premium. The policy will, of course, also cover the acupuncturist in his or her private practice.[220]

Therefore, the first item in our one year, two-hour-per-day, five-day-per-week program budget is:

Acupuncture Services	**@ $30/ hr***	**15,600**

    * $25 for the acupuncturist, and $5 for liability insurance.

Now, there may be more than one acupuncturist working in the program, sharing the hours. In the optimum setting, the goal will be to have at least two acupuncturists on duty at the same time for enhanced client services and safety, but it is not likely that you will be able to start with that in a demonstration program. Thus the budget item is "per hour," and the figure doesn't change even though more than one acupuncturist is sharing the work. What may change is the per-hour fee that each acupuncturist will need to charge if two (or more) acupuncturists have to purchase separate liability policies. But let's assume for purposes of this proposal that the acupuncturist is working alone.

The next budget consideration is determining how many clients we expect to treat. This is an important question, because it is here that we are going to be able to demonstrate to the agency, in theory at least, the cost-effectiveness of acupuncture as compared with other components of their treatment program. Therefore, it is important to budget this item to the *maximum number of clients that can be treated* in the clinic hours we are proposing.

Of course, if you are proposing a component to a "self-contained" program with a predetermined number of slots, such as the hypothetical 12-slot perinatal program, or the 45-client residential program suggested above, there will be a potential built-in limitation to the proposal. However, be creative in your program planning. Perhaps the 12-slot perinatal program is going on in an agency that also offers outpatient counseling services, or the residential program has an on-going waiting list of eligible clients who want to get in, or it has a graduate (aftercare) outpatient or residential facility or other related services. In either case, you can recommend that the clinic time be opened up to other clients of the agency or to the public at large (most agencies are eager to expand services to more clients if they can do so without much additional cost, and you are uniquely in a position to offer them an opportunity to do that). You will therefore want to budget your number of treatments to the *realistic maximum number of clients* that you will be able to treat in the time scheduled. In our hypothetical two-hour-per-day plan, this number is 40 clients per clinic session (20 per hour). If you are an acupuncturist accustomed to treating one or two people each hour in your private practice, this may seem an alarming figure. But with the NADA protocol in a public setting, it is surprisingly reasonable.

The next item in your budget will be "program supplies" based on the projected number of clients. Program supplies include:

>disposable needles;
>pre-packaged individual alcohol swabs;
>cotton balls and dispenser;
>dispensation of hazardous (contaminated) waste,
>rubber gloves;
>benedine or other cleansing soap for clinic staff;
>tea;
>cups.

The rule-of-thumb figure to use in budgeting these items is .95 per treatment. This is based on a needle cost of 5.5 cents per disposable needle (with ten needles per treatment), the meeting of basic Federal Office of Safety and Health Administration (OSHA) standards (see Appendix XI, Section B), and a bulk source for "sleep mix" detox tea.[221] As the clinic grows to allow you to purchase in greater quantities, these numbers will come down, but 95 cents is a safe figure for start-up because, in addition to the medical supplies listed above, you may want to purchase a blood pressure machine, dispensing trays, or other one-time-only clinical items.

In our hypothetical clinic, then, you are budgeting for 40 treatments per day, five days per week. The annual budget entry will look like this:

Program Supplies

Treatment Supplies	10,400 treatments @ .95	9,880

   * this program will provide a maximum of 10,400 acupuncture detoxification and relapse prevention treatments @ .95, and will provides clinic services two hours daily, five days per week.

You may be asked later for a final budget breaking this down, requiring contacting local vendors for cost estimates of supply items, but this general figure is likely to be acceptable at this stage. You are not in reality going to spend this much, because you won't be operating at full clinic capacity every day, or perhaps *any* days the first year, but it is far better to over-estimate than to come to the agency director before year's end to request more money for basic supplies. Your agency will be locked in to a fiscal year budget and won't look kindly on having to juggle to keep the program alive the last few weeks or months.

The next item in your budget is start-up costs. This is a standard budget item in all new programs, and it will cover consultant and training expenses, and administrative costs of initial program outreach such as printing, mailing, and the like.

Consultant and training expenses will apply to NADA's involvement in program start-up. This budget item should include a plan for a NADA Certification training before the program actually begins. This three-day certification training will prepare all principal program personnel for successful clinic operation, management, and outreach and networking. The cost of the certification training will be borne largely by the fees that individual acupuncturists in your area will pay to take the training. Their incentive will be to fulfill the partial requirements of NADA Certification.[222] Additionally, continuing education units (CEUs) are generally offered when applicable at NADA Certification trainings. The cost of the three-day training is usually around $250, and if you are to be the program's acupuncturist and are not yet NADA Certified, you will want to include your own enrollment fee in your budget as well as fees for two or three members of the counseling and program staff of the agency, depending upon agency size. If you are an acupuncturist and want to do a NADA internship at an existing program that charges an internship fee, you should also include that cost in your budget, but try and keep these fees low. NADA will stay with you following certification in the sense of continuing to offer free telephone consultation support, but budget an additional $500 in case the program encounters special clinical difficulties that might require a later on-site consultation fee. Most NADA regional coordinators would be willing and able to provide several on-site consultation hours within that budget if necessary.

For administrative start-up costs, figure an additional $500, which will cover the cost of printing a fairly nice brochure and the cost of distributing it to other agencies in the area.

These budget items will look like this:

Start-Up Costs

Consultant and Training	1,500
Brochure printing and distribution:	500

The next budget item is "printing and copying." This is the cost of reproduction of materials for basic clinic files that you will want to keep *in addition to* the client files that the agency will already likely be maintaining on their clients (see Appendix XI, Section C). These materials include treatment cards for client self-monitoring of symptoms and for recording daily treatments, and possibly a *brief* medical intake that you may want to do on clients in addition to medical information contained in the agency's regular client files. You will also want to provide for the duplication costs of a clinic "Welcome" statement (see Appendix XI, Section C), and of other articles or information you can give members of the public who make inquiries about the program (especially potential private donors!). This budget item should be approximately $500.

And, you need an office supplies budget of $150 for a client index card file, a cash box (if required for client fees), a client sign-in log book, pens, staples, etc. These items will look like this:

Administrative Supplies

Printing and copying	500
Office supplies	150

Annual Budget for One-Year (10,400 est. treatments)

Acupuncture Demonstration Project at [name of agency]

Item	Cost
Acupuncture Services	15,600
Program Supplies	9,880
Consultant and Training	1,500
Brochure printing and distribution:	500
Printing and copying	500
Office supplies	150
TOTAL	28,130

You don't need to be so ostentatious as to provide the arithmetic for them, but they will certainly do it themselves and find that 10,400 treatments at $28,130 provides a $2.70 per-treatment cost. If they have experience with a third-party-pay program, they are accustomed to figures closer to $55 and up per unit cost, and so your budget proposal will be impressive indeed. It will be a cost effective program even if the acupuncturist is paid at a higher rate, as may be indicated depending on demand.

You can use this budget as a base, and, using percentages, construct a comparable budget using higher or lower program hours and client numbers. For example, using comparative figures, the budget for our hypothetical 12-slot perinatal day treatment program, providing acupuncture one hour per day four days per week would look like this:

Annual Budget for One-Year

Acupuncture Demonstration Project at [name of agency] Perinatal
Substance Abuse Project [or program title]

Item	Cost
Acupuncture Services	**6,240**
Program Supplies	**2,371**
Consultant and Training	**1,500**
Brochure printing and distribution:	**500**
Printing and copying	**125**
Office supplies	**38**
TOTAL	**10,274**

  * this program will provide a maximum of 2,496
acupuncture detoxification and relapse prevention treatments, and
provides clinic services one hour daily, four days per week.
Treatment cost $0.95.

Our cost-per-client figure has gone up in this budget to $4.12
because only 12 clients will be treated per hour as opposed to the
maximum of 20 possible in the open clinic budget. This budget
assumes all 12 clients will receive treatment every time, which is
not likely. Seeds for treatment of infants[223] can be purchased well
within the $2371 program supplies figure. This plan allows for
four rather than five days per week. While five would be ideal, the
assumption is that the women are not in acute withdrawal; therefore, four treatments per week will provide a good benefit and
treatment outcome. This is minimum planning. Optimum planning in a perinatal program would provide an additional number of
hours of treatment availability for women who are on a postpartum
methadone detox regimen and, therefore, require twice-daily acupuncture during the critical days of their withdrawal. In planning
how many days should be anticipated, it is necessary to obtain
from the clinical director of the program a history of the number of
program days the previous year that women were detoxing from
methadone, and then double it to be sure you budget for ample

time to meet this critical need, because untreated clients in methadone withdrawal are at high risk of relapse.

Some items are lacking from these sample budgets, such as rent, utilities, accounting, auditing, and other administrative overhead. These are expenses that the agency will incur if they implement your program, but it will be at their discretion to determine these amounts and, in turn, charge them to whatever public or private source is ultimately providing the funds for your program through them. This is an internal agency budget matter, and it would be a little presumptuous of you to second-guess these expenses, and so it is better to leave them out and defer this part of the budget to the agency. This is standard procedure.

Also missing from these budget proposals is possible revenue generated by the acupuncture program. Possible acupuncture program revenue might include:

General client fees:

It is reasonable to expect that people will be able to pay something for their treatments, and many believe that it is important to recovery that people do indeed pay something, even if it is only a very small amount. Client fees are usually charged on a sliding scale (see Appendix XI, Section C for samples);

Smoking cessation:

Your agency may be interested in promoting the acupuncture program as an aid to cigarette smoking cessation. This practice has clear economic advantages since cigarette smokers often include individuals who are higher up on the fee schedule;

EAP Client Fees:

Acupuncture is popular with public and private employee assistance programs[224] (EAPs) because EAP clients may access treatment for relapse prevention without interruption in work. As with nicotine clients, these individuals are higher on the fee scale because they are employed;

Fee-For-Service Medicaid:

Policy on and the status of fee-for-service state Medicaid for acupuncture varies from state to state. In the past, California fee-for-service Medicaid[225] (Medi-Cal) has paid for two acupuncture treatments per month at a rate of around $14 per treatment. Billing for this in your program requires that the acupuncturist(s) apply to become state service providers, and the billing generally needs to be for attending health issues and not for substance abuse. However, depending upon the mechanism by which state Medicaid is administered in a particular region, there is sometimes local discretion in both allowable billable events and frequency. For example, if you live in a small county which has contracted with a medical service agency to provide substance abuse treatment in the county, it is possible that acupuncture can be billed along with other services through that agency.

The sample budgets presented above assume adding an acupuncture component to an existing program. But what if we are starting from scratch, and building a free-standing but integrated acupuncture-based chemical dependency treatment program? Designing such a program will reveal a number of important organizational aspects of the ideal acupuncture-based program.

Let's enter the ideal world, having just found perhaps a wealthy benefactor, an individual or a foundation or a new county contract, or some combination of these. If we were going to design a state-of-the-art acupuncture-based program from the ground up, what would the considerations be?

Let's conceptualize this ideal basic program. It will offer ample daily acupuncture clinic hours seven days per week in an outpatient setting. Counselors will be available for on-demand crisis and referral counseling during clinic hours, and they will also do individual and group counseling and case management following clinic. We'll also provide daily on-site urine testing for clients referred by probation, parole, and the courts. We'll anticipate a client capacity of 75 slots per day, and staff to that figure. We will also provide for an adequate level of Chinese medical primary care beyond detoxification. Beyond these basic services, the program may well provide other expanded acupuncture services to other sites in the community. These would be budgeted for as adjunctive services, using the budget guidelines described above. Our design here will be the budget for the basic services.

It is standard procedure to divide the budget into two categories: salaries and operations. Each of these categories later can be divided further into program, or direct client services costs, and administrative costs. Public and many private funders understandably want to see at least 80% of their money going to program or direct service costs rather than to pay administrators.

Nevertheless, the first item in our budget will be the administrator, the Program Director. Depending on the size of the program, this person may not be a full time administrator. He or she may personally do some acupuncture or counseling, in which case a percentage of the person's salary would be in the administrative category, and the balance in the program category.[226] But with 75 slots, let's assume a full-time director with overall responsibility for the program management.

Salaries for positions like these range from $30,000 to $60,000 and even more in very large programs with complex funding requirements. The person must be good at fund raising (for program expansion to other sites, and for the years to come). This person must also have extensive background in financial and personnel management, and in interfacing politically with the community, and a keen understanding of recovery. General knowledge about Chinese medicine is also very desirable (see Appendix XI, Section D, for sample job descriptions).

Our agency in Santa Barbara recently advertised state-wide for the position of director of a large prevention and treatment project and received hundreds of resumes from well-qualified and even over-qualified applicants, so it is, at the moment, a "buyer's market." But let's budget $45,000 for a starting salary.

For a program of this size, the Director will need assistance in both the administrative and in the program areas. Let's budget for a half-time Administrative Assistant and a half-time Program Assistant. If this were a Medi-Cal/Medicaid or comparably funded program, these would need to be full time positions because of the reporting requirements. Also, if the program begins to see a substantial number of criminal justice-referred clients for whom program participation and urinalysis tracking will be required, more administrative time may be needed. But for now we'll assume a program with minimum reporting requirements, and budget for two half-time positions.

Salary budgets are generally written in full time equivalents (FTE). The FTE is determined by dividing the number of hours worked per week by 40. So, if our two half-time people are working 20 hours per week in these positions, they will each be budgeted at a FTE of .5. Let's pay them at an annual full time rate of $21,000. To determine the annual budget amount, we simply multiply $21,000 by the FTE of .5, which gives us $10,500 for each position..

Now, the individuals we hire for these positions may do other things in the program. They may even be the same person. But, when we construct a budget, we construct it by positions rather than by individuals. Joe, for example, may be the program Assistant, and the counselor, and the program's outreach worker...

Position	% of FTE	Cost
Program Assistant	0.5	$10,500
Counselor*	0.25	5,250
Outreach Worker#	0.25	5,250

Joe, therefore, earning $21,000 per year 40 hours per week, theoretically appears in three places in the budget.

If we are providing up to 75 auricular treatments daily, with expanded general Chinese medical health services, it would be wise to have a Director of Acupuncture Services who can not only perform treatment but who can also act as clinical supervisor for the acupuncture and Chinese medical portion of the program. This person should have some clinical background in chemical dependency, would ideally be a certified chemical dependency counselor, would be NADA Certified, and would have been licensed as an acupuncturist long enough to provide legal supervision of interns from the local college of Oriental medicine. He or she should also have some administrative and personnel management talent or background, and should be a good public speaker for outreach demonstrations because we are going to project expansion into satellite programs, and this person will be the "point person" for the task of cultivating those opportunities. Let's budget this as a full time position at $40,000 per year.

The acupuncture clinic will be open for 30 hours per week, and, since we are planning an ideal arrangement, let's schedule 50% of the time when two acupuncturists are on duty at once so that we can do primary care as well as detox. As we have discussed, some states provide for detox specialists who perform auricular detox treatment only under the direct supervision of a licensed acupuncturist. While it is possible that this practice will become an eventual necessity in most regions of the country when the demand for these services exceeds the number of licensed acupuncturists able to deliver the service, for our purposes we'll hire licensed acupuncturists only for 45 hours per week, and we'll use the $30 rate used for the earlier programs we designed.

Position	% of FTE	Cost
Director of Services	1	40,000
Acupuncture Services	1.125	70,200

We should also provide for a Clinic Coordinator - a person to welcome clients, do intakes when counselors are busy, make and serve the tea, collect client fees, and take responsibility for overall management of the clinic. This is an entry-level position, but the person should have a background in recovery and probably at least be in pursuit of a drug and alcohol counseling certificate (see p. 214). Let's assume that our weekday clinic hours will be three hours in the morning - from 7:30 to 10:30, and three hours in the evening - from 4:00 to 7:00. This is a good schedule because it allows for clients who work various hours to come daily, and it provides a long enough time to do some general Chinese medicine as well as serving 75 detox clients. Clinic hours should also be designed to respect the schedules of homeless shelters and transition-type or drug and alcohol recovery houses nearby. Such facilities have time constraints for meals and other basic services, and we want to be sure in the planning that clients can come for afternoon treatment and still have ample time to meet shelter admission or meal deadlines.

Having established that our clinic will be open 30 hours per week, we should budget our Clinic Coordinator at 35 hours per week, allowing for a fifteen minute set-up and clean-up for each clinic time. Let's make this a full time position, since there will be lots of other odd jobs for this person to do, like managing our supply inventory, ordering and mixing tea, filing, etc. Let's pay an entry level salary of $16,000 - $7.69 per hour.

We need a position at the same level for a Urinalysis Technician to monitor the daily urines. Like the Clinic Coordinator, this person will have to work a split shift to cover both morning and evening clinic times, and will have to be scheduled with enough time to set up before clinic and to run the urinalysis results and clean up after clinic. This is another full time position, and we'll hire them at the same entry rate of pay as the Clinic Coordinator. Although it is not a high salary, it is not low for entry level, and our program is paying high competitive salaries in the other positions, and so we should be able to attract talented people. Let's hire a third person at this level to do both jobs on weekends. If we have the same clinic hours on weekends, this relief person will be working 18 hours on Saturday and Sunday. 18 divided by 40 is .45 FTE.

Let's also follow through on our example above and budget for an outreach worker at ten hours per week - .25 FTE.

Now let's consider the counseling part of the program. There are three levels at which one may employ chemical dependency counselors. Licensed Marriage, Family, and Child Counselors (MFCCs), or licensed Clinical Social Workers (LCSWs) are generally qualified beyond the requirements of early stage recovery counseling. However, in the contemporary population of chemical dependency clients, a large percentage are dual diagnostic, suffering from a psychiatric disorder as well as from chemical dependency.

Salaries:

Position	% of FTE	Cost
Program Director	1	45,000
Administrative Assistant	0.5	10,500
Program Assistant	0.5	10,500
Director of Services	1	40,000
Acupuncture Services	1.125	70,200
Clinic Coordinator	1	16,000
Urinalysis Technician	1	16,000
Relief Clinic Coordinator & Urinalysis Technician	0.45	7,200
Outreach Worker	0.25	5,250

There will be trauma issues as well, related to battering, incest, violence, etc., that will often justify the need for more in-depth counseling following the acute withdrawal phase. Therefore, if someone qualified to deal with these specialized needs is not on staff, there needs to be good assessment and referral counseling available so that these problems can be adequately referred to other agencies.

There are advantages to having someone with these qualifications on staff. First, of course, is the assurance that clients needing these services will have them *when* they are needed. The client needing such services may not make it to the agency to which he or she is referred, thus "falling through the cracks" and relapsing instead. There are advantages for the program as well. An MFCC or LCSW can provide licensed supervision to other staff members,[227] and also MFCC or LCSW interns can be recruited who are often willing and able to work without pay in order to meet the required number of clinically supervised hours for their licensure, opening the door to great potential talent at low cost. It also provides, through clinical supervision, enhanced quality of services for clients, opportunities for staff to deal with issues that could otherwise result in burn-out, and an enhanced reputation of your program in general with the treatment, health, mental health, and social services community. A further benefit of having such talent on-site is to provide support for the acupuncturists who, on the front lines of a busy clinic, don't have the time nor perhaps the expertise to deal with emotional crises that often come up during treatment.

The second level of counselor that can be employed is a certified alcoholism and drug Counselor (CAC). Many colleges and universities now have such certificate programs available, sometimes through their extension programs. These programs are generally 24 or 30 quarter units in length, and can be completed part time in an academic year. Some of these certificate programs also have intern programs. Some states have associations, such as the California Association of Alcoholism and Drug Abuse Counselors (CAADAC), which awards more formal certification for people completing these programs who meet internship requirements and who pass a written and oral exam. There is also a national certifying association (NAADAC). Though perhaps certified by these private associations, none of the counselors at this level are *licensed* by the state, nor can they enter private practice. They can usually, however, legally perform group education and individual counseling to the point of referral.

These activities can also be done by non-trained individuals who have a Twelve Step program background in connection with their own recovery. Many people in early recovery from alcoholism or other drug addictions often are interested in working in the field, but are sometimes not sure if they want to make it a career. It is good to have guidelines established requiring a minimum of sobriety for employment. For most agencies, the minimum sobriety requirement is two years although program volunteers may be recruited with less sobriety, and some programs hire staff with less sobriety depending on the level of client contact and clinical responsibility..

Since we are designing the "ideal" acupuncture-based program, let's include an MFCC or LCSW level counselor/therapist with enough experience to provide clinical supervision to other staff members. The role of this counselor, in addition to providing clinical supervision to other counselors and to acupuncture staff, will be to be available during clinic times for crisis counseling and assessment and to oversee the leading of groups.[228]

The salary requirements for our professional counseling supervisor will depend upon the region of the country. Let's budget the position at $37,000. Other counselors need not be licensed, and let's budget those positions at $12 per hour.

Position	% of FTE	Cost
Counseling Supervisor	1	37,000
Counseling Staff	1	24,960

Having completed the salaries portion of our budget, next we determine the cost of employee benefits, including the cost of worker's compensation insurance, other health insurance benefits, vacations, and sick leave coverage. Benefits are typically calculated at 22% of salaries. Let's see what the "Salaries" portion looks like:

Position	% of FTE	Cost
Program Director	1	$45,000
Administrative Assistant	0.5	10,500
program Assistant	0.5	10,500
Director of Services	1	40,000
Acupuncture Services	0.125	70,200
Clinic Coordinator	1	16,000
Urinalysis Technician	1	16,000
Relief Clinic Coordinator & Urinalysis Technician	0.45	7,200
Outreach Worker	0.25	5,250
Clinic Coordinator	1	16,000
Counseling Supervisor	1	37,000
Counseling Staff	1	24,960
SALARIES TOTAL		327,060
Item	**% of Gross**	**Cost**
Benefits	22%	71,953
TOTAL - SALARIES &	**BENEFITS**	399,013

This is a well-staffed and well-balanced program. In the world of current funding levels, compromises would likely need to be made, but it is important to keep the highest standards in mind in terms of delivery of program services to clients. We hope to continue to move toward this ideal in the real world as our program success continues to be demonstrated.

In a program of the size we have imagined, budget considerations, under the category of "Operations," would include the following:

Acupuncture program Supplies

Treatments	Unit Cost	Cost
27,375	0.75	20,531

We are planning this clinic for an average of 75 treatments per day, 365 days per year. We have reduced the price-per-treatment from .95 to .75 because we are now going to be able to buy in greater quantity and hence realize discounts for herbs, needles, and other supplies.

Urinalysis tox screen chemicals[229]

Tests	Unit Cost	Cost
10,000	2.50	25,000

This figure anticipates 25 tests per day, which is probably high. Not every client will require or wish to be tested. The price of tests will vary depending upon the quantity. Tests will be conducted on site by our urinalysis technician.

We are providing 75 acupuncture treatments daily in addition to a complete array of individual and group counseling, education,and case management services. If 25 of the 75 clients access some type of counseling, education, or case management

Item	Cost
Consultant & Training-NADA Certification	7,500
Brochure printing and distribution	2,500
Program Supplies	20,531
Urinalysis tox	25,000
Rent	36,000
Building maintenance	2,000
Utilities	1,600
Administrative Supplies	3,000
Phone	2,000
Copier/Printing	5,000
Postage	750
Conferences	5,000
Program materials (educational materials)	2,500
Insurance/bond (no acupuncture liability included)	3,500
Accounting/Audit	5,000
Medical screen (includes TB and Hep vaccine/screen for staff	2,500
TOTAL OPERATIONS	124,381
TOTAL Salaries and Benefits	399,013
Grand Total	523,394

service daily, five days per week, we will be delivering a total of 33,875 units of service per year for $523,394 - a per-unit cost of 15.45. This is a very reasonable service delivery, and very favorable program outcomes will be assured with this level of service being provided.

We hope that we have furnished information adequate to the development of program proposals and budgets in a variety of situations that may arise. Additional information and assistance is available through NADA resources (see Appendix III).

Having developed a free-standing program in our last scenario, independent of a pre-existing agency, our attention should finally be drawn to the issue of community-based *linkages*. Treatment agencies historically have functioned autonomously, often as isolated entities. However, this practice is changing. Increasingly, the measure of competence in treatment (and indeed a primary funding criteria) is the *degree to which an agency functions as an integral part of the community that it serves.* Such networking requires the creative development of alliances with many other community-based agencies and organizations. These linkages will serve in two directions. First, these other agencies will serve as "feeders," providing the way by which clients hear about our services and are referred to us. Second, these other agencies will provide more specialized ancillary services to which our clients will in turn be referred for services beyond those which we provide on-site. There are many additional dividends as well in forming such linkages that come from the synergy created by combining talent and resources from a variety of individual providers.

This network of services will include:

private and public *health care service providers*:
    mental health services;
    community health clinics;
    public health nurses;
    public health homeless outreach services;
    HIV/AIDS:
      testing;
      case management;
      treatment services;
      needle exchange programs;
      etc.
private and public *social service providers*:
    general public assistance;
    homeless shelters;
    public housing agencies;
    public disability insurance programs;
    food services;
    legal assistance;
    veteran centers;
    family counseling agencies;
    women's shelter services;

  rape crisis and trauma centers;
  child protective services agencies;
  geriatric assessment services;
  etc.
educational service providers:
  vocational rehabilitation;
  job training networks;
  literacy programs;
  community college services;
  etc.
criminal justice system:
  courts;
  departments of probation and parole.

It will also include the network of *other substance abuse providers*, public and private, adult and youth.

We will, as we have discussed, not be expecting to find all of these agencies firmly centered in recovery. Many will be functioning addictively, "hooked" on a particular ideology, or in a way that enables or denies alcohol and drug addiction. To this degree, these systems become our clients, because they are in drastic need of a new paradigm, and we can influence that movement toward recovery with our own success and support, and with our generosity, for while these programs often function from a perspective of *scarcity*, we will have learned that the healing energy of the *qi* is in great *abundance*!

This is the spirit of NADA.

When we attempt a definition of the term recovery, we find ourselves on the other side of the elusive elephant we attempted to describe in the first two chapters. From a semantic point of view, those in the Eastern, Traditional, or so-called "holistic" health fields, for example, may understandably inquire, why do we use the term *recovery* when in fact we mean *health*? Or, as some have suggested, why not use the word *un*covered rather than *re*covered? It is likely that as this frontier is explored further, the concepts and processes we wish to describe will find more and more apt and precise descriptive language. For the moment, however, three things appear important in settling for the term *recovery* as a useful transition concept.

The first is revealed in a subtle and interesting semantic controversy that persists among people in the Twelve Step programs. Am I a *recovering* or a *recovered* alcoholic/addict? The book *Alcoholics Anonymous* uses the language "have recovered" and "can recover" throughout, and yet, from the beginning of Alcoholics Anonymous, alcoholics have identified themselves in the fellowship with the word *recovering*. This is an important distinction. The newcomer's first tacit (though burning) question is, "When will I be *well*? When will I cross the line that separates me from wellness/wholeness/health so that I will at last be 'out of the woods'"?

In the very practical terms of relapse, the seemingly gloomy answer is, "never," because alcohol and other drug addiction is, mysteriously, a disease that progresses *independently of use*, and the alcoholic/addict may never drink or use again in *any* quantity in *any* circumstance or they will rapidly find themselves not just where they were when they last became abstinent, but in fact *worse*. This fact implies a life-long vigilance that is repugnant to both the newcomer and to the critic for whom it smacks of either/or thinking. For the newcomer, this saddening news is intended to be softened with the cliché, "one day at a time." But even though "one day at a time" is not a philosophy but rather a simple observation concerning the way in which one's life passes, it is a truth generally resisted by the newcomer who sees it as little more than a facade for the fearful ultimatum of lifelong abstinence.

The seriously expressed notion that "I am well now" in the Twelve Step theology borders on heresy, for it is unequivocally understood by more seasoned members that it is precisely that attitude that forebodes relapse for newcomers who have not yet accepted their alcoholism/addiction. "I am well/recovered" often translates: "I can drink/use again." It signals the restoration of original denial, and an undoing of the first of the Twelve Steps in which powerlessness over the drug has been admitted. And we can substantiate the point in more clinical terms with the knowledge that the neurological mechanisms that are altered as a result of chronic use, so far as we know, do not return through abstinence to their original state. What, then, do we suppose was meant by the words in *Alcoholics Anonymous*, "we have recovered..." ? Elsewhere in the book, it says that "We are not cured of alcoholism. What we really have is a daily reprieve contingent on the maintenance of our spiritual condition." [230] Perhaps in hindsight (and at the risk of additional heresy) we can say that, had more sophisticated medical terminology been available in 1939, the book's authors would have chosen the phrase "in remission from..." rather than "have recovered from..." for it is indeed the *chronic use of the substance* from which one has recovered, and not the addiction. "We have recovered," in other words, from alcohol *use*, from *chemical intoxication*, but not from alcohol*ism*, not from the *process of addiction*.

For some people in recovery, the entire issue is settled quite simply by the experiences of seeing others, sometimes with five, ten, fifteen, or twenty years of sobriety relapse, perhaps fatally. Hence, the case for vigilance, and for the presumably melancholy prospect of forever identifying one's self in reference to the disease. These seasoned recoverers embrace with religious zeal the proposition that they will *never* be "out of the woods;" they will never be fully "recovered;" they will never be "well."

This does not, however, as one might suspect, equate with living forever in the *fear* of relapse. Quite the opposite. Vigilance, alertness, and consciousness are not the same as fear. In recovery, the drug of choice becomes neutral, morally inert. Those in true recovery embrace *faith*; so long as they keep "working their program" and adhering to the principles of the Twelve Steps, they will maintain sobriety.

The second issue follows from this. We can see, based on our exploration of this landscape in Part I of this book, that addiction involves far more than one's relationship with a chemical. If we follow with Ernest Kurtz the notion that modernity is inherently addictive, conceived of as a cunning, baffling, powerful, patient, and seductive process that is endemic in the culture in which we live, pervading all of its institutions, then we can see that recovering addicts, like the frontier-folk of our earlier discussion, are transition figures. Recovering addicts are in a process far larger than their specific *clinical* addictions. Like all frontier survivors, they remain vigilant, alert, and conscious as a matter of wise choice. They strive for the posture characteristic of surviving warriors: *impeccably centered.*

We suggest, then, that the notion that individual wellness or health can precede a greater wellness (such as the healing of the institutions in which we live, or the culture that produced them, or even the planet itself) is more than tenuous; it places us, by definition, squarely back in denial of our *collective* disease by disconnecting us from the reality of life in the late Twentieth century. Acceptance of the *process* of recovery requires acceptance of our disease not as a pathological entity or static event that occurred sometime in the past, but as an ongoing process that is, as Anne Wilson Schaef has said, "in the air we breath."

Daily vigilance is, in this sense, indispensable. Also, we see then that recovery ultimately implies a certain political posture, which leads to the third issue of why we choose the word *recovery* rather than the word *health.* The popular phrase "holistic health" reveals an ambivalence about the cultural meaning of health. The phrase is, literally, a redundancy in that the words *holistic* and *health* share the same root meaning, and the political agenda implied by the phrase is to reclaim the original, traditional, non-contemporary significance of the concept of health. The assumption, of course, is that modern, Western, health is not *healthy* at all. To the degree that the concept means successful adaptation to the addictive system, it is, of course, the antithesis of wholeness.

Western medicine didn't begin that way - certainly not with Hippocrates, nor even with general medicine as it was practiced in Europe and America before the 19th century, nor indeed by significant numbers of heroic individual Western health practitioners who have continued to resist the compartmentalization and reductionism which has come to characterize the institution of Western medicine.

However, Western physicians as a class have become the High Priests of the Theology of Exclusionary Rationalism (see *n.* #62). This theological system has co-opted health in the same manner that the dominant rational political and philosophical systems, as we have described earlier, co-opted Romanticism, Populism, and Progressivism. This co-opting phenomenon on the part of the addictive system is functional denial; it is the classic scenario of the practicing alcoholic buying a round of drinks for everyone else in the bar, or of the cocaine addict passing the mirror and straw to the visitor, coercing others through generosity to "do as I do" in order to deflect the reality of his or her condition.

Perhaps we can eventually discover a new context for using the word health, a context that will suggest what we mean by recovery. In the meantime, there is something very noteworthy going on with the Twelve Step programs as institutions or systems in our culture. Though their *exterior trappings* have been usurped by the Western treatment establishment, they themselves have tenaciously remained autonomous from any outside affiliation. They have not been co-opted. They remain non-rational, counter-cultural phenomena, substantially because of the "Twelve Traditions" that govern them.[231] The development of these Twelve Traditions by Bill Wilson prompted Aldous Huxley to proclaim Wilson "the greatest social architect of the century." [232]

The relevant question is, what are the dynamics that allow organizations and/or systems to maintain their functional and radical integrity and center in recovery in the midst of a flourishing addictive system? What makes it possible for a system or organization to remain in the eye of the storm? One obvious answer is that the individuals within them are able to remain centered in the principles of recovery. But how do the *institutions* forged by these individuals also remain radically centered? And, what of the more political, economic, and social concerns that demand critical attention at this moment in history? Should not movements which address issues of ecological imbalances, of racial, ethnic, class, and gender oppression, also be considered as recovery paradigms? Are not the internalized and externalized forms of repression and oppression that these movements address, in fact, the most salient manifestations of exclusionary Rationalism and the patriarchal values which it serves? Do not feminism, the men's movement, the green movement, and movements which target the empowerment of people of color and their cultures, and so on, speak to the heart of recovery?

There is great paradox here, for while the resolution of these issues is the center we seek, the pursuit of that resolution can *divert and divide* us from that same center. Perhaps the healing of the issues of class, race, gender and ethnicity is the *implication* and not the *origin* of recovery. We have seen that the central dilemma of the addict is *power*. The paradoxical issue of power/powerlessness is pivotal in the recovery process at every phase. When we begin to consider recovery on a larger systemic and organizational scale, the issue of power intensifies. Empowerment is recovery's highest goal, yet the seeking of it can be the greatest barrier to recovery as well. While, as we have said, recovery ultimately implies a political posture, the current intensity of racial, ethnic, class and gender exclusion and oppression; the tumultuous degree of emotional, physical, and sexual violence; the degree of institutional decay, and the epidemic of diseases presented by our traumatic communities, scarcely allow us time to make the same mistakes that have been made historically time and again, mistakes which have resulted in the seduction and occlusion and co-opting of healing energy by the addictive system which these healing movements intended to overcome.

Therefore, with a keen sensitivity to all of these critical issues that face us, we seek these new emerging paradigms, a new place to stand, a new looking glass, a new and radical center. We seek not to be beguiled by symptoms, but to discover the root. This challenge will surely require all of the vigilance, humility, wisdom, love, and healing we can marshal.

What are these emerging forms? What will they be like? How will we recognize them? Perhaps they are already present.

We have used the descriptive phrase "acupuncture-based" to describe the program development we seek. This is an important phrase. It implies that the auricular acupuncture treatment functions *at the center* of everything else that goes on in the clinic. This is not to say that the acupuncture is more important than the counseling, more important than the education, more important than the case management or vocational training or urine testing or relations with probation or funding sources. Instead, the acupuncture is simply the *center* around which all of this other activity takes place. The base. It makes everything else reasonable, possible, sane. Everything else, to use a word we have used before, *nestles* in and around the acupuncture.

Here is the significance of Michael Smith's words that we used to open this section: *Remember, your program is always sicker than your sickest client!* The tendency in the treatment program, like the tendency in the addictive society raging outside, is to place greater importance upon the rational or exterior forms of the program than upon that which the acupuncture represents, stimulates, moves. We are back to a simple and ancient truth of Chinese philosophy and Chinese medicine: *the qi - that which is essential - is invisible.* The *qi* is to the treatment program as anonymity is to the Twelve Step program. It is the invisible quality on which the program is based that no one notices. If the *qi* of the clients becomes honored as the *qi* of the clinic, then what the clinic becomes *is* recovery.

One form this idea has taken has been called *Community health with a recovery focus.* This emerging recovery paradigm, still in its assertive infancy as a concept, is an organic and malleable structure with roots in the efforts of Puerto Ricans and African Americans who learned and practiced Chinese medicine at Lincoln Hospital in the South Bronx of New York in the early 1970s. Elements of the form remain at Lincoln, and have appeared in spirit at the El Rio program in the South Bronx, and at Bayview Hunters Point Clinic in San Francisco.

The original notion of Community or Public Health in general is analogous to the Romantic, Populist, and Progressive movements. A revolutionary and splendid notion, born of the 1960s, Public Health has been expropriated by the ever-occluding addictive system of Western exclusionary Rationalism. The radical intuitions of Dr. David Smith, founder of the Haight-Ashbury Free Clinic, and other Great Society physicians and public health professionals of the 1960s, sought counter-cultural relevance in the notion of community health by integrating addiction and drug treatment into the basic fabric of these community-based clinics. But these and other similar clinics, while acknowledging addiction and hence moving against the current of addiction-denial that is endemic in other Western medical institutions, became as the tail wagging the dog; what was implemented were the essentially Rationalist treatment strategies of drugs and psychotherapy. By emphasizing drug treatment *per se*, they became seduced by the symptoms and lost the recovery focus.[233]

The El Rio and Bayview Hunters Point programs have turned the focus around. Instead of attempting to integrate drug treatment into a general health setting, all general health issues are approached here from the point of view of community (systemic) recovery. With Chinese medicine as the template, complemented by Western medicine as necessary, and holding the clinical focus on recovery, we find a social infrastructure capable of healing community and public health with integrity and elegance.

The unique interface of Chinese medicine and acupuncture with addiction recovery allows us to begin to look at traditional public health care in the United States in a new way. Many of us have asked why, in Manfred Porkert's words, acupuncture has so "stubbornly and successfully resisted assimilation" into Western medical science. The answer of course is that we have two paradigms that appear, from the Western Rationalist perspective, to be inherently *non* complementary. The criticism that Western medicine frequently makes of Chinese medicine is that *it treats only symptoms*; the criticism that Chinese medicine frequently makes of Western medicine is that *it treats only symptoms*!

This is a seemingly irreconcilable paradox from the Western point of view, for which it is not enough to say that the organizing principles of Chinese medicine are *energic* while those of Western medicine are *somatic*. In China, of course, Western medicine has been integrated quite successfully and well into Chinese medicine because, from the Chinese point of view, what appear to the Western Rationalist as irreconcilable opposite organizing principles are in fact two aspects of the same thing and are very complementary indeed.

It is understandable from our present vantage point on the frontier we have been exploring that it is the Western modern pathology of *addiction* that now allows us to build a conceptual framework for the mutually supportive integration of these two systems in the Western medical setting. Like the Twelve Step program, this framework will become a new paradigm, centered in the principles of recovery as we have been describing them.

To build this framework, we will begin metaphorically. The character in Chinese that depicts the idea of a disease running its course is the representation of a leaf falling into a stream. Once the leaf is in the stream, once the disease has manifested at the level of tissue, the great efficacy of Chinese medicine weakens, and it becomes, guilty as charged, able to offer only symptomatic relief. And it is at this crisis stage of disease, of course, where Western medical intervention is most effective, employing no less a symptomatic intervention at that point.

Assuming that there is pathology (and that it is not simply Autumn!), the Chinese interest is in the conditions that caused the leaf to drop from the tree, an interest which leads from leaf to twig to branch to trunk to root to soil and so on. Here, Western medicine is ineffective, because there is no pathology at the level of tissue in the early phases of the disease process. For all of the high technology in his or her arsenal, the Western physician's best response to the patient for whom the leaf has not yet fallen is the standard, "take two aspirin and call me in the morning." In the morning, either things will be better, or there will be pathology. It is easy to see metaphorically, then, that these two systems are not inherently incompatible; quite the opposite, they are, as the Chinese practitioner well knows, very compatible indeed, existing on a very logical continuum.

In a majority of the diseases that are presented in the modern urban or semi-urban public health clinic, we can follow the leaf to the root and return to our original thesis that the systems of *nuclear family*, of *extended family*, and of *community* in which our patient functions daily, are, as we have described, *dysfunctional*, or *inherently addictive*. Let us review this environment, repeating what we described in Chapter Two: It is a barren, stress-inducing environment, non-validating of health, characterized by loneliness and isolation, an environment in which the individual has been cut off from what is conventionally thought of as a social support system, which we translate as external sources of validation of life-enhancing feelings and behaviors. Examples of such an environment are urban slums, war zones, prisons, schools, and primary social systems such as families which function to alienate rather than validate or reinforce living processes, particularly trauma such as loss, death, abuse, violence, homelessness, repression, or political, economic, or sexual exploitation, a culture characterized by alienation and criminalization.

This is the epidemiological staging ground for infectious diseases such as HIV, AIDS, and TB; for chronic drug and alcohol dependence; for affective disorders such as PTSD, depression, anxiety, sleep disorders, etc., for chronic pain and traumatic injury ... We could extend the list indefinitely, and find ourselves covering a very substantial percentage of the pathologies that are presented in community health clinics and emergency rooms across the country.

Consequently, basing community health delivery on the philosophical organizing principles of Western medicine will fail to address etiologically virtually all of these root syndromes. If those organizing principles are based upon traditional Chinese medicine as it is practiced in the West, there will still be vast shortcomings in addressing etiology because the patient will arrive too late. Conventional Western health consciousness is not oriented to prevention but to crisis. If the two systems were integrated, we would have some advantages. But, if the two systems were integrated around an organizing template of the *principles of recovery* as we have described them, we would have a new form, capable of bringing unprecedented significance to the notion of *community health.*

To envision this marriage of East and West, let us look again for a moment at the principles of efficacy in the Twelve Step recovery movement, which functions and flourishes in the addictive culture.

This movement functions through the Twelve Step meeting network. There are different kinds of meetings and meeting formats, but certain organizing principles are universal in the Twelve Step movement, as follows:

1.Meetings are *accessible.* There are no requirements for membership or attendance.[234] There are no appointments or screening required, and no expectations are placed upon those in attendance. People are free to come in and out at any phase of their disease. Hence, the meeting network, in general, is an *open, barrier free system.*

2. Meetings function as *extended families.* Not only does the Twelve Step network as a whole include meetings for all members of the addictive family system (Al-Anon, Nar-Anon, Ala-Teen, Ala-Tot, Codependents Anonymous, etc.), but if an individual is alone in a new city, he or she can go to a meeting and find the same degree of communality, acceptance, and emotional support that in saner times characterized the extended family system.

3. Though the essential function of the network is the group process, there is a highly individualized system of guidance/assessment provided by *peer sponsorship*. Implicit in the system (through the Twelfth Step) is a willingness on the part of members to spend time and energy with anyone in need. This willingness may even extend, though certainly not universally, to providing temporary material assistance, but always extends to providing emotional validation and a way of connecting with others on a short-term crisis basis or in more formal, long term sponsorship.

4. *Addiction is the referent* for addressing all problems and issues on every level. While it is acknowledged that many life issues emerge in recovery that are not directly involved with addiction recovery, these issues are always addressed in the context of *addiction recovery consciousness*. Most conversations, in other words, always come back to the Twelve Steps: "You are having relationship/financial problems (etc.)? What Step are you on? " There is an implicit bias that, while diverse needs may require expanded solutions, the priority is always to remain centered in the process of one's own recovery.

5. While recovery activities are formally organized around the meeting, the recovery process is fluid, extending out into the "real world," where "the rubber meets the road." The principles of recovery permeate the community that surrounds the formal organization. There are not only many "mini meetings" informally held in grocery store check-out lines, on street corners, and in other informal settings, but the Twelfth Step ("practiced these principles in all our affairs") causes a ripple effect outward through the recoverer and the lives he or she touches.

6. The act of coming together around recovery contains an emphasis upon ritual and celebration of passages through recovery. Meetings have a ritualized structure that has grown out of the group experience and which provides a context and meaning to newcomers and to people who may be new to that particular meeting.

What would community health look like if organized around these principles? In the healing of communities, as in the healing of the individual, we can envision the same three general phases we discussed to Chapters Six and Seven: *transition, stabilization*, and *empowerment*.

Our basic auricular chemical detoxification protocol will provide an ideal entry point and central organizing principle. We can conceive of transforming the traditional waiting room of the public health clinic into a "Treatment room" in which the basic five-point acupuncture treatment is available on demand. This *yin*-nurturing, five-point protocol is a generic protocol, "good for what ails you," designed to support the body in the elimination of stress and toxicity. It is a treatment that will assist in maintaining balance in a life of imbalance. It addresses generic craving. Administered in a group setting, it creates and demonstrates a healthy environment, generating *jing* energy. The herbal tea served in the detox clinic provides a nice social amenity, and also helps the body to cleanse, and promotes relaxation, all of which helps to create a positive, ritualistic environment. People don't need an appointment. They are welcome at any time that the treatment is available, and, barring acute medical emergency, assessment or screening need not be required prior to receiving this treatment. In other words, people don't need a stated reason for being there. In fact, for new clients, the administration of this treatment can be itself the opportunity for assessment and screening on an informal basis as the person performing the treatment begins to collect information and make observations.

In addition, the treatment not only demonstrates a healthy environment in the larger ambience of the clinic setting, but it also demonstrates health on an individual basis by inviting the attention of the client inward to the sources of healing. A secondary benefit it provides is a gentle introduction to acupuncture, serving to prepare people who are unaccustomed to Chinese medicine for acceptance of more expanded acupuncture treatment.

The focus of the clinic would be expansive. Inquiries would be politely made concerning one's relatives and friends and living situation, and people would be encouraged to bring others with them to the clinic next time they come in. Children would be particularly welcome. Some of them would receive treatment with their parents, and intelligently managed adjunctive nursery and child care facilities would also be available where additional assessments and clinical recommendations might be formulated concerning the child's health needs.

The individuals administering treatment would be *specialists in initial assessment*. They would be trained by and work under the direct supervision of a clinical team representing expertise in both Chinese and Western medicine, psychotherapy, and perhaps social expertise in such areas as parenting, vocation, housing, law, and so on, although many of these latter needs will be addressed by a volunteer network of "Twelve Steppers" interested in helping others in order to themselves remain in recovery. There would be ongoing opportunities for the recruitment and training of clients into positions of peer counselors and auricular treatment specialists.

This would be the entry or transition point into the health care delivery system, a "Level 1" to which people would wish to return no matter where else they may find themselves in the system later on. It would be the basic identifying core of the clinic's structure.

The full participation of "clients" in the atmosphere and spirit of the room in which this would happen would be encouraged. The room would be an expression of the ethnic values of the participants, decorated with art work or other gifts people would bring. There might perhaps be a non-denominational "altar" for the celebration of births, marriages, and other rites of passage.

A second level of activity in the clinic would include more intensive crisis intervention treatment on demand, involving both Chinese and Western medicine and counseling, an amplification of the crisis counseling available in the detox clinic. A third level would perhaps begin to resemble a more traditional Western treatment setting, addressing crisis and pathology that required a more acute level of treatment. These second and third levels, of course, would include both Chinese and Western herbal/pharmaceutical therapies.

Ideally, other kinds of activities could take place on site. These might include a variety of Twelve Step meetings and support groups, parenting and neonatal classes, nutrition education and *qi gong* classes. Ideally, this would be in interface with the local community college or adult education institution. And, the clinic environs would also serve as a community cultural center, with such activities as food, music, and art fairs, weddings, and other community events.

Accessing health care, in short, would become not the result of pathological crisis, but rather a form of celebration and participation in life, culture, and community.

In this rather expansive vision, we can see community health as embracing the principles of recovery for individuals, but we can also begin to see the possibility of true *community* health, in which the systemic healing of families and the culture of their communities becomes possible through remaining centered in the participatory principles of inclusion, cultural validation, and empowerment. This vision may be idealistic and perhaps "futuristic," especially if it is envisioned as being implanted "from above." However, it may be a natural outgrowth of our work if we pay attention to the deep linkages that form in our communities as a result of our work.

And then allow the *qi* to go where it wants to go.

Appendix I: United States Federal Drug Policy

Section A: History of Drug Regulation in the United States

1875	City of San Francisco adopts ordinance prohibiting the smoking of opium in smoking houses.
1882	New York City bans opium smoking.
1885	Federal law limits manufacture of opium for smoking.
1906	Pure Food and Drug Act passes, requiring labeling quantities and constituents from of drugs.
1909	Opium Exclusion Act prohibits importation of opium or its derivatives for non-medicinal use. (expanded in 1942)
1909	Shanghai International Opium Conference and
1911	Hague International Opium Conference shifted opium control focus to an international level, directed primarily at opium problems in the Far East and the Philippines.
1912	Townsend Act penalizes opiate use.
1914	Harrison Narcotic Act makes possession of narcotics without a prescription illegal.
1919	Eighteenth (alcohol prohibition) Amendment.
1920	a law preventing physicians from giving opiates to addicts. (This began the black market, and by 1925 the price of morphine was 50 times the legal price. This law was ultimately repealed.)
1924	Importation of heroin banned.
1925	Linder v. the United States establishes drug dependency as an illness.
1929	Porter Narcotic Farms Law passes establishing federal "treatment" farms for jailed opiate dependents.
1930	Federal Bureau of Narcotics established (replaced in 1968 by the Bureau of Narcotics and Dangerous Drugs).
1933	Twenty-first amendment repeals prohibition.
1937	Marijuana Tax Act passes taxing physicians and marijuana distributors for marijuana prescription.
1938	Food, Drug, and Cosmetic Act requires proof of product safety.

1942   Opium Exclusion Act requires domestic growers to register.

1956   Narcotic Drug Control Act.

1962   Kefauver-Harris Amendment to Pure Food and Drug Act requires proof of product safety and effectiveness.

1963   Community Mental Health Center Act passes emphasizing rehabilitation for mental problems.

1965   Drug Abuse Control Amendments to 1938 Food Drug and Cosmetic Act pass classifying depressant, stimulant, and hallucinogenic drugs as "dangerous drugs."

1966   National Addiction Rehabilitation Administration established.

1968   Bureau of Narcotics and Dangerous Drugs established replacing the Federal Bureau of Narcotics.

1970   Comprehensive Drug Abuse Prevention and Control Act passes, liberalizing penalties for drug-abuse offenders.

1972   Presidential Council on Marijuana and Drug Abuse recommends decriminalization.

1972   Drug Abuse Office and Treatment Act.

1973   Oregon becomes first state to decriminalize marijuana.

1974   Narcotic Addict Treatment Act.

1974   Alcohol and Drug Abuse Education Act.

1976   Amendments to National Security Act of 1947 prohibit CIA experimentation with drugs on unknowing or unwilling human subjects. PL 94-237 establishes the Office of Drug Abuse Policy within the executive office of the president.

1979   S-1075 revises FDA procedures and authority concerning new-drug introduction, testing, marketing, packaging, and recall and litigation powers.

1988   Drug Abuse Act creates cabinet level position of "Drug Czar."

Section B: Legal Classifications

Following is a partial list of psychoactive drugs as they are rated by federal law:

SCHEDULE I DRUGS

potential for abuse: high; medical use: none; production controlled: yes

heroin	mescaline
marijuana	opiates (generally)
THC	opium and opium derivatives
LSD	hallucinogenic substances

SCHEDULE II DRUGS

potential for abuse: high; medical use: yes; production controlled: yes

morphine	amobarbital
cocaine	pentobarbital
methadone	meperidine
opium	methaqualone
codeine	all amphetamine type stimulants
secobarbital	

SCHEDULE III DRUGS

potential for abuse: some; medical use: yes; production controlled: no

nonamphetamine type stimulants
some narcotic preparations
some barbiturates

paregoric

SCHEDULE IV DRUGS

potential for abuse: low; medical use: yes; production controlled: yes

barbital   diazepam
chloral hydrate   chlordiazepoxide
phenobarbital   propoxyphene
certain nonamphetamine stimulants not listed in previous schedules

SCHEDULE V DRUGS

potential for abuse: low; medical use: yes; production controlled: no

compounds, mixtures and preparations with very low
amounts of narcotics
dilute codeine and opium compounds

Appendix II: Pharmacological Resources

Suggested for Clinic Reference:

There are an abundance of Western Medical resources on all aspects of the pharmacology of psychoactive drugs. Following is a suggested short list of general resources for at-hand clinic reference. A more extensive and technical list of books can be found at the end of this section.

A helpful brief medical guide is Peter Johnson, *et. al.*, "Hints for the Identification of Alcohol and Other Drug Problems," published by the Robert Wood Johnson Foundation's Fighting Back program, and available from Fighting Back, Lexington/Richland Alcohol and Drug Abuse Council, Post Office Box 50597, Columbia, South Carolina 29250, (803) 733-1390. More extensive is the U. S. Department of Health and Human Services' Seventh Special Report to the U. S. Congress, *Alcohol and Health*, especially Chapter V., "Medical Consequences," available from Public Health Service, Alcohol, Drug Abuse, and Mental Health Administration, 5600 Fishers Lane, Rockville, Maryland.

We also particularly recommend:

Beasley, Joseph D. *Diagnosing and Managing Chemical Dependency*, Essential Medical Information Systems, 1990.

Gilman, Alfred G., et al, *Goodman & Gilman's the Pharmacological Basis of Therapeutics*, New York: McGraw Hill, 1990.

Inaba, D., and Cohen, W., *Uppers and Downers and All Arounders,* Ashland, Oregon: Cinemed, Inc., 1989.

Julien, Robert, *Primer of Drug Action*, 6th edition, New York: W. H. Freeman & Co., 1991.

Schuckit, M. A., Drug and Alcohol Abuse: A Clinical Guide to Diagnosis and Treatment, New York: Plenum Press, 1989.

Helpful for updates is the California Society for the Treatment of Alcoholism and Other Drug Dependencies News, published triennially and available from California Society for the Treatment of Alcoholism and Other Drug Dependencies, 3803 Broadway Suite 2, Oakland, CA 94611, (415) 428-9091.

Other updated Western medical resources are available from:

American Society for Addiction Medicine
5525 Wisconsin Avenue, N.W.
Washington, D.C. 20016
(202) 244-8948

National Clearinghouse for Alcohol and Drug Information
National Institute of Health
P.O. Box 2345
Rockville, MD 20852
(800) 729-6686
(301) 468-2600

National Council on Alcoholism and Drug Dependence, Inc.
(NCADD)
12 West 21st Street
New York, NY 10010
(800) 475-HOPE
(212) 206-6770

(NCADD publishes the "Medical Scientific Advisory" and a host of other materials available through their 200 state and local affiliates.)

Holistic Resources:

SAAVE neurophysiological and supplemental nutritional information:
Matrix Technologies, Inc.
A Subsidiary of Neurogenesis, Inc.
1020 Bay Area Boulevard
Houston, TX 77058
(800) 345-8912

Other resources concerning biochemical and nutritional supplements and holistic clinical approaches to chemical dependency treatment include Robert Erdmann's *The Amino Revolution*, Green Tiger Press, 1989 (second printing), and Joan Matthews-Larson's *Alcoholism: The Biochemical Connection*, Villard Books, 1992.

Treatment programs which have developed holistic nutrition-oriented approaches:

Health Recovery Center (HRC)
3255 Hennepin Avenue, South
Minneapolis, MN 55408
(612) 827-7800

California Recovery Systems
147 Lomita Drive, Suite D
Mill Valley, CA 94941
(415) 383-3611

Milam Recovery Program
12845 Ambaum Blvd., SW
Seattle, WA 98146
(206) 241-0890

Comprehensive Medical Care
149 Broadway Place
Amityville, NY 11701
(516) 598-2960

(The above are cited in Susan Kissir's "Treat Alcoholism with Nutrition: A Pioneering Program has Early Successes," *Natural Health*, January/February, 1993.)

Medical/Pharmacological Bibliography:

Blum, K. Alcohol and the Addictive Brain: New Hope for Alcoholics from Biogenetic Research, New York: Free Press, 1991.

Bowman, W. C., and Rand, M. J., Textbook of Pharmacology (2nd Edition), London: Blackwell Scientific Publications (1980).

Carlton, Peter L, A Primer of Behavioral Pharmacology, New York: W. H. Freeman & Co., 1983.

Cohen, Sidney, The Chemical Brain, Minneapolis: CompCare, 1987.

Ellison, J. M., The Psychotherapist's Guide to Pharmacotherapy, Chicago: Year Book Medical Publishers, 1989.

Fitzgerald, K. W., Alcoholism: The Genetic Inheritance. NY: Doubleday, 1988.

Gerstein, D. R., and Harwood, H. J., editors, Treating Drug Problems, Volume I, Washington D. C.: National academy Press, 1990.

Gitlen, M. J., The Psychotherapist's Guide to Psychopharmacology, New York: The Free Press, 1990.

Jonas, Jeffrey, M.D., and Schaumburg, Ron, Everything You Need to Know about Prozac, New York: Bantam, 1991.

Julien, Robert, Drugs and the Body in Health & Disease, New York: W. H. Freeman & Co., 1987.

Kramer, Peter D., Listening to Prozac, New York: Viking Press, 1993.

LaDu, B. N., Mandel, H. G., and Way, E. L. (Editors), Fundamentals of Drug Metabolism and Drug Disposition, Baltimore: Williams and Wilkins, 1971.

Lamble, J. W. (Editor), Towards Understanding Receptors, Amsterdam: Elsevier: North Holland Publishing Company, 1981.

Lawson, Gary, Clinical Psychopharmacology for Non-Medical Therapists, Aspen Press, 1987.

Lawson, Gary W. & Cooperrider, Craig C., Clinical Psychopharmacology: A Practical Reference for Nonmedical Psychotherapists, Gaithersburg, Maryland: Aspen Publishers, 1988.

Levine, R. R., Pharmacology: Drug Actions and Reactions (3rd Edition), Boston: Little, Brown and Company, 1983.

McKim, W. A., Drugs and Behavior, Englewood Cliffs, New Jersey: Prentice Hall, 1986.

Palif, Tibor & Jankiewicz, Henry, Drugs & Human Behavior, Madison, Wisconsin: Brown & Benchmark, 1991.

Snyder, S. H.. Drugs & the Brain: A Scientific American Book, New York: W. H. Freeman & Co., 1986.

Spitz, Henry, M.D., and Rosecan, Jeffrey S., M.D., eds., Cocaine Abuse: New Directions in Treatment and Research, New York: Brunner/Mazel, 1987.

Stimmell, Barry, and the editors of Consumer Report Books, The Facts About Drug Use, New York: Haworth Press, 1993.

Appendix III: Acupuncture Resources

NADA Resources:

National Acupuncture Detoxification Association
3115 Broadway #51
New York, NY 10027
(212) 579-5138

NADA California
2417 Castillo Street
Santa Barbara, CA 93105

NADA Literature Clearinghouse *(see catalogue at the end of this section)*
P.O. Box 1927
Vancouver, WA 98662-1927
(206) 254-0186

Partial List of NADA Clinic Commercial Vendors and Suppliers to:

Tea and herbs:

Nutri-Control
Box 1199, Old Chelsea Station
New York, New York 10011
(212) 929-3780

K'an Herb Company
2425 Porter Street, Suite 18
Soquel, CA 94501
(408) 462-9915

Needles and supplies:

OMS Medical Supplies
1950 Washington Street
Braintree, MA 02184
(617) 331-3370

TCM Supply Corporation
15588 East Gale Avenue
Hacienda Heights, CA 91745
(818) 333-5222

Urine Testing:

Syva Company
3403 Yerba Buena Road
San Jose, CA 95161
(800) 322-7982

Insurance Services:

Lincoln Associates
188 Industrial Drive, Suite 226
Elmhurst, IL 60126
(800) 860-8330

Educational Services:

Med-Serve of Illinois
P. O. Box 20232
Chicago, IL 60620
(312) 445-0043
(Med-Serve publishes the newsletter *Acu-News*. Monthly. $6/yr.)

Chinese Medicine and Acupuncture Professional Associations:

American Foundation of Traditional Chinese Medicine
1280 Columbus Avenue, Suite 302
San Francisco, CA 94133
(415) 776-0502

AFTCM publishes the newsletter *Gateways: Exploring New Horizons in East/West Medicine*. Quarterly. $3/copy.

The California Acupuncture Association publishes the *CAA Phoenix: The Journal of the California Acupuncture Association,* and the *CAA Bulletin*, 12335 Santa Monica Blvd., Suite 135, West Los Angeles, CA 90025, (213) 390-7911. Monthly. Free with membership.

Chinese Medical Bibliography:

Beinfield, Harriet and Korngold, Efrem, *Between Heaven and Earth: A Guide to Chinese Medicine*, New York: Ballantine Books, 1991.

Bensoussan, Alan, *The Vital Meridian*, Edinburgh: Churchill Livingstone, 1990.

Eisenberg, David, M.D., *Encounters with Qi: Exploring Chinese Medicine*, New York: W. W. Norton, 1985.

Kaptchuk, T., *The Web that Has No Weaver: Understanding Chinese Medicine*, New York: Congdon and Weed, 1983.

Mann, F., *Acupuncture: The Ancient Chinese Art of Healing and how it Works Scientifically.* New York: Vintage Books, 1973.

Porkert, Manfred, and Ullman, Christian, *Chinese Medicine - Its History, Philosophy and Practice*, translated and adapted by Mark Howson, New York: William Morrow and Co., 1988.

Sivin, Nathan, *Traditional Medicine in Contemporary China (Science, Medicine, and Technology in East Asia, Volume 2)*, Ann Arbor: Center for Chinese Studies, University of Michigan.

NATIONAL ACUPUNCTURE DETOXIFICATION ASSOCIATION, INC.
NADA Literature Clearinghouse -
(Prices in effect December 1, 1993 to March 31, 1994)

NADA Literature Clearinghouse
PO Box 1927
Vancouver WA 98668-1927
Phone/Fax (206) 260-8620

Item	Section 1: CHEMICAL DEPENDENCY TREATMENT	Authors	Date	Desc	Pgs	Min	Price
1000	SELECTED PACKAGE (includes numbers with "x"--save 10% on items if bought separately)	various	na	man	na		36.00
1001x	Acupuncture Treatment for Alcoholism -- An early and comprehensive statement of the NADA principles of treatment	Smith, M.; Pittman, L.; Oliveira, A.	1986	man	7		3.50
1002	Acupuncture Treatment for Alchoholism-- Brief summary	Smith, M.	1986	man	2		1.00
1003	Acupuncture Treatment for Substance Abuse -- Extension of the NADA principles to drugs other than alcohol	Smith, M.	1986	man	2		1.00
1004	Lincoln Acupuncture Clinic Outcomes -- Findings from daily urinalysis program	Smith, M.	1992	man	1		1.00
1005	Portland Addictions Acupuncture Center Court Program Outcomes -- Charts and graphs on drug court clients	Smith, M.	1992	man	8		4.00
1006	Miami Drug Court Outcomes -- Statistical update after two years	Smith, M.	1992	man	3		1.50
1007	Acupuncture and Natural Healing -- Re-print from American Journal of Acupuncture	Smith, M.	1979	man	11		5.50
1008	Acupuncture Programme for the Treatment of Drug Addicted Persons -- Re-print from UN Bulletin on Narcotics	Smith, M.; Khan, I.	1988	re-print	7		3.50
1009x	Controlled Trial of Acupuncture for Severe Recidivist Alcoholism -- Landmark article from The Lancet	Bullock, M; Culliton, P; Olander, R.	1989	re-print	5		2.50
1010x	Acupuncture Treatment of Chemical Dependency and Violence -- Practical clinical observations	Smith, M.	1985	man	7		3.50
1011x	Acupuncture Detoxification and Relapse Service -- On effective bundling of supportive services for long-term recovery	Webb, A; Puccio, P.	1991	man	8		4.00
1012	Lincoln Hospital Acupuncture Drug Abuse Pgm.-- Testimony to US House of Rep.	Smith, M.	1989	man	18		9.00
1013x	Use of Acupuncture in the Criminal Justice System -- Basic statement of the proper role of the treatment provider	Smith, M.	1988	man	7		3.50
1014x	Chinese Theory of Acupuncture Detoxification -- Brief statement of underpinnings of auricular therapy	Smith, M.	1985	man	2		1.00
1015x	Ethics of Acupuncture Detox Specialists -- Defines scope of practice and behavioral standards of ADS-trained staff	Smith, M.	1985	man	2		1.00

Item	Section 1: CHEMICAL DEPENDENCY TREATMENT (cont)	Authors	Date	Desc	Pgs	Min	Price
1016	The Clinical Impact of Tai Chi Treatment for Alcoholism -- The un-exercise approach to improved fitness and recovery	Pittman, L.	1983	man	10		5.00
1017x	Auricular Acupuncture Treatment for Chemical Dependency -- Comprehensive summary and survey of all relevant literature to date	Ackerman, Ruth	1993	man	34		17.00
1018	Acupuncture Detox Specialists: Benefit to the Acupuncture Community -- Case for ADSes as valuable outreach agents for acupuncture	Mercier, D.	1993	man	6		3.00
1019	A Counselor's Guide to Acupuncture in the Treatment of Addiction NEW ITEM	Acupuncture Recovery Assocs.	1993	man	15		7.50
1020	Testimony to Office of Alternative Medicine of NIH re: Efficacy of Acupuncture in Varied Sites -- NEW ITEM	Smith, M.	1993	man	7		3.50
1021x	Acupuncture: New Perspectives in Chemical Dependency Treatment -- Widely quoted from Journal of Substance Abuse Tx. NEW	Brumbaugh, A.	1993	re-print	9		4.50
1022	Mental Health Treatment Outcome Report from Biscailuz Jail, Los Angeles -- Documents dual diagnosis impact -- NEW ITEM	Taub, C.	1993	man	18		9.00
1023	Outcome Report on Hooper Detoxification Center, Portland, OR -- Final Evaluation -- NEW ITEM	Lane, C.	1989	man	24		12.00
1024	Relationship of Acupuncture Treatment to Completion Rate in Hooper Detoxification Center -- NEW ITEM	Lane, C.	1990	man	11		5.50
1025	Acupuncture Detoxification for Homeless Substance Abusers -- NEW ITEM	Pittman, L.	1991	man	28		14.00

Item	Section 2: WOMEN'S ISSUES	Authors	Date	Desc	Pgs	Min	Price
2000	SELECTED PACKAGE (All items this section -- save 10% on price of items bought separately)	various	na	na	na		36.90
2001	Raising Healthy Babies for the 90's -- Lincoln Hospital's response to maternal crack use	Lincoln Hospital staff	1991	man	2		1.00
2002	American Hospital Assoc. Case Study No. 10 -- Lincoln Hospital Perinatal Program	AHA staff	1991	re-print	5		2.50
2003	Relation of Maternal Involvement in Drug Treatment and Prenatal Care to Infant Birth Weight -- Results of Lincoln program	Lincoln Hospital staff	1993	man	1		1.00
2004	Acupuncture as a Treatment for Drug Dependent Mothers -- Testimony to the New York City Council	Smith, M.	1988	man	9		4.50
2005	Violence, Trauma and Posttraumatic Stress Disorder Among Women Drug Users -- Documents high frequency of trauma and PTSD	Fullilove, M. ; et al.	1992	man	15		7.50
2006	Auricular Acupuncture Treatment for Chemical Dependency During Pregnancy -- Reviews all relevant literature to date	Ackerman, R.	1993	man	49		24.50

	Section 3: OTHER DISORDERS	Authors	Date	Desc	Pgs	Min	Price
3001	Chinese Medical Treatment for AIDS-- Results of Five Years' Experience at Lincoln and other US sites including cases	Smith, M.	1987	man	8		4.00
3002	Acupuncture Treatment of AIDS -- Sample of specific clinical techniques including points	Smith, M; Rabinowitz, N.	1986	man	8		4.00
3003	Psychiatric Functions of Acupuncture -- Clinical observations on anxiety, psychotropics, schizophrenia, depression, stress, hysteria	Smith, M.	1983	man	4		2.00
3004	Acupuncture Treatment of Multiple Sclerosis: Two Detailed Clinical Presentations	Smith, M.	1985	man	4		2.00
3005	Acupuncture as Treatment for the Borderline Personality Disorder	Smith, M.	1982		15		7.50
3006	Case History Treatment of AIDS, ARC and HIV with Acucpuncture, Moxibustion and Ch. Herbs -- NEW ITEM	Pittman, L.	1988	man	16		8.00
3007	Acupuncture May Prevent Relapse in Chronic Schizophrenic Patients -- Texas experiences with group home residents -- NEW ITEM	Smith, M.; Atwood, T; Turley, G.	1993	man	5		2.50
3008	Managing Hypertension with Tai Chi Chuan, Meditation and Nutrition -- NEW ITEM	Pittman, L.	1982	man	17		8.50
	Section 4: TEACHING OUTLINES: RELATED GENERAL TOPICS						
4000	SELECTED PACKAGE (All items this section -- save 10% on price of items bought separately)	various	na	na	na		31.05
4001	Introduction to General Care Treatment and Famous Body Points	Pittman, L.	1983	man	6		3.00
4002	Acupuncture Points and Midline Balance	Smith, M.	1983	man	7		3.50
4003	Observations, Palpation, Questioning	Smith, M.	1983	man	9		4.50
4004	General Questioning	Smith, M.	1983	man	6		3.00
4005	Diagnosis of Digestive Problems	Smith, M.	1983	man	3		1.50
4006	Diagnosis of Women's Conditions	Smith, M.	1983	man	6		3.00
4007	Wu Xing (Five Elements)--Outline relating especially to Symbolism and Psychological Pattens	Smith, M.	1983	man	3		1.50
4008	Basic Realities--On Qi and Acu-locations	Smith, M.	1983	man	3		1.50
4009	Diagnosis by Internal Organs--With treatment points listed	Smith, M.	1983	man	6		3.00
4010	Patterns of Life--On Yin and Yang	Smith, M.	1983	man	3		1.50
4011	Basic Patterns of Psychological Imbalance	Smith, M.	1983	man	2		1.00
4012	Effects of Acupuncture on the Immune System	Smith, M.	1983	man	3		1.50
4013	The Healing Crisis	Smith, M.	1983	man	1		1.00
4014	Does Chinese Energy Flow Theory Conflict with Western Medical Theory?	Smith, M.	1983	man	1		1.00
4015	Abuse Patterns--According to Chinese Diagnosis	Smith, M.	1983	man	2		1.00
	Section 5: MISCELLANEOUS RELATED ISSUES						
5001	Legal Heroin: A Problem Disguised as a Solution	Smith, M.	1977	man	12		6.00
5002	I Ching and Time	Smith, M.	1985	chart	1		1.00
5003	Cell Salts	Smith, M.	1983	man	2		1.00
5004	Herbal Formulary	Lincoln Hospital Staff	1981	man	6		3.00
5005	Acupuncture Treatment for Cigarette Smoking	Smith, M.		man	4		2.00

	Section 5: MISCELLANEOUS RELATED ISSUES (cont)	Authors	Date	Desc	Pgs	Min	Price
5006	What is Acupuncture? -- Lincoln Hospital Patient Education Handout	Lincoln Hospital Staff	1989	man	3		1.50
5007	Acupuncture Helps Programs More Than Patients -- Comments on the pathology of the system -- NEW ITEM	Smith, M.	1993	man	9		4.50
5008	Informed Consent for Acupuncture-- (English and Spanish) -- NEW ITEM	Kavanagh, E.	1993	man	4		2.00
5009	Methadone Maintenance Report by United States General Accounting Office -- Documents chronic failures of methadone -- NEW	GAO	1990	re-print	37		18.50

	Section 6: VIDEOTAPES		Date	Desc	Time	Min	Price
6001	Miami Court Diversion and Treatment Program -- Good tool for community education on drug courts		1991	video	15	15	30.00
6002	Overview of Basic Lincoln Hospital Treatment Program -- Daily realities of Lincoln come through despite weak production values		1987	video	11	11	25.00
6003	Jersey City Program		1991	video	7.5	7.5	15.00
6004	Qi Gong for AIDS--Dr. Jia Jinding		1988	video	27	27	45.00
6005	Maternal Program at Lincoln Hospital--S. Lundine TV tape		1990	video	18	18	35.00
6006	Acupuncture for Chemical Dependency in Pre and Post Natal Periods-- Detailed review of sites in California, Minnesota and New York		1992	video	41	41	45.00
6007	Project Recovery -- Depicts pioneer public health program in Santa Barbara		1989	video	23	23	45.00
6008	Acupuncture and Computers in Treating Chemical Dependency--M. Smith lecture at U. of MD. -- NEW ITEM		1986	video	60	90	45.00
6009	Acupuncture and Oriental Medicine I -- First in a series of three lectures by L. Pittman -- NEW ITEM			video		90	45.00

	Section 93: AUDIOTAPES FROM NADA CONFERENCE 1993 -- ALL NEW	Speakers	Date	Desc	#	Min	Price
9301	Welcoming Messages; Nurturing Public Health Thru Acupuncture; The Spirit of NADA	Andrew, Pung, Oliveira, Eisen	1993	audio	1		7.00
9302	Keynote Addresses: Beyond Substance Abuse--The Challenge of the 90's; Turning Point Programs	Robert Olander; Margie Clay	1993	audie	1		7.00
9303	Getting Started--The yin and the yang of getting a program going	Culliton, Eisen, Haber, Rossanno	1993	audio	2		11.00
9304	Dual Diagnosis Programs--Special Needs and Opportunities	Tom Atwood; John Blank; Carol Taub	1993	audio	1		7.00
9305	Residential Programs--How to Set up a Program	Kelly Simms; Mark Sutherland	1993	audio	1		7.00
9306	Methadone Clients--Integrating Acupuncture Into Their Care	W. Jumbe Allen; Rachel Diaz	1993	audio	1		7.00
9307	Integrating Services--On demand oriental medical care for criminal justice, homeless and HIV+ populations	Osborne Association Staff	1993	audio	1		7.00
9308	HIV, Tuberculosis and Hepatitis	Cohen, Beyendorff, Daly, Eisen, Goh	1993	audio	1		7.00

	Section 93: AUDIOTAPES FROM NADA CONFERENCE 1993 -- ALL NEW	Speakers	Date	Desc	Time	Min	Price
9309	Men's Programs	Jesse Morgan	1993	audio	1		7.00
9310	International Programs--France, Germany, Hungary, Sweden	McKenna, Wahlstrom, Zmiewski	1993	audio	2		11.00
9311	Maintaining Your Program--Clinical, behavior management, staff burnout, cultural issues, treatment design	Patty Klucas; Charlie Singer	1993	audio	1		7.00
9312	Serving Communities of Color	Feliciano, Allen, Kolenda, Weston	1993	audio	1		7.00
9313	Clinical Issues--Discussion for acupuncturists of clinical problems and successes in a group treatment setting	Moderator: Cally Haber	1993	audio	2		11.00
9314	Pregnant Women--Easing access to perinatal care; midwives; peer counselors and recovered staff	Rizak, Slater, Yearde	1993	audio	1		7.00
9316	Infants and Children--Assessing, early intervention, stimulation, daycare, massage, acupressure, heat tx.	Feliciano, Maye, Smalls	1993	audio	1		7.00
9318	Criminal Justice and Prison Programs-- Sex offender outcomes, parole and probation perspective, drug courts	J. Forman; L. Leef; T. Murray; L. Simmons	1993	audio	2		11.00
9319	Feeling the Qi-- Practical techniques for demonstrating and experiencing qi	Stephen Birch	1993	audio	1		7.00
9320	Family Systems-- Designing programs for family involvement in residential and non-residential settings	Ruth Ackerman	1993	audio	1		7.00
9321	The Pathology of the System--How acupuncture helps programs more than patients	Michael Smith	1993	audio	1		7.00
9322	Trauma/Incest Survivors--Unique issues of assessment, motivation and treatment	Mindy Fullilove	1993	audio	1		7.00
9323	Acupuncture Research-- Clinical, methodological and political issues	Birch, Culliton, Clemence, Diaz, Kiresuk	1993	audio	1		7.00

Sec 1: CD TREATMENT			
Item	Price	Qty	Cost
1000	$36.00		
1001	$3.50		
1002	$1.00		
1003	$1.00		
1004	$1.00		
1005	$4.00		
1006	$1.50		
1007	$5.50		
1008	$3.50		
1009	$2.50		
1010	$3.50		
1011	$4.00		
1012	$9.00		
1013	$3.50		
1014	$1.00		
1015	$1.00		
1016	$5.00		
1017	$17.00		
1018	$3.00		
1019	$7.50		
1020	$3.50		
1021	$4.50		
1022	$9.00		
1023	$12.00		
1024	$5.50		
1025	$14.00		
Sec 1 subtotal			
Sec 2: WOMEN'S ISSUES			
2000	$36.90		
2001	$1.00		
2002	$2.50		
2003	$1.00		
2004	$4.50		
2005	$7.50		
2006	$24.50		
Sec 2 subtotal			

Sec 3: OTHER DISORDERS			
Item	Price	Qty	Cost
3001	$4.00		
3002	$4.00		
3003	$2.00		
3004	$2.00		
3005	$7.50		
3006	$8.00		
3007	$2.50		
3008	$8.50		
Sec 3 subtotal			
Sec 4: TEACHING OUTLINES			
4000	$31.05		
4001	$3.00		
4002	$3.50		
4003	$4.50		
4004	$3.00		
4005	$1.50		
4006	$3.00		
4007	$1.50		
4008	$1.50		
4009	$3.00		
4010	$1.50		
4011	$1.00		
4012	$1.50		
4013	$1.00		
4014	$1.00		
4015	$1.00		
Sec 4 subtotal			
Sec 5: MISCELLANEOUS			
5001	$6.00		
5002	$1.00		
5003	$1.00		
5004	$3.00		
5005	$2.00		
5006	$1.50		
5007	$4.50		
5008	$2.00		
5009	$18.50		
Sec 5 subtotal			

Sec 6: VIDEOTAPES			
Item	Price	Qty	Cost
6001	$30.00		
6002	$25.00		
6003	$15.00		
6004	$45.00		
6005	$35.00		
6006	$45.00		
6007	$45.00		
6008	$45.00		
6009	$45.00		
Sec 6 subtotal			
Sec 93: AUDIOTAPES '93			
9301	$7.00		
9302	$7.00		
9303	$11.00		
9304	$7.00		
9305	$7.00		
9306	$7.00		
9307	$7.00		
9308	$7.00		
9309	$7.00		
9310	$11.00		
9311	$7.00		
9312	$7.00		
9313	$11.00		
9314	$7.00		
9316	$7.00		
9318	$11.00		
9319	$7.00		
9320	$7.00		
9321	$7.00		
9322	$7.00		
9323	$7.00		
Sec 93 subtotal			

Enter items cost (total of all sections above)

Enter Postage/Handling Fee (12% of items cost, 15% foreign -- $5.00 minimum)

Enter Billing Fee If Applicable ($8.00). MY PURCHASE ORDER NO. IS: _____

TOTAL DUE THIS ORDER

MAIL THIS ENTIRE PAGE WITH PAYMENT TO:
NADA Literature Clearinghouse, PO Box 1927, Vancouver WA 98668-1927

A comprehensive guide to all private and public funding trends and sources is the *Community Health Funding Report*, published by CD Publications, 8204 Fenton Street, Silver Springs, MD 20910, 800/666-6380. Bi-monthly. $229/yr; $15/issue.

Section A: Private Resources

Alcohol and Other Drug Information
Hazelden Foundation
Center City, MN 55012
800/257-7800

Hazelden publishes the *Hazelden News and Professional Update*, available from the Hazelden Foundation, 1400 Park Avenue, Minneapolis, MN 55405-1597. Triennial.

American Society for Addiction Medicine
5525 Wisconsin Avenue, N.W.
Washington, D.C. 20016
(202) 244-8948

National Association for Perinatal Addiction Research and Education
11 E. Hubbard Street, Suite 200
Chicago, IL 60611
312 / 329-2512

National Council on Alcoholism and Drug Dependence, Inc. (NCADD)
12 West 21st Street
New York, NY 10010
(800) 475-HOPE
(212) 206-6770

NCADD publishes the "Medical Scientific Advisory" and a host of other materials available through their 200 state and local affiliates.

Private Funding Sources - Publications:

Annual Register of Grant Support (Wilmette, Illinois: National Register Publishing Company, published annually).

Corporate 500: The Directory of Corporate Philanthropy (San Francisco: Public Management Institute).

Coggins, Christiana, *A User's Guide to Proposal Writing, or How to get Your Project Funded* (New York: International Planned Parenthood Federation, 1990).

Corporate Foundation Profiles (New York: The Foundation Center).

The Foundation Center Directory (New York: The Foundation Center, published annually).

Foundation Grants to Individuals, 7th edition (New York: The Foundation Center).

Hall, Mary, *Getting Funded: A Complete Guide to Proposal Writing,* 3rd edition (Portland, Oregon: Continuing Education Publications, 1988).

Margolin, Judith B., ed., *Foundation Fundamentals: A Guide for Grantseekers*, 4th edition (The Foundation Center, 1991).

National Data Book of Foundations: A Comprehensive Guide to Grantmaking Foundations (New York: The Foundation Center, published annually).

Computer Resources:

There is a NADA bulletin board conference network just starting on the "Whole Earth 'Lectronic Link" (WELL). The WELL may be accessed through Internet.

Email:
alexb@well.sf.ca.us
for more information.

WELL Voice Phone Number: 415-332-4335
WELL (300/1200/2400 baud):   415-332-6106
WELL (9600 baud):   415-332-8410
WELL Status Hotline: 800-326-8354
WELL FAX Phone Number: 415-332-4927
WELL Postal Address:
The WELL
27 Gate Five Road
Sausalito, CA 94965

Section B: Government Resources

Federal Resources:

National Clearinghouse for Alcohol and Drug Information (NCADI)
Publications Catalogue
P.O. Box 2345
Rockville, MD 20852
301 / 468-2600
800 / 729-6686

NCADI is the source for many free materials, including the monthly periodical *Alcohol Alert,* published by the National Institute on Alcohol Abuse and Alcoholism. NCADI is also the access point for all literature disseminated by the National Institute on Drug Abuse (NIDA).

State Resources:

Federal funds for drug and alcohol treatment are typically awarded to the states, and states themselves generate additional revenue for treatment services. Small states may administer these funds themselves, but more often they are administered locally. Following is a list of state departments who are responsible for the allocation of these resources. These offices will be able to describe the mechanisms by which funds are allocated and administered in your locale. This list was published by the National Association of State Alcohol and Drug Abuse Directors (NASADAD), 444 North Capitol Street NW., Suite 642, Washington, DC. 20001, (202) 783-6868.

NASADAD MEMBERSHIP LIST

ALABAMA
Division of Substance Abuse Services
Department of Mental Health & Mental Retardation
200 Interstate Park Drive
P.O. Box 3710
Montgomery, AL 36193
(205) 270-4650
FAX: (205) 240-3195

ALASKA
Div. of Alcoholism and Drug Abuse
AK Department of Health & Social Services
P.O. Box 110607
Juneau, AK 99811-0607
(907) 465-2071
FAX: (907) 465-2185

ARIZONA
Alcoholism and Drug Abuse
AZ Department of Health Services
Office of Community Behavioral Health
2632 East Thomas
Phoenix, AZ 85016
(602) 255-1025 or 1030
FAX: (602) 255-1042

ARKANSAS
AR Office of Alcohol and Drug Abuse Prevention
Donaghey Plaza North, Suite 400
P.O. Box 1437
Little Rock, AR 72203-1437
(501) 682-6650
FAX: (501) 682-6610

CALIFORNIA
Governor's Policy Council on Drug & Alcohol Abuse
1700 K. Street, 5th Floor
Executive Office
Sacramento, CA 95814-4037
(916) 445-1943   FAX: (916) 323-5873

COLORADO
Alcohol and Drug Abuse Division
CO Department of Health
4300 Cherry Creek Drive, South
Denver, CO 80222-1530
(303) 692-2930   FAX: (303) 782-4883

CONNECTICUT
CT Alcohol and Drug Abuse Commission
999 Asylum Avenue, 3rd Floor
Hartford, CT 06105
(203) 566-4145   FAX: (203) 566-6055

DELAWARE
DE Division of Alcoholism, Drug Abuse & Mental Health
1901 N. DuPont Highway
Newcastle, DE 19720
(302) 577-4461
FAX: (302) 577-4405

DISTRICT OF COLUMBIA
DC Health Planning and Development
1660 L. Street, NW.
Washington, DC 20036
(202) 673-7481
FAX: (202) 673-4318

FLORIDA
Alcohol and Drug Abuse
FL Department of Health & Rehabilitation. Services
1317 Winewood Blvd., Bldg. 6, Room 182
Tallahassee, FL 32301
(904) 488-0900
FAX: (904) 487-2239

GEORGIA
GA Alcohol and Drug Services Section
878 Peachtree Street, NE
Suite 318
Atlanta, GA 30309
(404) 894-4200
FAX: (404) 853-0778

HAWAII
Alcohol & Drug Abuse Division
HI Department of Health
P.O. Box 3378
Honolulu, HI 96801
(808) 586-3962
FAX: (808) 586-4016

IDAHO
Division of Family and Children Services
ID Dept. of Health & Welfare
450 West State Street, 3rd Floor
Boise, ID 83702
(208) 334-5935
FAX: (208) 334-5694

ILLINOIS
IL Dept. of Alcoholism and Substance Abuse
222 South College, 2nd Floor
Springfield, IL 62704
(217) 785-9067
FAX: (217) 785-0954

INDIANA
Division of Mental Health
Bureau of Addiction Services
W-353, 402 W. Washington Street
Indianapolis, IN 46204-2739
(317) 232-7816
FAX: (317) 233-3472

IOWA
Division of Substance Abuse
IA Department of Public Health
Lucas State Office Building
3rd Floor
Des Moines, IA 50319
(515) 281-3641   FAX: (515) 281-4952

KANSAS
KS Alcohol and Drug Abuse Services.
300 SW Oakley, Biddle Building
Topeka, KS 66606-1861
(913) 296-3925   FAX: (913) 296-0511

KENTUCKY
Division of Substance Abuse
KY Department of Mental Health & Mental Retardation Services
275 East Main Street
Frankfort, KY 40621
(502) 564-2880   FAX: (502) 564-3844

LOUISIANA
Division of Alcohol and Drug Abuse
Department of Health and Hospitals
1201 Capitol Access Road
P.O. Box 2790
Baton Rouge, LA 70821-3868
(504) 342-9354   FAX: (504) 342-4419

MAINE
Office of Substance Abuse
State House Station #159
24 Stone Street
Augusta, ME 04333-0159
(207) 287-2595
FAX: (207) 626-5555

MARYLAND
MD State Alcohol & Drug Abuse Administration
201 West Preston Street
Baltimore, MD 21201
(301) 225-6925
FAX: (301) 333-7206

MASSACHUSETTS
MA Division of Substance Abuse Services
150 Tremont Street
Boston, MA 02111
(617) 727-7985
FAX: (617) 727-9288

MICHIGAN
Center for Substance Abuse Services.
MI Department of Public Health
3423 N. Logan/M.L. King Blvd.
P.O. Box 30195
Lansing, MI 48909
(517) 335-8808
FAX: (517) 335-8837

MINNESOTA
Chemical Dependency Program Division
MN Department of Human Services
444 Lafayette Road
St. Paul, MN 55155-3823
(612) 296-4610
FAX: (612) 296-6244

MISSISSIPPI
Division of Alcohol and Drug Abuse
MS Department of Mental Health
Robert E. Lee State Office Bldg., 11th Floor
Jackson, MS 39201
(601) 359-1288   FAX: (601) 359-6295

MISSOURI
Division of Alcohol & Drug Abuse
MO Department of Health
1706 E. Elm Street
Jefferson City, MO 65109
(314) 751-4942
FAX: (314) 751-7814

MONTANA
Alcohol and Drug Abuse Division
Department of Corrections and Human Services
1539 11th Avenue
Helena, MT 59601-1301
(406) 444-2827
FAX: (406) 444-4920

NEBRASKA
Division of Alcoholism & Drug Abuse
NE Department of Public Institutions
P.O. Box 94728
Lincoln, NE 68509-4728
(402) 471-2851, Ext. 5583
FAX: (402) 479-5145

NEVADA
Bureau of Alcohol and Drug Abuse
NV Department of Human Resources
505 East King Street
Carson City, NV 89710
(702) 687-4790
FAX: (702) 687-4733

NEW HAMPSHIRE
NH Office of Alcohol & Drug Abuse Prevention
105 Pleasant Street
Concord, NH 03301
(603) 271-6104
FAX: (603) 271-6116

NEW JERSEY
Division of Alcoholism, Drug Abuse and Addiction Services
NJ Department of Health, CN 362
Trenton, NJ 08625-0362
(609) 292-5760   FAX: (609) 292-3816

NEW MEXICO
Department of Health
Behavioral Health Service Division/SA
Harold Runnels Bldg., Room 3200 N.
1190 St. Francis Drive
Santa Fe, NM 87501
(505) 827-2601
FAX: (505) 827-0097

NEW YORK
NY State Office of Alcoholism and Substance Abuse
P.O. Box 8200, Executive Park
Albany, NY 12203-8200
(518) 474-5417 or (518) 457-2061
FAX: (518) 473-7652

NY Division of Substance Abuse Services
Bureau of Government Relations
Executive Park South, Box 8200
Albany, NY 12203
(518) 457-7629
FAX: (518) 485-7198

NORTH CAROLINA
Alcohol and Drug Abuse Section
NC Division of Mental Health and Mental Retardation Services
325 North Salisbury Street
Raleigh, NC 27611
(919) 733-4670
FAX: (919) 733-9455

NORTH DAKOTA
Division of Alcoholism & Drug Abuse
ND Department of Human Services
Professional Building
1839 East Capitol Ave.
Bismarck, ND 58501
(701) 224-2769   FAX: (701) 224-3008

OKLAHOMA
Substance Abuse Services
OK Department of Mental Health and Substance Abuse Services
P.O. Box 53277, Capitol Station
Oklahoma City, OK 73152
(405) 271-8653   FAX: (405) 271-7413

OHIO
OH Department of Alcohol & Drug Addiction Services
Two Nationwide Plaza, 12th Floor
Columbus, OH 43216
(614) 466-3445
FAX: (614) 752-8645

OREGON (Not a NASADAD member)
OR State Alcohol and Drug Office
1178 Chemeketa N.E.
Salem, OR 97310
(503) 378-2163

PENNSYLVANIA
Office of Drug & Alcohol Programs
PA Department of Health
P.O. Box 90
Harrisburg, PA 17108
(717) 787-9857
FAX: (717) 772-6959

RHODE ISLAND
RI Office of Substance Abuse
P.O. Box 20363
Cranston, RI 02920
(401) 464-2091
FAX: (401) 464-2089

SOUTH CAROLINA
SC Commission on Alcohol and Drug Abuse
3700 Forest Drive
Columbia, SC 29204
(803) 734-9527
FAX: (803) 734-9663

SOUTH DAKOTA
Division of Alcohol and Drug Abuse
Department of Human Services
Hillsview Plaza, East Hwy. 34
% 500 E. Capitol
Pierre, SD 57501-5090
(605) 773-3123
FAX: (605) 773-5483

TENNESSEE
Bureau of Alcohol & Drug Abuse Services
TN Department of Health
Cordell Hull Building, Room 255
Nashville, TN 37247-4401
(615) 741-1921   FAX: (615) 741-2491

TEXAS
TX Commission on Alcohol and Drug Abuse
720 Brazos Street, Suite 403
Austin, TX 78701
(512) 867-8802   FAX: (512) 867-8181

UTAH
Department of Social Services
UT Division of Substance Abuse
120 North 200 West, 4th Floor, P.O. Box 45500
Salt Lake City, UT 85145-0500
(801) 538-3939   FAX: (801) 538-4016

VERMONT
VT Office of Alcohol and Drug Abuse Programs
103 South Main Street
Waterbury, VT 05676
(802) 241-2170, 241-2175   FAX: (802) 244-8103

VIRGINIA
Office of Sub. Abuse Services
VA Dept. of Mental Health, Mental Retardation & Substance Services
109 Governor Street, P.O. Box 1797
Richmond, VA 23214
(804) 786-3906   FAX: (804) 371-0091

WASHINGTON
Division of Alcohol and Substance Abuse
WA Department of Social and Health Services
P.O. Box 45330
Olympia, WA 98504-5330
(206) 438-8200   FAX: (206) 438-8078

WEST VIRGINIA
WV Division of Alcohol & Drug Abuse
State Capitol Complex
1900 Kanawha Boulevard Building 3, Room 451
Charleston, WV 25305
(304) 558-2276   FAX: (304) 558-0045

WISCONSIN
WI Office of Alcohol & Other Drug Abuse
1 West Wilson St., P.O. Box 7851
Madison, WI 53707
(608) 266-3719   FAX: (608) 266-0036

WYOMING
WY Alcohol and Drug Abuse Programs
Hathaway Building
Cheyenne, WY 82002
(307) 777-6494

AMERICAN SAMOA
Public Health Services
LBJ Tropical Medical
Pago Pago, AS 96799

AMERICAN SAMOA
Social Services Division
Alcohol and Drug Program
Government of American Samoa
Pago Pago, 96799

GUAM
Department of Mental Health and Substance Abuse
P.O. Box 9400
Tamuning, GU 96911
(671) 646-9262-69   FAX: (671) 649-6948

PUERTO RICO
PR Dept. of Anti-Addiction Services
Box 21414, Rio Piedras Station
Rio Piedras, PR 00928-1414
(809) 764-3795   FAX: (809) 765-5895

VIRGIN ISLANDS
VI Division of Mental Health
Alcoholism and Drug Dependency Services Department of Health
Charles Harwood Memorial Hospital
Christianstead, St. Croix, VI 00820
(809) 773-1992   FAX: (809) 774-4701

Appendix V: Criminal Justice Resources

Public:

> United States Department of Justice
> Office of Justice Programs
> Washington, DC 20531

See the U.S. Department of Justice Office of Justice Programs Bureau of Justice Statistics (1992). *A National Report: Drugs, Crime, and the Justice System*, December, 1992, NCJ-133652, U.S. Government Printing Office, Washington DC.

> National Institute of Justice (NCJRS)
> National Criminal Justice Reference Center
> Box 6000
> Rockville, MD 20850
> (800) 851-3420

The National Institute of Justice (NIJ) is the research and development agency of the United States Department of Justice. Their goals include research and evaluation of programs in the criminal justice system. The NIJ publishes, among many other documents, *Research in Brief.* Monthly. Free.

> National Institute of Justice
> Data Resources Program
> 633 Indiana Avenue NW., Room 847
> Washington, DC 20531
> (202) 307-2961

> Drugs and Crime Data Center and Clearinghouse
> Box 6000
> Rockville, MD 20850
> (800) 666-3332

Private:

> The National Association of Criminal Justice Planners
> 1331 H Street N.W., Suite 401
> Washington, D.C. 20005

The National Association of Criminal Justice Planners is a private association that has been a very supportive lobbying force for acupuncture at the federal level.

See also the *Drug Policy Newsletter*, Drug Policy Foundation, 4801 Massachusetts Avenue, N.W., Suite 400, Washington, D.C. 20016-2087, (202) 895-1634. Bi-monthly. $25/yr.

Six Month Jail Demonstration Program
(Santa Barbara, California)
Preliminary Analysis   *August 12, 1991*

by Alex Brumbaugh and Susan Wheeler

Background:

On April 1, 1991, Project Recovery began offering daily (six days per week) acupuncture treatments at both the men's and women's Honor Farms, which are minimum security annexes of the Santa Barbara County Jail.

Funding for this project was private. Subjective responses to the program from jail personnel have been very positive, with reports of fewer discipline problems and improved attitude on the part of inmates receiving treatment. Inmates report consistent relief from post-acute drug/alcohol withdrawal, including improvements in sleep and energy levels and reduced fear and anxiety. They report feeling a deeper resolve to continue sobriety upon release.

The intent of the program was to demonstrate a reduction in recidivism among inmates who volunteered for the daily acupuncture treatment for the thirty days prior to their release (an optimum total of 24 treatments).

Although treatment was voluntary, inmates often pursue treatment while incarcerated in order to achieve favorable parole hearings and, hence, an earlier release. This agency has been in dialogue with the judges, with the public defender, and with the district attorney as well as the jail administration concerning the possibility of making acupuncture treatment while in jail a condition of either sentencing or probation. This has not been possible during this project since not all inmates are eligible for Honor Farm placement and our treatment was available only at the Honor Farm sites.

This preliminary study is of the re-arrest rates of those inmates who volunteered for acupuncture treatment during their incarceration and who were subsequently released. A greater lapse of time and more statistical analysis is required for a more precise evaluation of this program.

Re-arrest in general among the Santa Barbara County Jail population is pervasive. The most recent inmate study showed that 91% of those incarcerated have been incarcerated before. It is also estimated that 85% of the inmates have a history of substance abuse which was a precipitating (if not sole) factor in the criminal behavior that resulted in incarceration.

Statistical Outcomes:

Between April 1 and July 29, 1991, one hundred and six male and female inmates volunteered for acupuncture. Of these one hundred and six inmates, this study concerns the seventy-six who had been released as of July 29. These seventy-six had received a total of 1,256 acupuncture treatments - ranging from one treatment to sixty-nine - for an average of 16.5.

According to the county jail administrative department, of these seventy-six inmates who received treatment and were subsequently released, fourteen (18%) were re-arrested.

As we examined the treatment records of these fourteen re-arrests, we discovered that twelve of them (86%) had not completed the recommended daily treatment for the thirty days prior to their release.

The following chart shows the treatment distribution among inmates and the corresponding re-arrest rates:

An attempt was made to find a correlation between release date and re-arrest - in other words, were those inmates released earlier in the program more apt to be re-arrested?

In the highest "success category" of inmates receiving eight or more treatments and having the lowest re-arrest rate, we found no correlation. 47% of inmates in this group were released before June 1. Another 29% were released before July 1, and the remaining 23% were released before July 29.

Treatments	Inmates	Re-arrested
1	7	2
2	9	2
3	4	2
4	9	3
5	3	-
6	2	-
7	3	1
8	1	-
9	4	-
11 - 17	8	-
19 - 24	7	2
25 - 30	8	-
31 - 36	5	2
37+	8	-
Total	**78**	**14**

No data are available from the jail on "average turnaround time" - on the time typically elapsing between release and re-arrest. Individual cases indicate that this time is often short: our most prominent treatment "failure" - an individual who received 34 treatments - was homeless upon release and continued outpatient treatment for two weeks. Then he moved to the Faulding Hotel, resumed daily heroin use, and was re-arrested within one week.

One inmate received 24 treatments in custody, and was re-arrested for jumping bail three days following release.

Conclusions and Recommendations:

Receiving a significant number of acupuncture treatments during the thirty days prior to release appears to have a positive influence on re-arrest rates.

Further study is required as to whether those inmates receiving treatment will continue to have lower rates of re-arrest than non-treated inmates over a longer period of time. Subsequent research will be conducted to make this determination.

This preliminary data, however, indicates that continuation and expansion of this program is clearly indicated. The cost of the program is $36,000 per year per site. Providing this service at both Honor Farms and at the main jail would therefore cost $108,000. The number of inmates who would be treated for this amount is estimated at 600.

The average cost of incarceration is $14,000 per inmate per year. If only eight of the 600 inmates treated achieved recovery as a result of the program and hence avoided re-arrest, the total cost of the program would be justified from a cost point of view.

Funding:

The annual $14,000 per inmate cost of incarceration is a theoretical figure in that costs of operations of the county jail are fixed costs and remain relatively constant whether or not the jail is substantially overcrowded. Like all county services, the jail is currently under severe budget constraints.

However, substantial inmate reduction using this treatment modality is likely over time. This reduction in recidivism will ultimately impact not only the cost of incarceration but also the entire spectrum of criminal justice service delivery from arrest, adjudication, public defense and prosecution, to probation services, all of which are dramatically overburdened at this time.

Funding from the private sector is required to extend this service for an additional year to more clearly demonstrate the ultimate impact on our community. More definitive outcome statistics can then be used to influence the state to adopt this treatment protocol in order to effect substantial savings throughout the criminal justice system, not only in Santa Barbara but throughout California, and hopefully in the State Prison system as well, where the average cost of incarceration is $22,000 per year per inmate.

Project Recovery Women's Honor Farm Jail Research Project
Status Report   October 28, 1992
Prepared by Alex Brumbaugh

A research project was initiated in October, 1992, to study re-incarceration rates of female inmates of the county jail's Honor Farm, comparing, with a non-acupuncture control group, re-incarceration rates of those women who received acupuncture treatment over a 13 month period.

Project Recovery administrative staff, in cooperation with the county jail's administrative staff, selected, at random, 29 women who were incarcerated at La Mirada during early 1989, before the acupuncture program was initiated. The jail administrative staff then determined, from their computer data base, re-incarceration data for these 29 women.

There were no identifiable variables at this facility between 1989 and 1992. The facility is a minimum security annex of the county jail, providing no on-site drug treatment except weekly Twelve Step meetings. A number of inmates are on a work furlough program, and virtually all inmates have a history of substance abuse regardless of the reason for their incarceration. Nor was there any significant change in sentencing philosophy on the part of the court, nor changes in arrest priorities on the part of the city or county law enforcement agencies, between the period during which the control group and the treatment group were subject to re-incarceration.

CONTROL GROUP		
Days After Release	**Re-Arrest**	**%**
30	3	10
90	10	30
120	15	52
TOTAL	**21**	**72**

Project Recovery then provided Jail administration with the names of 29 women who had volunteered for at least ten acupuncture treatments while at La Mirada during 1991 and 1992. We selected only those women who had been subsequently released prior to June 1, 1992 - 120 days prior to the date of the study. Jail administration did a search of their computer data base to determine re-incarceration data for these 29 women, finding that:

	ACUPUNCTURE		CONTROL	
Days after release	**Re-Arrest**	**%**	**Re-Arrest**	**%**
30	2	7	3	10
90	7	25	10	30
120	7	25	15	52
TOTAL	**16**	**55**	**21**	**72**

The treatment protocol used was a basic five-point auricular protocol developed by the National Acupuncture Detoxification Association. Since clients were not generally detoxifying, expanded treatment protocols were used from time to time in response to inmate complaints of insomnia, anxiety, irritability, depression, menstrual difficulties, viral infections, or digestive problems.

Women in the acupuncture group all received ten or more treatments, with an average of 32 treatments each. Sixteen received fewer than 32 treatments, and 13 received more than 32 treatments. Of the group who had fewer than 32 treatments, ten (63%) were re-incarcerated following release; of the group receiving more than 32 treatments, six (46%) were re-incarcerated.

Treatments	**Re-Arrest**	**%**
less than 32	10	63
greater than 32	6	46

Summary of Findings:

1. Women receiving acupuncture had a 17% lower re-incarceration rate overall than the controls.

2. Women in the control group were twice as likely to be re-incarcerated during the first 120 days following release than women in the acupuncture group.

3. There seemed to be a relationship between re-incarceration rates and the number of acupuncture treatments received. Women receiving 32 or more treatments while in custody had an overall re-incarceration rate 26% lower than the controls, and a rate 17% lower than those receiving fewer than 32 treatments.

Appendix VI: Recovery Resources

These groups may be contacted at the addresses or telephone numbers listed in order to find a meeting close to you. If there is not a meeting close to you, these organizations will help you begin one.

Adult Children of Alcoholics (ACA)
(Twelve-Step program for adults who had an alcoholic parent.)
P.O. Box 3216
2522 W. Sepulveda Boulevard, Suite 200
Torrance, CA 90505
(213) 534-1815

Al-Anon Family Group Headquarters, Inc.
(Twelve-Step program for people for whom a friend or relative has an alcohol problem.)
P.O. Box 862
Midtown Station
New York, NY 10018-0862

Alateen
(Al-Anon for teens.)
Al-Anon Family Group Headquarters, Inc.
P.O. Box 862
Midtown Station
New York, NY 10018-0862

Alcoholics Anonymous (A.A.)
(Twelve-Step program for people who have a problem with alcohol.)
P.O. Box 454
Grand Central Station
New York, NY 10017
(718) 686-1100

Co-Anon
(Twelve-Step program for families and friends of cocaine addicts.)
P.O. Box 64742-66
Los Angeles, CA 90064
(213) 859-2206

Cocaine Anonymous (CA)

(Twelve-Step program for cocaine addicts.)
World Service Office
3740 Overland Avenue, Suite G
Los Angeles, CA 90034
(213) 559-5833

Co-Dependents Anonymous (CoDA)

(Twelve-Step program to help people maintain functional relationships.)
P.O. Box 33577
Phoenix, AZ 85067-3577

Codependents of Sex Addicts (Co-SA)

Minnesota Co-SA
P.O. Box 14537
Minneapolis, MN 55414

Debtors Anonymous

General Service Board
P.O. Box 20322
New York, NY 10025-9992

Drugs Anonymous

P.O. Box 473
Ansonia Station
New York, NY 10023

Emotions Anonymous (EA)

(Twelve-Step program to help people recover from a variety of emotional difficulties and/or mental illnesses.)
International Services
P.O. Box 4245
St. Paul, MN 55104
(612) 647-9712

Families Anonymous, Inc. (FA)

(FA operates different group formats, including Twelve-step groups, for people who have a concern about substance use or behavioral problems of a relative or friend. FA is especially concerned with substance abuse in children.)
P.O. Box 528
Van Nuys, CA 91408
(818) 989-7841

Fundamentalists Anonymous (FA)
(Support system for people who are recovering from an experience with a fundamentalist religious group.)
P.O. Box 20342
Greeley Square Station
New York, NY 10001
(212) 696-0420

Gam-Anon International Service Office, Inc.
(Twelve-Step program for families of compulsive gamblers.)
P.O. Box 157
Whitestone, NY 11357
(718) 352-1671

Gamblers Anonymous
P.O. Box 17173
Los Angeles, CA 90017
(213) 386-8789

Incest Survivors Anonymous (I.S.A.)
(Support for people recovering from all manner of childhood sexual abuse. Perpetrators, victimizers, and initiators are excluded.)
P.O. Box 5613
Long Beach, CA 90805-0613

Marijuana Anonymous
1527 North Washington Avenue
Scranton, PA 18509

Nar-Anon
(Twelve-Step program for people who have a relative or friend dealing with narcotic addiction.)
P.O. Box 2562
Palos Verdes, CA 90274
(213) 547-5800

Narcotics Anonymous
P.O. Box 9999
Van Nuys, CA 91409
(818) 780-3951

National Association of Children of Alcoholics
31582 Coast Highway, Suite B
South Laguna, CA 92677
714 / 499-3889

O-Anon

(Twelve-Step program for the families and friends of compulsive eaters.)
General Service Office
P.O. Box 4350
San Pedro, CA 90731

Overeaters Anonymous

P.O. Box 92870
Los Angeles, CA 90009
(213) 542-8363

Parents Anonymous

22330 Hawthorne
Torrance, CA 90505

Pill Addicts Anonymous

P.O. Box 278
Reading, PA 19603
(215) 372-1128

Rational Recovery Systems

Box 100
Lotus, CA 95651
(916) 621-4374

Recovering Couples Anonymous (RCA)

(Support system for couples who are in recovery together.)
P.O. Box 27617
Golden Valley, MN 55442

S-Anon International Family Groups

(Support group for families and friends of sex addicts.)
(for families and friends of sex addicts)
P.O. Box 5117
Sherman Oaks, CA 91413
(818) 990-6901

Save Ourselves or Secular Organization for Sobriety

P. O. Box 5
Buffalo, NY 14215-0005
(716) 834-2921

Sex Addicts Anonymous
P.O. Box 3038
Minneapolis, MN 55403
(612) 339-0217

Sexaholics Anonymous
P.O. Box 300
Simi Valley, CA 93062
(805) 581-3343

Sex and Love Addicts Anonymous
Augustine Fellowship
P.O. Box 119
Newtown Branch
Boston, MS 02258
(617) 332-1845

Smokers Anonymous
2118 Greenwich Street
San Francisco, CA 94123

Survivors of Incest Anonymous (SIA)
(For persons over eighteen years of age who have been sexually abused by a family member or other trusted adult. The word "abuse" is defined broadly.)
P.O. Box 21817
Baltimore, MD 21222-6817
(301) 282-3400

Women for Sobriety and Men for Sobriety
P.O. Box 618
Quakertown, PA 18951
(215) 536-8026

Periodicals:

Sober Times, P. O. Box 40259, San Diego, CA 92164, 619 / 295-3030. Monthly. $17.50/yr. (not affiliated with any Twelve Step program.)

Anne Wilson Schaef conducts private "living process" recovery workshops and retreats. For information, contact:
Wilson-Schaef Associates, Inc.
P. O. Box 18686
Boulder, CO 80301

Recovery Bibliography

Alcoholics Anonymous. 3rd Ed., Alcoholics Anonymous World Service, New York, NY, 1976.

Beattie, Melody, *Codependent No More: How to Stop Controlling Others and Start Caring for Yourself,* Minneapolis: Harper/Hazelden, 1987.

Beattie, Melody, *Codependents' Guide to the Twelve Steps,* New York: Prentice Hall/Parkside, 1990.

Black, Claudia, *It Will Never Happen to Me.* Denver: Medical Administration Co., 1982.

Bowden, Julie and Gravitz, Herbert, *Genesis,* Pompano Beach, FL: Health Communication, Inc. 1988.

Bradshaw, John, *Bradshaw on the Family,* Pompano Beach, FL: Health Communication, Inc. 1988.

Bradshaw, John, *Healing the Shame that Binds You,* Pompano Beach, FL: Health Communication, Inc. 1988.

Bradshaw, John, *Homecoming,* Pompano Beach, FL: Health Communication, Inc., 1990.

Brown, Stephanie, *Safe Passage: Recovery for Adult Children of Alcoholics,* New York: John Wiley and Sons, Inc., 1991.

Gravitz, Herbert L., and Bowden, Julie D., *Guide to Recovery: A Book For Adult Children of Alcoholics,* Holmes Beach, FL: Learning Publications, Inc., 1986.

Gravitz, Herbert L., and Bowden, Julie D., *Genesis,* Pompano Beach, FL: Health Communication, Inc. 1988.

Kasl, Charlotte, *One Journey, Many Paths: Beyond the Twelve Steps,* New York: Harper, 1992.

McClure, Mary Beth, *Reclaiming the Heart: A Handbook of Help and Hope for Survivors,* Warner Books.

Mellody, Pia, Miller, Andrea J., and Miller, Keith, *Facing Codependence: What It Is, Where It Comes From, How It Sabotages Our Lives,* San Francisco: Harper & Row, 1989.

Peck, M. S. *The Road Less Traveled,* New York: Simon and Schuster, 1978.

Ricketson, Susan, *The Dilemma of Love: Healing Co-Dependent Relationships at Different Stages of Life,* Pompano Beach, FL: Health Communications, Inc., 1989.

Schaef, Anne Wilson, *Co-dependence: Misunderstood, Mistreated,* Minneapolis: Winston, 1985.

Appendix VII: The Twelve Steps and Twelve Traditions of Alcoholics Anonymous

Alcoholics Anonymous Twelve Steps of Recovery

1. Admitted we were powerless over alcohol - that our lives had become unmanageable.
2. Came to believe that a power greater than ourselves could restore us to sanity.
3. Made a decision to turn our will and our lives over to the care of God *as we understood Him.*
4. Made a searching and fearless moral inventory of ourselves.
5. Admitted to God, to ourselves, and to another human being the exact nature of our wrongs.
6. Were entirely ready to have God remove all these defects of character.
7. Humbly asked Him to remove our shortcomings.
8. Made a list of all persons we had harmed, and became willing to make amends to them all.
9. Made direct amends to such people wherever possible, except when to do so would injure them or others.
10. Continued to take personal inventory and when we were wrong promptly admitted it.
11. Sought through prayer and meditation to improve our conscious contact with God *as we understood Him*, praying only for knowledge of His will for us and the power to carry that out.
12. Having had a spiritual awakening as the result of these steps, we tried to carry this message to alcoholics, and to practice these principles in all our affairs.

The Twelve Steps are reprinted with permission of Alcoholics Anonymous World Services, Inc. Permission to reprint the Twelve Steps does not mean that A.A. has reviewed or approved the content of this publication, not that A.A. agrees with the views expressed herein. A.A. is a program of recovery from alcoholism - use of the Twelve Steps in connection with programs and activities which are patterned after A.A., but which address other problems, does not imply otherwise.

Alcoholics Anonymous Twelve Traditions

1. Our common welfare should come first; personal recovery depends upon A.A. unity.
2. For our group purpose there is but one ultimate authority - a loving God as He may express himself in our group conscience. Our leaders are but trusted servants; they do not govern.
3. The only requirement for A.A. membership is a desire to stop drinking.
4. Each group should be autonomous, except in matters affecting other groups or A.A. as a whole.
5. Each group has but one primary purpose - to carry the message to the alcoholic who still suffers.
6. The A.A. group ought never endorse, finance, or lend the A.A. name to any related facility or outside enterprise, lest problems of money, property, and prestige divert us from our primary purpose.
7. Every A.A. group ought to be fully self-supporting, declining outside contributions.
8. A.A. should remain forever non-professional, but our service centers may employ special workers.
9. A.A., as such, ought never to be organized; but we may create service boards or committees directly responsible to those they serve.
10. A.A. has no opinion on outside issues; hence, the A.A. name ought never to be drawn into public controversy.
11. Our public relations policy is based on attraction rather than promotion; we need always maintain personal anonymity at the level of press, radio, and films.

12. Anonymity is the spiritual foundation of all our Traditions, ever reminding us to place principles before personalities.

Appendix VIII: "Acupuncture: New Perspectives in Chemical Dependency Treatment" [235]

by Alex G. Brumbaugh

Chinese medicine has been characterized as "an intellectual treasure throve." [236] That is to say, apart from whatever specific clinical efficacy it may have, which is still not well understood in the West, a study of Chinese medicine in general, and its most publicized component, acupuncture, can be most instructive in the nature of life, disease, and recovery. This ancient wisdom is now coming to shed much needed light upon the field of drug and alcohol treatment.

Acupuncture has, in the words of medical historian Manfred Porkert,[237] "stubbornly and successfully resisted assimilation" into Western medical science. This is less the case in Europe. In fact, auricular (ear) acupuncture, which is used in the chemical dependency treatment setting, is as much a European as it is a Chinese development. Acupuncture as it came to be used in Europe is itself a hybrid of Chinese acupuncture, which is only a small part of traditional Chinese medicine, whose primary emphasis is upon herbs. Acupuncture protocols were passed along in Europe beginning in the early 17th century in pamphlets that were filled with contradictory information concerning point location and diagnoses. Curiously, during the post World War I period, when the popularity of acupuncture was spreading in Europe and gaining the attention of European medical societies, Western medicine itself was replacing Oriental medicine in China. During this Westernizing "open door" Nationalist Period in China, under Chiang Kai-shek and the influence of the Rockefellers, acupuncture and other ancient Chinese medical traditions came under attack as primitive and their practice became temporarily outlawed. Clinical knowledge went "underground" until, with Mao Tse-tung's Cultural Revolution of the 1940's and 50's, there was a revision and a revitalization of traditional Chinese medicine.

These revised texts poured into Europe and gained a degree of popularity in France, where, in 1955, Dr. Paul Nogier,[238] using an instrument to measure the level of electrical activity on the surface of the skin, discovered that all of the traditional Chinese acupuncture meridians or arterial pathways were accessible at points of the ear. Clinical experimentation and research in China soon confirmed this, and both Chinese and "Nogier" ear charts began to appear and find clinical application. This was fortuitous for treatment in a public setting, since a large group of individuals can be treated simultaneously without the need for private treatment rooms which are required for the full body treatment normally associated with acupuncture.

It is of some historical irony that this very specialized hybrid form of acupuncture as it has evolved in the drug and alcohol treatment setting in the United States is now being "exported" to Japan and Hong Kong to address the growing drug problem in that part of the world where acupuncture originated over 2,500 years ago.[239]

Interest in acupuncture in general in the United States was piqued by an article written by the syndicated American newspaper columnist James Reston.[240] He had visited China and been stricken with acute appendicitis. He underwent surgery there, and acupuncture was used as an anesthetic. His experience with this very specialized application of acupuncture, and that of physicians and others who visited China with President Richard Nixon in 1972, resulted in a sprinkling of Western research involving pain,[241] and in the eventual discovery that acupuncture prompts the production of beta- endorphins - the body's "endogenous opiates" - in animals. The transmitter or "information" substances for which research data has established a connection with acupuncture include alpha- and beta-endorphins, leu- and met-enkephalins, dynorphin A and B, substance P, serotonin, epinephrine, noradrenalin, dopamine, acetylcholine, adrenocorticotrophic hormone (ACTH), glycine, glutamic acid, the prostaglandins, and cyclic AMP and GMP.[242] Despite the fairly extensive research in this area, precisely how acupuncture works remains a mystery, at least to the Western scientific mind.[243]

Perhaps most simply, it can be said that acupuncture moves energy. In the Chinese view of the body, life energy, or chi, circulates through pathways that are called, in the West, "meridians." "Disease" is seen as a stagnation or blockage of this movement of energy. The acupuncturist places needles which, based upon diagnosis, will stimulate an opening of and therefore a movement of energy through the appropriate pathways.

The effect is homeostatic. For example, a person with an excess of stomach acid who is needled at a point called "Stomach 36" will experience a decrease in the amount of acid in the stomach; a person with a stomach acid deficiency, needled at the same point, will experience an increase in stomach acid. [244]. Again, the mechanism of action involved in this phenomenon is not known.

Acupuncture is not a panacea, and it loses much of its efficacy in the treatment of chemical dependency when practiced in isolation from the more traditional Western modalities of counseling, pharmaceutical therapies, Twelve Step programs, and urine testing. It is best seen as an adjunct or a complement to these other forms, and, in this regard, it is an exceedingly fluid modality. We are beginning to see that, properly used, it can enhance and support the program goals of virtually any traditional chemical dependency treatment setting.

When used in an inpatient detoxification setting, alcoholic seizures virtually disappear, even without the use of pharmaceutical intervention. One of the first residential detox programs to implement acupuncture was Portland, Oregon's Hooper Memorial Detox Center in 1987. Clients entering this five day residential detox-to-referral program were six times less likely to return in the following six months than clients who entered the facility prior to the implementation of twice-daily acupuncture, and the program's overall completion rate increased from 60% to 92%.[245] A residential, social model, detox-to-referral program operated by Santa Barbara, California's Council on Alcoholism and Drug Abuse opened in June of 1991, offering twice-daily acupuncture. Only two alcoholic seizures were reported out of the first 150 clients, the majority of whom were late stage, chronic alcoholics, and completion rates for the program are comparable to Hooper's. In the treatment of acute 284 withdrawal, acupuncture is also effective, the symptoms of "kicking" often resembling a mild flu. And the cravings, anxiety, and depression of crack cocaine withdrawal become manageable.

Subjectively, acupuncture treatment offers to the client support during acute withdrawal through relief of classic withdrawal symptoms. According to Michael Smith, M.D.,[246] the body's response to acute withdrawal from toxic drugs is a "crisis in elimination," which is seen as a "healing crisis." He suggests that "acupuncture works by releasing blockages of energy and correcting imbalances of energy flow," and that its physiologic effects also likely involve homeostatic action on the autonomic nervous system, various neurotransmitters, and elements in the pituitary subcortical axis.[247]

In an outpatient, residential, or day treatment setting, counseling sessions are greatly enhanced by the relaxed and non-hostile ambience created by the acupuncture treatments, and it provides a useful tool in dealing with the otherwise virtually non-treatable symptoms of "protracted abstinence syndrome" or "post-acute" withdrawal. Used as a basis for treatment in conjunction with daily urine testing in the outpatient setting, it provides a higher ground for the counselor in dealing with the perplexing issues of relapse and relapse prevention.

Acupuncture is also well suited as an entry point to treatment and/or recovery in such diverse non-treatment settings as jails, public defender's offices, homeless and battered women's shelters, and neighborhood community centers and medical clinics. In this latter arena, it is providing not only an entry point into treatment/recovery for the chemically dependent client, but also a long awaited entry point into general medicine for acupuncture itself.

For example, a program of the Multicultural Inquiry and Research on AIDS (MIRA) Clinic located in Bayview-Hunter's Point, San Francisco, under the auspices of the University of California San Francisco Center for Aids Prevention and San Francisco General Hospital, was started to study the effects of acupuncture on the detoxification of heroin addicts, and has subsequently expanded to include general medicine. Acupuncture is also now in use in general medical treatment at Lincoln Hospital in The Bronx, New York, where it began as a treatment for acute drug withdrawal.

It is important to note in this regard that acupuncture offers the unique feature of more expansive protocols to address physical and psychological conditions that may have been precipitating factors in the chemical dependency, such as chronic pain or depression, conditions which may have discouraged clients in chemical dependency recovery. With acupuncture, integrated and drug-free treatment options are immediately available for such "relapse trigger" pathologies that may become unmasked as chemical abstinence is achieved. This can be especially helpful in the treatment of dual diagnosis clients, since traditional Chinese medicine has been shown to be effective in the treatment of depression, chronic anxiety, mania, insomnia, schizophrenia, and other mental disorders.[248]

The use of auricular acupuncture in treating acute drug withdrawal began in Hong Kong in 1972. It was used sporadically throughout the United States during the 1970's, and some experimentation with the method was done at the Haight-Ashbury Free Clinic in San Francisco.[249] But it has been at Lincoln Hospital in New York, under the guidance of Michael O. Smith, M.D., Director of the hospital's Division of Substance Abuse, that the protocol has been refined, expanded, and has taken its firmer root.

Lincoln is located in the South Bronx where alcoholism and drug addiction have been endemic for many years. Smith's clinic was primarily a methadone program in 1973 when he first read of Dr. H. L. Wen's research in Hong Kong[250] concerning the treatment of heroin withdrawal with acupuncture. Dr. Wen, a neurosurgeon, had made his initial discovery while administering acupuncture anesthesia to a patient who happened to be in heroin withdrawal. The withdrawal symptoms disappeared, and Wen subsequently conducted a formalized study. By 1980, Wen had replicated the positive outcomes of his research and published no fewer than ten additional studies[251] concerning narcotic withdrawal symptoms and acupuncture, including research on the adjunctive use of the opiate block naloxone to essentially flush opiates from receptor sites in the brain to speed up the detoxification process. It was discovered that naloxone also partially blocked the effects of acupuncture itself. This led to additional research on the relationship of acupuncture to the production of endogenous opiates.

Smith, interested in potential alternatives to methadone treatment, began employing Chinese doctors at Lincoln to experiment with different protocols in the treatment of heroin addiction. Wen's research had involved electrical stimulation as well, and Lincoln Hospital experimented extensively with electrostimulation protocols, eventually discontinuing its use when it was discovered that manual acupuncture resulted in more consistent clinical outcomes. A five-point auricular protocol was eventually established, consisting of four to five points in each ear, including kidney, liver, lung (or heart), sympathetic, and *shen-men*. By 1975, acupuncture had become a permanent feature at the Lincoln program, not only for heroin dependence but for alcoholic patients as well. And, in 1985, when the "crack" cocaine epidemic reached New York, it was discovered that the same protocol was effective in addressing the cravings, anxiety, and dysphoria accompanying "crack" withdrawal.[252]

In 1985, Smith founded the National Acupuncture Detoxification Association (NADA), an organization representative of experts in chemical dependency as well as Oriental medicine. NADA's function is to provide training and consultation to treatment programs that have begun throughout the world and to assure specific clinical and ethical standards in the certification of "acupuncture detox specialists."

Though much of NADA's focus as well as the research has been upon the acute detoxification phase of withdrawal, clinical experience since NADA was established has shown that acupuncture has applications as well for post-acute or "latent" withdrawal. Clients return to the acupuncture clinic months and even years into recovery for "tune-ups." Many clients find the far more expansive application of traditional Chinese medicine to be a valuable tool in treating the anxiety-depression-craving phenomenon that Edward Brecher[253] termed the "post-addiction syndrome." These symptoms, as well as the majority of Terence Gorski's symptoms that forebode alcoholic relapse[254] correspond with "disorders of the spirit" in the classic Chinese medical texts and are very responsive to traditional Chinese medical treatment, which includes herbs as well as acupuncture.[255]

Oriental medical schools, however, in which acupuncturists receive their education and training, are generally as deficient in chemical dependency curricula as are their Western counterparts. Therefore, a primary role of NADA is to provide acupuncturists with basic education in chemical dependency and recovery through intensive 3-day NADA Certification trainings coupled with a clinical internship. Chemical dependency professionals working in the acupuncture program also benefit from these trainings, since clinical success requires a complementary relationship between the counseling and acupuncture aspects of the treatment program.

The NADA protocol has a precise focus, elegant in its simplicity. In its original application in the outpatient, drop-in setting, the clinic is to be, like the Twelve Step program, "barrier-free" in that there are no motivational or other screening requirements for entering or continuing acupuncture treatment. Clients are instructed to come as "clean and sober as they can" for treatment, and treatment is recommended daily, in the same "one day at a time" rhythm as recovery, so that the treatment, as Michael Smith has said, "will be as reliable as the drug was." While Twelve Step meetings are frequently held in proximity to the clinic, and while group and individual counseling is generally available on site, participation in these activities is not a condition of receiving acupuncture treatment.

The clinic protocol is to be "empowering" in that clients do everything they can for themselves, such as "prepping" their own ears with an alcohol solution and cotton. In some NADA clinics, clients select their own personal autoclaved or pre-packaged disposable needles. Often, clients even use a mirror to remove their own needles upon leaving. The acupuncture staff are counseled not to "fuss" with clients, question them as to relapse, or lecture or confront them in any way. Clinic rules are minimal, and clients are barred from treatment only for disruptive behavior. Such instances are rare in this setting.

The NADA protocol includes "sleep mix" tea, a recipe also developed at Lincoln,[256] using the Western herbs chamomile, hops, catnip (sometimes substituted with valerian root), scullcap, peppermint, and yarrow. Clients drink it during or following treatment and are encouraged to take it home to help them sleep.

Clients are treated for 45 minutes in a group setting, seated. Talking - especially drug-talk and "war stories" - is discouraged. In observing this process, where there are no behavioral or cognitive expectancies, where clients are "free to do nothing," one gets a sense of some of the more discreet resonances between this modality and the form and structure of the Twelve Step meeting. There is an implicit trust established in the client's ability to find his own way in recovery, and the responsibility of the clinic is to make available the most helpful tools for the task.

This clinical ambience is often unsettling at first for new clients, especially the more "treatment-seasoned" ones. They may spend the first few days of treatment waiting for "the program" to begin. They will perhaps "test" the program by "chipping" or coming under the influence, and find that they are welcomed back just the same. While traditional alcohol and other drug treatment strategies require an external focus, here, in the NADA clinic, the attention of the client is invited inward, where the ultimate responsibility for recovery lies.

According to John D. McPeake, et.al.,[257] a shortcoming of traditional alcohol and drug treatment is that it ignores a primary motivation for drug use, which is mood modification. One aspect of the efficacy of acupuncture may be that, to degrees that vary with individual clients, the treatment elicits an experience of altered consciousness. Heroin addicts often self-report euphoria as an altered mood response to acupuncture, induction of which has shown a tendency to reduce baseline withdrawal and craving.[258] An additional subjective effect of the treatment is a feeling of relaxation and stress-reduction. For this reason, it is not unusual in acupuncture clinics to see counselors or other staff receiving treatment with the clients!

NADA held its first annual convention in February, 1991, in Santa Barbara, California. The roster was dominated not by chemical dependency professionals nor by acupuncturists but by representatives of the criminal justice community, including Superior Court Judge Herbert Klein, former "Drug Czar" of Dade County, Florida, Mark Cunnif, Executive Director of the National Association of Criminal Justice Planners in Washington, D.C., and Orville Pung, Commissioner of Corrections and James Bruton, Director of Adult Release, of the Minnesota State Department of Corrections. Local presenters included the Santa Barbara Chief of Police, and the Director of Administrative Services for the Santa Barbara County Department of Probation. They came, as advertised in the Conference brochure, to herald the arrival of a "new beacon on the dark landscape of chemical dependency treatment."

That the strongest advocates for acupuncture treatment for chemical dependency are members of the criminal justice community is echoed by the fact that much of the funding for acupuncture-based chemical dependency programs in the United States comes not through traditional drug and alcohol but through criminal justice sources. There are clinical reasons for this, and they reveal a great deal about the efficacy of acupuncture, and have resulted in a growing bias among practitioners in this field that the premier "window of opportunity" for intervention in drug treatment lies on the continuum of arrest, adjudication, incarceration, and probation or parole of the drug offender.

The standard skepticism about drug and alcohol treatment in general in the law and justice community derives from the fact that law enforcement and treatment have traditionally labored under conflicting definitions of alcoholism and drug addiction. The clinical (and recovering) community has long accepted the disease of alcoholism/addiction as a chronic relapsing disorder in which recovery is typically achieved only through a process of "slips and starts." For this reason, there has been a shift in chemical dependency treatment away from the concept of detoxification and toward relapse prevention or "sobriety maintenance." Clinical experience is clear that rare is the addict or alcoholic who negotiates the transition from use to non-use in a single movement.

While individual judges, probation, or parole officers may indeed be personally aware of this relapsing nature of typical early recovery, the criminal justice system itself has not been able to tolerate relapse since its charge is not to bring about recovery per se, but to prevent the resumption of the criminal behavior that relapse precipitates. This "hard line" either/or definition of recovery as requiring total and continuing abstinence has been justified, for in traditional drug and alcohol treatment, relapse is generally catastrophic, resulting in treatment drop-out. This is true of course in residential intensive or social model treatment, often the "treatment of choice" for the most chronic addicts and alcoholics, because a "clean and sober" living environment is tantamount to the program's success. But it is also true of outpatient treatment modalities because of the special difficulties of the chemical dependency counselor in dealing with the problems of relapse.

In the highly successful acupuncture-based drug diversion programs, however, in such varied locations as New York City, Miami, Portland, Oregon, and Santa Barbara and Santa Maria, California, a higher ground can be taken by the judge or probation or parole officer, because the acupuncture-based program is able to keep the client in treatment during the early relapsing period. Relapses here tend to be shallow and non-catastrophic. Clients "keep coming back," and, over time, abstinence is achieved. Dade County Judge Stanley Goldstein, who presides in Miami over a "drug court" which hears only first and second cocaine offenses, began diverting all offenders to a three phase treatment program in October, 1989. The first phase of the program involves daily acupuncture and urine testing. Defendants return to court during this phase, and Judge Goldstein reviews their urinalysis records. His response to intermittent positive tests is not punitive; rather, he encourages defendants in their struggle and commends them for the "clean" days they have achieved. This unusual posture of relapse tolerance is well justified, for of the first 1,200 defendants to complete the first phase of the program, only seven were re-arrested during the first six months.[259]

The concept of daily urine testing as it is used in Miami was also a development of the Lincoln Hospital program. The notion of urine testing in a therapeutic setting may seem at first an anathema, since urine testing is traditionally punitive, a clear manifestation of judgmentalism, giving the treatment program the role of critic rather than supporter of the client's recovery process. In practice, however, quite the opposite turns out to be the case. The goal is not punitive disclosure but education and therapeutic feedback. Unlike urine testing in a law enforcement setting, clients assume much of the responsibility for self-monitoring the urinalysis process. Fear that clients will provide fraudulent test results under these conditions have not been justified. As Michael Smith has aptly said, "drug addicts lie, but they don't lie every day." Once the daily treatment rhythm has been established, and once the client has learned that a positive urine test will not result in program expulsion, attempts to deliver "false negatives" are uncommon.

To fully understand the utility of such testing, a brief examination of the dynamics of relapse may be helpful. In the traditional relationship between a chemical dependency counselor and client, there is an implicit trap surrounding the issue of relapse. In the Rogerian and other generally accepted models of chemical dependency counseling, the appropriate posture of the counselor is one of non-judgmental acceptance. The overt agenda is to validate the experience and feelings of the client. Trust is, of course, a necessary prerequisite for this stance. Honesty, particularly self-honesty, is the hallmark of recovery. The counselor wants the client to be honest about his or her feelings and behavior.

And, if the counselor is skilled, the trust and honesty will come early in the relationship, because the client desires it as well. It will become part of what is called in recovery the "honeymoon" period - generally the first 30 days.

The difficulty, of course, is that both counselor and client know that addiction is a disease characterized by relapse. The counselor cannot, in good conscience, validate relapse when it happens because the overriding covert agenda in the relationship is for the client to stop relapsing. This agenda implies, of course, judgment, which is contrary to the goal of therapy.

This is a bind, and one to which the client is not insensitive. If the counselor has done a particularly good job and has won the trust of the client, then, when the generally inevitable relapse occurs, the client's usual move will be to drop out of treatment so as to protect the counselor from disappointment.

Daily urine testing in a therapeutic acupuncture-based setting discharges this dilemma. At Lincoln, and in other similar programs, the computer software interfaces with an on-site urine testing machine. With substantial client numbers, the cost of urinalysis for the single drug for which the client has been referred to treatment can be reduced to as little as a dollar and a half per test. Multiple client urines are tested at once, and the data is downloaded to the client's attendance file. A print-out of urine toxicity patterns over the period of the client's treatment attendance can be generated while the client is having acupuncture. A subsequent counseling session that begins with the client having this print-out in hand can commence at an entirely different therapeutic level, free from the potentially codependent "how are you doing? ", because "how the client is doing" is already objectively established. The content of the answer to the question, "how are you doing? " is not being elicited by the counselor. Nor does the answer depend upon the clients best recollection of when he or she last used, but rather has been provided by the client's own body, so one important element of denial is also dispelled. Clinical experience shows that clients come to enjoy this daily feedback. It can perhaps be likened to a person who is trying to lose weight stepping on the scale each morning.

A significant barrier to treatment in criminal justice settings is that acupuncture is designated by federal law as an "experimental procedure," thus precluding mandated application among incarcerated, probated, and paroled populations. Its current use is therefore limited to those who "volunteer" for treatment. Even so, the use of the auricular acupuncture protocol in incarcerated settings illustrates its application beyond the detoxification phase and its potential for addressing some of the social and economic problems attending chemical dependency.

In Minnesota, it has been integrated into four state prison treatment programs, one of which is a research program. Elsewhere, the protocol has been to treat inmates with a history of chemical dependency daily for 30 days prior to their release. In the Dade County Stockade in Miami, from late 1989 to the present, approximately 140 inmates have been treated in this manner, but no outcome or reincarceration studies have been done. Similar programs have begun in Santa Clara, San Luis Obispo, and Santa Barbara counties in California. A preliminary study of Santa Barbara county jail inmates indicates that those receiving 24 or more treatments during the last 30 days of their incarceration are two-thirds less likely to be re-arrested in the two months following release than those receiving six or fewer treatments.[260] In that an acupuncturist can treat as many as 35 inmates in an hour, this treatment modality shows great promise as a cost-effective method of inmate reduction in our vastly overcrowded jails.

Also promising is the use of acupuncture in homeless shelters, where alcohol and drug treatment is often resisted due to the unmanageability of withdrawal symptoms in such a setting, and where shelter client safety has become an increasing concern. A Santa Barbara program operates an acute detoxification program with clients who are under the custodial care of a homeless shelter at night. Clients receive two acupuncture treatments daily, and the program has had a minimum of withdrawal-related medical emergencies, seizures, or social altercations. Shelter staff report that the program has had a positive effect on management of the facility in general. The program has a 90% program completion and aftercare program placement rate.[261]

Acupuncture treatment has also found successful application in the treatment of chemically dependent pre- and post-partum women, and a variation of the protocol is being used to treat chemically exposed infants.[262] Clinics which use acupuncture as part of the treatment design and which are specifically focused on the needs of pregnant women are now in operation at Lincoln Hospital,[263] at the MIRA Clinic at Bayview-Hunter's Point in San Francisco[264], in Miami at the Metro/Dade Office of Rehabilitation Services, and in St. Paul, Minnesota at the Maternal Child Project.[265]

Acupuncture is of particular efficacy with pre-natal women, because, while it is well known that the common substances of abuse such as alcohol, cocaine, heroin, amphetamines, PCP, and marijuana have documented teratogenic potential for the fetus,[266] medications used to accomplish detoxification are also teratogenic.[267] There is concern that abrupt withdrawal during pregnancy may be damaging to the mother and fetus. Acupuncture reduces this risk by supporting the process of withdrawal and avoiding the impact of sudden abstinence.

The enthusiastic law enforcement speakers at the 1991 NADA conference were, unfortunately, "preaching to the converted," for the small audience was comprised largely of people already working in this frontier field. Although there are now over 175 acupuncture-based chemical dependency programs operating in the United States, and dozens more elsewhere in the world, acceptance of acupuncture as a legitimate treatment component by the chemical dependency community has been, at best, guarded. In the areas of the country where acupuncture has flourished, it is highly localized. While it has a firm foothold, for example, in the chemical dependency treatment delivery systems in the cities and regions mentioned above, it has failed to gain acceptance with the departments of drugs and alcohol in any of the states where these programs exist. The single exception as of this writing is New York, where the State's Division of Substance Abuse Services recently released a concept paper strongly advocating acupuncture as a "threshold technology," most effective in "assisting cocaine and/or alcohol addicted clients who resist initial treatment." Acupuncture, according to the paper, "works in concert with traditional drug abuse treatment approaches (and) transcends the barriers to all treatment components." [268]

Acceptance at the federal level is also reserved. A February, 1991 memo from the National Institute on Drug Abuse (NIDA) to the U. S. Congress Select Committee on Narcotics Abuse, states that they feel this treatment modality "shows some promise," but that more research is required.[269] The only acupuncture research they are currently funding is a new cocaine treatment research project in Minneapolis, and a three year study in Miami focused on IV needle use. At less than $1,000,000 each, these are among the smallest of NIDA's current research grants. Miami is a three phase grant. The first phase has been completed, and the experimental group receiving acupuncture has demonstrated a faster rate of delivering clean urines than groups receiving counseling only. Also of interest is that, with acupuncture, court referred clients responded more favorably than self-referred clients.[270]

The Federal Office of Treatment Improvement (OTI), in their first funding cycle in 1990, received one application that included acupuncture. They denied the application by a five-to-four vote, questioning "the efficacy of the use of acupuncture in (the treatment of high-risk narcotics addict probationers)." [271] Due in part to the lobbying efforts of the National Association of Criminal Justice Planners, OTI's director Beny Primm has since been quoted as stating that future funding applications to OTI will not be denied "solely on the basis that they contain acupuncture components." [272] Charles Rangel,[273] Chairman of the Select Committee on Narcotics Abuse and Control, in a letter to Beny Primm in July of 1990, perhaps contributed to the softening of OTI's position by stating that "acupuncture (though) not, as yet, fully understood...should not be overlooked or rejected off-hand." Citing the dramatic success of the cocaine diversion program in Miami, Rangel went on to say that "This is precisely the kind of innovative experiment that Congress has provided for through demonstration grant funds. I strongly urge you to look into this program, to consider it objectively, with an open mind and without prejudgment."

But again, such support is isolated. In the voluminous triennial report of the Department of Health and Human Resources to Congress, in their cataloging of innovative new drug treatment modalities, mention is made of such experimental treatment tools as pocket computers by which nicotine addicts can keep track of the number of cigarettes smoked during the day, but there is no mention of acupuncture in the document.[274]

This resistance, often tacit, like the Western cultural resistance to acupuncture in general, is understandable. Acupuncture, and the "invisible circulatory energy" paradigm of the organism upon which it is based, is implicitly non-rational.   In that its basic premises about the body are based upon energetic rather than somatic considerations,[275] it is in fundamental conflict with Western medical and scientific philosophy, from which current drug treatment strategies and theories have developed.   Like Alcoholics Anonymous, itself a historical and cultural reaction against Western "scientism,"[276] acupuncture addresses addictive disorder on a "non-Rationalistic" and subjective plane where the issues of recovery lie not in the relationship of the addict with the external world or "fix" but rather in relationship with self, in the possibility of healing from within. Oriental medicine characterizes addiction in terms such as "yin deficiency," "stuck liver chi, and "empty fire syndrome." Such unfamiliar and "non-medical" tautology is not easily embraced by the "rational" Western drug treatment establishment.

However, in addition to the studies already cited, some research under the parameters of Western scientific investigation has been achieved. In 1987 in a medically supervised study of chronic homeless alcoholic men in Hennepin County, Minnesota, 80 subjects were divided into two groups matched for drinking history and prior treatment experience. The control group were given sham acupuncture, needled at non-therapeutic points a few millimeters away from standard treatment points. 53% of the treatment group completed the eight week treatment regimen, compared with 2 1/2% of the control group. During the six month follow-up of the two groups, the control group had more than twice as many drinking episodes and had to be re-admitted to detox more than twice as often as the experimental group.[277] These same researchers are currently comparing acupuncture with Valium in treating the symptoms of acute alcohol withdrawal, and are the recipients of the new NIDA cocaine treatment research grant.

A similar placebo-type study was done at Bayview Hunter's Point Clinic comparing methadone and acupuncture in the detoxification from heroin. This 3-phase, one and a half year study was commissioned by the California legislature. A report to the legislature indicates that acupuncture clients were more likely to have clean urinalysis and reported longer periods of abstinence with fewer problem days than their methadone controls.[278]

One of the non-criminal justice speakers at the 1991 NADA Conference was Robert Olander, Commissioner of Chemical Health for Hennepin County, Minnesota, and one of the active NIDA researchers there. He suggested that there have been three "benchmarks" in the history of alcohol and drug treatment in the United States, three things that have revolutionized the way we do alcohol and drug therapy: first was the founding of Alcoholics Anonymous in 1935; second was the development of pharmaceuticals in the late 1950's and early 60's, and the third is acupuncture.

Whether acupuncture indeed deserves a place on this exclusive list remains to be seen. Given the economic and social devastation of the current drug and addiction problem in the United States, however, we are perhaps well advised to reflect upon Rangel's urging, "to consider it objectively, with an open mind and without prejudgment."

Appendix IX: Auricular Acupuncture Treatment for Chemical Dependency" - A Literature Review

by Ruth W. Ackerman, Ph.D., L.C.S.W.
reprinted with permission

The crack/cocaine epidemic raging in this country has evoked one hopeful response from an otherwise overwhelmed treatment community: a renewed interest in acupuncture treatment, for detoxification, preparation for counseling, and relapse prevention.

Usually administered in an outpatient setting, with needles inserted on the outside of the ear - therefore the term "auricular" - auricular (ear) acupuncture is an accessible treatment which allows individuals to withdraw from drugs and/or alcohol and to pursue recovery without having to leave their families, equipping them to maintain abstinence in the face of everyday pressures. Acupuncture is a valuable entry point for chemical dependency treatment and provides a bridge from active substance abuse to readiness for counseling and other support services via its calming and focusing effects.

Acupuncture Treatment for Chemical Dependency

Developed by the Chinese more than 2,500 years ago, acupuncture is a technique to relieve pain and stress by inserting needles into specific points on the body believed to correspond to structures and functions within the body.

Auricular acupuncture was first applied as a treatment for opiate addiction in 1972 by H.L. Wen, M.D. in Hong Kong. (Smith & Kahn, 1988; Wen & Chueng, 1973). Acupuncture procedures based on Wen's initial protocol which used electroacupuncture on two ear points have become varied and diverse. Different numbers of acupuncture points and types of stimulation have been used. These include needling with and without electrical stimulation, surgical staples or tacks, and transcutaneous electrical nerve stimulation (TENS) using surface electrodes without needles

(Katims, Ng & Lowinson, 1992). Although ear points have been used predominantly, body points have been used as well.

Lincoln Clinic

Acupuncture detoxification was first used on a large scale beginning in 1974 at Lincoln Clinic, Bronx, New York. The community sought an alternative to straight methadone detoxification. Acupuncture promised an alternative to the "demoralizing and stupefying effects of trying to solve a problem of drug abuse by administrating more abusive drugs" (Smith, 1979, p. 98). When acupuncture was first introduced into the program, the protocol established by Wen was followed using electroacupuncture. Budgetary restraints preventing replacement of broken equipment and an extended power shortage led to the discovery that manual needling on auricular acupuncture points was more effective than electroacupuncture. It was more successful, easier to administer, and less expensive. Lincoln clinic has continued to use manual acupuncture and has developed a standardized three to five-point protocol that is the most commonly used treatment protocol (American Hospital Association [AHA], 1991).

Auricular points (kidney, liver, lung, sympathetic and *shenmen*) located on the outer ear are manually stimulated with half inch stainless steel sterile/disposable needles which remain in place 45 to 60 minutes. In the case of pregnant women, only three points are used: liver, lung and sympathetic. Treatment is administered to clients seated in a quiet group setting. Withdrawal symptoms gradually improve within 15 minutes. Patients initially receive daily treatment for two weeks, then decrease the frequency.

After a treatment session, patients seem more alert, relaxed, and report the ability to think clearly. They also tend to be more verbal. These effects last from many hours to several days, depending on the severity of addiction. Once beyond the immediate symptoms of withdrawal, they receive regular counseling and are encouraged to attend Twelve Step meetings. Daily urine samples are collected. The cost per patient averages $21 per treatment including counseling and urinalysis (AHA, 1991).

National Acupuncture Detoxification Association

A nonprofit organization has been established to teach and annually recertify practitioners who utilize the auricular acupuncture detoxification protocol developed at Lincoln Clinic. The National Acupuncture Detoxification Association [NADA] is known by the acronym NADA, which means "nothing" in Spanish and symbolizes the commitment to a drug free response to addiction. NADA consults with communities and other groups interested in starting similar treatment programs, provides training and certification in the treatment protocol developed at Lincoln, and provides cross training for chemical dependency specialists and acupuncturist to enhance treatment collaboration.

Since the founding of NADA anecdotal reports on the application of NADA protocol acupuncture have been consistently encouraging (Smith & Kahn, 1988). More than 100 publicly funded clinics in 14 states and another 25 in Europe, Eastern Europe, Latin America and Asia have been established explicitly on the model of the South Bronx clinic (AHA, 1991). The treatment settings are diverse and include psychiatric outpatient clinics, chemical dependency inpatient and outpatient programs, homeless shelters and criminal justice settings (Pittman, 1992; Smith, 1987; Smith, 1990; Smith, Alvarez & Small, 1987; Smith & Kahn, 1988).

Acupuncture Treatment for Pregnant Substance Abusers

Since 1974 more than 1000 pregnant women have received manual auricular acupuncture, without incidence of uterine seizures or spontaneous abortion (M. O. Smith, personal communication, November 23, 1990).

Ignorance about acupuncture leads many to assume that any acupuncture treatment administered during pregnancy places the fetus at risk (Becke, 1988). In fact, acupuncture has been used for thousands of years to treat morning sickness, premature labor, malposition of fetus, toxemia, and labor pain (Academy of

Traditional Chinese Medicine, 1975; Shanghai College of Traditional Medicine, 1981). Electroacupuncture is contraindicated during pregnancy, however manual stimulation of acupuncture points has long been used beneficially for conditions related to pregnancy.

Lincoln Clinic has treated more than 750 pregnant women since 1988 in its special program for pregnant substance abusers (N. Smalls, personal communication, February 23, 1991). The program combines the services of an obstetrician-gynocologist, psychiatrist, acupuncturist, and nurse-midwife as well as counseling support staff (Smith, 1988,c; Smith, 1990c). Similar programs have been established in many locations in the United States and abroad.

By providing supportive acupuncture during the process of gradual reduction of the use of addictive substances, this treatment mitigates elements of drug and alcohol withdrawal during pregnancy which may be damaging to the mother and/or infant such as seizures (Fitzgerald, 1988).

Acupressure for Newborns and Infants

Babies exposed to drugs during gestation have been treated with acupressure with dramatic success (Keenan, 1990). The infants were treated for withdrawal symptoms with acupressure to the outer ear. Herbal seeds (*semen vicarae*) were taped to one to three ear points specific to addiction and selected according to the degree of the infants' development. The mothers and/or other care givers were instructed to press the seeds several times a day. In this way the mother could contribute directly to the recovery of her baby. This procedure afforded an opportunity to address maternal guilt about having used substances during pregnancy. By relieving withdrawal symptoms and reducing the "dulling" seen in substance effected newborns, acupressure stimulation enhanced "focusing" and maternal-infant bonding. Acupressure may be an important tool to assist the newborn through the neonatal abstinence syndrome and should be evaluated as soon as possible. Now widely described as "seed therapy" this method of treating infants is being used in many locations in this and other countries (P. Keenan, personal communication, August, 1992).

Methadone Treatment

Methadone, a synthetic opiate which decreases the craving for heroin, is commonly recommended for all heroin addicts including pregnant addicts in spite of its known toxic effects (Finnegan, Connaughton, Emich & Wieland, 1972). A dose level of 20 milligrams (mg) or less per day is currently recommended to avoid teratogenic effects (Kosten, 1989). In practice, pregnant women are regularly maintained on doses of 40 mg or higher.

The addict who is detoxified from heroin, even if maintained on methadone, is very likely to increase his or her use of alcohol and/or cocaine (Anglin, 1989) or to continue to use heroin and/or larger doses of methadone. Studies have shown that half of all addicts on methadone maintenance test positive for other substances of abuse and more than 50% of methadone maintenance clients typically drop out of treatment (Clark, 1990). One obvious problem with methadone treatment is that only one substance, heroin, is being addressed. This is problematic, since most addicts are polyabusers (Lipton & Miranda, 1983; Zuckerman & Alpert, 1988). Acupuncture has been found to be as clinically effective and more cost efficient than methadone treatment (Clark, 1990). Acupuncture relieves withdrawal symptoms for all substances of abuse simultaneously. "Acupuncture relieves withdrawal symptoms and craving, promotes general relaxation, systemic rebalancing, and enhances mental and physical functioning" (Smith & Kahn, 1988).

Current Therapies for Addiction

Numerous therapies for addictive problems exist, each claiming success (Frances, 1989). The cost effectiveness and accuracy of these claims is questionable and generates much debate in the field of chemical dependency (Shaffer, 1986). Rival positions from inpatient as opposed to outpatient settings (Hayshiada et al, 1989) and from 12-Step and social model to aversion therapy claim success. However, they are difficult if not possible to compare because there is no uniformity in standards for outcome measures (Frawley, 1990). For a comprehensive overview of current therapies see Donovan and Marlatt (1988) and Lowinson, Ruiz, Millman and Langrog (1992).

According to Trachtenberg and Blum (1989), therapeutic approaches can be categorized as follows: (1) traditional verbal psychotherapy and/or 12-Step group processes, education and activity; (2) medication or neurochemical support with little education or therapy; (3) Verbal therapy with medication; and (4) aversion therapy, with or without medication.

In the first category, most are inpatient programs which had typically scheduled for thirty days, the amount of time previously supported by insurance. Recently, the average length of stay funded by insurance has been reduced to five to ten days. These programs typically require that the client complete detoxification before admission. Such detoxification is usually medication based, using a three-day inpatient protocol which entails sedation. Whether 28-day inpatient programming is more successful than other methods is doubtful since it is estimated that 40-50% of alcoholics are believed to relapse within a one year and 50-80% of cocaine abusers relapse in the first year (Gawin & Ellinwood,1988). The effects of psychotherapy have been favorably reported in spite of conflicting outcomes in studies of opiate addicts. See Kaufman and McNaul (1992) for a thorough review of recent findings.

Medication and/or neurochemical support modalities with minimal education and counseling comprise the second category. The chemical agents utilized include antidepressants, neuroleptics, anti-Parkinson agents, and amino acids. Trachtenberg and Blum (1988) reviewed the use of antidepressant medication and concluded that generally antidepressant medications have not been significantly successful in preventing relapse to cocaine addiction. Although researchers are clearly looking for "cocaine's methadone" (Scientists say...., 1993) the search for cocaine antagonists has not been successful (Gawin & Kleber, 1986; Kosten, Kleber & Morgan, 1989). Medications are prescribed for cocaine withdrawal to ward off a cocaine "crash." Problems stemming from these medication are the generation of side effects and the risk of drug dependence. Studies in this area have shown inconclusive outcomes (Cosser, Brower & Bresford, 1990; Dackis & Gold, 1985; Dakis, Gold, Sweeney, Byron & Climko, 1987).

Whether medication is really necessary during withdrawal from a variety of substances is itself controversial. For example, in a report on cocaine treatment in 12-month follow up study (Summer,1990) cocaine withdrawal without medication was found successful.

Alternate therapies including acupuncture are incorporated in the category of neurochemical support. This would also include modalities such as biofeedback, Vitamin C therapy and amino acid supplementation. A summary of alternate modalities can be found in Lowinson, Ruiz, Millman and Langrod (1992), Kleber (1977), Kleber and Riordan (1982).

In the third category, verbal therapy plus medication and/or nutritional and neurochemical support modalities, psychotherapy alone was found to have disappointing results: only 17% of the group studied were able to abstain and improvement was limited to only half of the group (Gawin and Kleber, 1986).

Aversion therapy with and without medication and/or nutritional and neurochemical support is the final category. Usually administered in a two week inpatient setting, there has been controversy regarding the claims for its success (Barbor, Stephens & Marlatt, 1987).

Theories of Addiction

While the issues regarding conditions which increase risk for substance abuse such as poverty, unemployment, severe deprivation in childhood, and physical and sexual abuse all need to be addressed (Hellert, 1988), it is not within the scope of this overview to do so. However, many theoretical models have been created to explain the phenomena of addiction and heavy drinking. These theories include anthropological, availability, conditioning aversion, economic, genetic, neurobehavioral, neurobiological, personality, psychoanalytic, social learning and social systems (Chaudron & Wilkinson, 1988; Fingarette, 1988). An excellent summary of these and other theoretical models can be found in Chaudron and Wilkinson (1988).

Biopsychosocial Theory

Although this literature review is focused primarily on detoxification and prevention of relapse on a physiologic basis during pregnancy, thus falling into the category of neurobiological theory, the theoretical model that more accurately applies to the phenomenon of acupuncture detoxification is the biopsychosocial model (Wallace, 1989). As the name implies, the biopsychosocial theory suggests that this illness involves biological, psychological and sociocultural factors. For a comprehensive discussion of the implications of this model, see Donovan (1988).

The value of acupuncture as a preparation for psychological and social change has been suggested by clinicians (Clark, 1990; Kao & Lu, 1974; Newmeyer, Johnson & Klot, 1984; Smith, 1988a; Smith, 1988c; Smith, 1989b; Smith, 1990a). It is essential that social and psychological aspects in addition to neurobiochemical issues be addressed both theoretically and clinically to obtain maximum results in chemical dependency treatment. Acupuncture is best understood as an entry point into a larger system of recovery that requires psychological and social change to prevent relapse. Further research regarding these aspects related to acupuncture detoxification is needed.

Genetic Theory

Support for studies on the genetic and biological basis of alcoholism has increased from $41 million in 1989 to $53 million for 1991 (Goleman, 1990). Researchers have identified a gene linked to the receptors for dopamine, a brain chemical involved in the sensation of pleasure. In the chronic alcoholics autopsied in the study, 77% were identified as having this genetic marker compared to none of the controls (Blum, 1990a; Blum et al, 1990b).

Research on alcoholism also suggests that imbalance in the brain's receptors for the neurotransmitter gamma-aminobutyric acid [GABA] result in increased anxiety; the less GABA present, the greater the anxiety. It has also been shown that sons of alcoholic fathers had lower levels of GABA and higher tension levels than men whose fathers were not alcoholic. When given a glass of vodka, the GABA levels of the first group rose to levels equivalent to those of controls and their tension levels declined. It was hypothesized that GABA irregularity is a trait marker link to the genetic vulnerability for alcoholism (Blum, 1990b).

Genetic research relevant to drug abuse is just beginning to be studies in five critical areas: animal selective breeding studies, adoption studies, twin studies, family studies and high risk situations. See Kaufman & McNaul, (1992) for a thorough review.

Neurobiochemical Theory

A neurobiochemical theory illustrating cocaine dependency suggests that the stimulating effects of cocaine are the result of its potentiation of the catecholamine neurotransmitters norepeneph-rine [NE] and d-phenelalynine [DA] (Trachtenberg & Blum, 1988). To understand how this addiction model works, it is first necessary to understand how brain neurotransmitters normally operate. Cells using NE and DA as neurotransmitters occur in discrete locations in the brain stem and project to higher brain areas including the basal ganglia (effecting motor dysfunction), limbic system (effecting arousal and basic appetite drives and aggression), and hypothalamus (effecting hormone function). These diffuse projections of nerve cell axons contribute to the general state of arousal. These neuronal systems exert their effects by releasing DA or NE into the synapse, the very narrow space between the neurons. Once released into the synapse, the neurotransmitter interacts with specific DA or NE receptors on the next neuron to exert central physiological effects. Under normal conditions, DA or NE is rapidly removed from the synapse by an uptake mechanism, resulting in the neurotransmitter having a brief pulsatile effect on the target receptors (p. 5).

Cocaine has powerful effects on the DA and NE synapses and inhibits the reuptake of DA and NE (Gawin,1988). By blocking the normal mechanism, the impact of these neurotransmitters is increased many times over. Instead of the brief pulse of transmission there is continued stimulation which is associated with cocaine intoxication.

Serotonin is a neurotransmitter providing many functions including arousal, mood, and endocrine regulation. Repeated use of cocaine effects the serotonin system by reducing the concentration of serotonin and its metabolites (Gold, Washton & Dackis, 1985). Recidivism may reflect adaptive, long lasting central nervous system [CNS] change which physiologic withdrawal fails to reverse (Katims, et al, 1992).

With this in mind, the impact of acupuncture on the process of addiction may be better understood.

Theory of Acupuncture Detoxification

Western Medicine Model

Kroening and Oleson (1985, p. 5) offered this succinct description of the neurochemical theory of acupuncture detoxification:

The mechanism by which the acupuncture effects withdrawal from narcotic addiction is not yet fully understood but similar theories have been proposed by several observers....In drug addiction exogenous opiates bond with receptor sites normally occupied by endogenous endorphins. The occupation of these opiate receptor sites by narcotic drugs leads to the inhibition of natural endorphins while the body's own internal mechanisms oppose the external drug therapy, resulting in intolerance and addiction. Abrupt withdrawal from the exogenous drug leaves the body's defense mechanism still geared to offset the narcotic action. Acupuncture may facilitate withdrawal by activating the release of previously suppressed natural endorphins which can then occupy the receptor sites formally dominated by the narcotic drug."

Western medicine has been reluctant to accept acupuncture (Diamond, 1971; Kroeger, 1973; Lau, 1976; Moyers, 1993), although basic science research has documented the phenomenon. Recordings have been made of the electrical flow along the meridians (Becker & Selden, 1985) energy flow along the meridians (Dumitrescu & Kenyon, 1983), and radioisotope flow along meridians (Darras & De Vernejoul, 1986). The physics of "Chi" energy continues to be researched in the West (Fetzer, 1989; Navach, 1989).

An increasing number of physicians outside of China are using acupuncture to treat chronic pain. Approximately 50,000 physicians in Germany, 30,000 in France, and 60,000 in Japan use acupuncture along with drugs, nerve blocks, and other approaches to treat patients with chronic pain. The numbers are much lower in Great Britain and North America, but have increased since the discovery of the acupuncture-endorphine relationship which provided evidence for the neurochemical theory of acupuncture (Pomeranz, 1987). As early as 1973, Lei had proposed the neurological basis of pain and its possible relationship to acupuncture analgesia. Omura (1976, 1978) demonstrated the pathophysiologic mechanisms of acupuncture while Jacobs, Anderson, Bailey, Ottaviano and McCarthy (1977) described the analgesic phenomenon in the limbic and thalmic responses in the brain. Wen and his associates conducted a series of studies which also demonstrated the connection between acupuncture and neurotransmitters (Wen, 1977; Wen, 1980; Wen et al, 1978; Wen et al, 1979; Wen, Ho, Ling & Choa, 1979). A rise in levels of endorphins in human narcotic addicts was shown as early as 1979 (Clement-Jones et al).

The work of Pomeranz and Chieu (1976) provided early evidence of the endorphine mechanisms in acupuncture. Mice, given electrical stimulation at "real" acupuncture points, exhibited higher pain thresholds than mice given "sham" electroacupuncture - stimulation of non-specific points. When "real" acupuncture was followed by naloxone -an opiate antagonist - the analgesic effects were absent, while powerful analgesic effects were found when electroacupuncture was followed by saline (Kroening & Oleson, 1985).

There is a growing body of scientific evidence to explain the behavioral and physiologic effects of acupuncture (All China Society of Acupuncture and Moxibustion, 1984). Since acupuncture reduces opiate withdrawal symptoms in rodents (Ng, Donthill, Thoa & Albert, 1975; Ng, Thoa, Donthill & Albert, 1975) these effects cannot be attributed to suggestibility or placebo effects in human subjects. The action of acupuncture was described in a study entitled "Endorphine release: a possible mechanism of acupuncture analgesia" (Peng, Yang, Kok & Woo, 1978) This was subsequently documented when researchers injected brain and blood serum extracted from rabbits which had received acupuncture into rabbits which had not been acupunctured (Wu & Hsu, 1979). This produced a marked analgesic effect on the recipient rabbits as shown by a significant increase in their pain threshold. The effect was counteracted by naloxone. It was then hypothesized that the release of endorphins is increased by acupuncture stimulation, thereby inhibiting pain. This is similar to the reciprocal relationship between heroin and naloxone.

Electrical stimulation at acupuncture body points has been shown to release endorphins and enkephalins in animals (Pomeranz, 1981). Studies have indicated that serum ACTH and cortisol levels were significantly reduced in human addicts after acupuncture treatment (Wen et al, 1978). Similarities between the mechanisms of acupuncture and morphine analgesia have also been shown (Han, Li & Tang, 1981).

In 1979, endorphine levels were directly measured during acupuncture, demonstrating the elevation of endorphins in cerebral spinal fluid (Han, Tang, Huang, Liang & Zhang, 1979). Cheng and Pomeranz (1979) demonstrated that amino acid and acupuncture produced greater analgesia than either treatment alone and naloxone reversed those effects.

Similar findings have been demonstrated regarding the release of endorphins in humans following auricular acupuncture (Pert et al, 1981). This evidence supports earlier findings that the blockade of the analgesic effect of acupuncture by naloxone establishes the relationship of acupuncture to the endorphine system (Liao, Seto, Saito, Fugita & Kawakami, 1979; Mayer, Price & Raffi, 1977; Peets & Pomeranz, 1978).

Oriental Medicine Model

Acupuncture is part of an Eastern tradition which embraces a systemic/holistic perspective (Macek, 1984; Mann, 1973). Drug dependence is seen as a symptom of a system or society which is out of balance. For a comprehensive overview of the philosophical and historical context of Oriental Medicine, see The Web That Has No Weaver (Kaptchuk, 1983).

The mechanisms of acupuncture detoxification from the perspective of Oriental Medicine can be described metaphorically. The lack of inner calm tone due to intense and frequent use of chemical substances is described as a condition of "empty fire" (Smith, 1985) wherein heat of aggressiveness overcompensates and the calm inner tone is lost.

It is easy to be confused by empty fire and to conclude that the main treatment goal should be sedation of excess fire. Addicts themselves take this approach to the extreme by using sedative drugs. The empty fire condition represents the illusion of power, an illusion that leads to more desperate chemical use and senseless violence. Acupuncture helps patients with this condition by stimulating "yin" points to restore inner calm tone (Smith & Ra, 1985). "Patients often consider these prolonged symptoms as permanent results of their past activities. They are amazed that fresh, clear, youthful life is still possible" (Smith, 1985, p. 3).

According to Traditional Oriental Medicine, the same acupuncture points seem to be effective for various substances of abuse suggesting that the critical energy disturbance is similar regardless of the substance of abuse (Smith, 1989b).

The procedure of stimulating points on the external ear links the ear which is shaped like a fetus or a kidney to kidney function. Frequent repetition of kidney-related ear (auricular) treatments works even with severely debilitated alcoholics and addicts. When the kidney energy has been damaged, the recovery period is slow and undulating in intensity. Even patients with severe paranoia respond well to this protocol. Paranoia involves fear - a kidney related and yin depleted emotion - and a hollow, aggressive ego structure that is an expression of empty fire. The more desperate antagonistic patients who have suffered more yin depletion seem to benefit most from these treatments. "In addition, many socially functioning empty fire patients who may or may not be abusers benefit greatly from these treatments" (p. 2).

Patients with moderate chemical dependency or who have completed most of their recovery from severe addiction do not respond as well to the kidney-ear protocol alone and often need additional body point acupuncture according to the conventional principles of Chinese medicine. The distinction of treatment protocols between moderate and severe abusers is critical. Smith observed (1985) that severe abusers are most in need of better health care and are most resistant to virtually all forms of intervention. By strengthening the kidney, these deficient patients are rehabilitated to return to the commonly expected level of yin function. Severely addicted clients need auricular-kidney treatment before they are able to respond to other forms of acupuncture or psychological and social interventions.

Acupuncture Detoxification Studies

Anecdotal Reports and Clinical Trials

The usefulness of auricular acupuncture to reduce withdrawal symptoms during opiate detoxification was accidentally discovered in 1972 by H.L. Wen (Wen & Cheung, 1973). While administering auricular acupuncture for pain control to a surgical patient who was an opiate addict, the patient reported relief from opioid withdrawal symptoms (Katims et al, 1992). Wen then studied forty opium addicts who were treated with electrostimulation of the lung points on both ears. Sessions ran 15-30 minutes, two or three times a day for the first two or three days and once daily for the next four to five days. Patients were freed of most of the characteristic symptoms of withdrawal such as irritability, runny nose, nervousness, aching bones, and cramps. They were discharged after eight days. Standard medical practice at that time was to gradually withdraw addicts over a three to five month period to prevent occurrence of withdrawal symptoms (Kleber, 1977). Abrupt cessation of opiates -kicking the habit cold turkey - takes several days and is usually accompanied by severe flu-like symptoms (Whitehead, 1978) Therefore, the 8-day length of treatment time was not by itself remarkable. However, of the 22 patients for whom urine samples were available, only two were positive for heroin at follow up. These urine sample results were remarkable as was the observation that craving for opium ceased after acupuncture stimulation.

The discovery that acupuncture with its 3000 year history now had a new application coincided with the several events that marked the opening of the United States to acupuncture. President Richard Nixon traveled to China in 1972. The work of the French physician, Paul Nogier who developed the technique known as auricular medicine utilizing acupuncture points on the ear became available in English. Nogier's discovery of auricular medicine had reached China and was substantiated and embraced there (Kenyon, 1983; Nogier, 1983). The "war on drugs" under Nixon was initiated, focusing on "the heroin plague" (Ford-Geiger, 1986). The reaction to the news of acupuncture as a treatment for heroin addiction was mixed: enthusiasm from those who projected a cure for heroin addiction (Patterson, 1974, 1976), curiosity (Lau, 1976) and wide spread skepticism (Whitehead, 1978).

Following the initial studies by Wen, there were many anecdotal reports of auricular electroacupuncture for detoxification from settings world-wide: Australia (Sainsbury, 1974), Canada (MacQuarrie, 1974), Great Britain (Patterson, 1974, 1976), Italy (Cocchi, Lorini, Fusari & Carrossino, 1979; Lorini, Fazio, Cocchi, Fusari & Roccia, 1979), Malaysia (Heggenhoughen, 1984), Mauritius (Shaowanasai, 1975), Pakistan (Shaiub, 1976), Southeast Asia (Spencer, Heggenhougen & Navaratam, 1980), Thailand (Shaowanasai & Visuthima, 1975), and the United States (Kao & Lu, 1974; Severson, Markhoff & Chun-Hoon, 1977; Smith et al,1979-90; Tennant, 1977).

In an attempt to duplicate the work of Wen and Cheung (1973), a clinical trial of 23 cases was conducted (Kao and Lu, 1974). All patients had previously been on methadone for at least one year and were considered well motivated to terminate methadone maintenance. Detoxification treatment included direct needling of auricular points for cramps, headache, backache, and anxiety. Bilateral electrostimulation was also applied to the lung and heart points. After the first few days of treatment, patients were taught to use the electrical stimulator themselves and could thus regulate the intensity and frequency of their own treatments. As was true in most early studies, treatment was administered in an inpatient hospital setting. Daily urine testing was done to insure that no drugs were being used surreptitiously. The procedure was found to be "extremely successful" (p. 207). However, no summary data was presented. This research was the first to elaborate the concern for the psychological and social aspects required for continued abstinence. The model proposed a multi-faceted program aimed at helping the drug addict achieve a 'lasting cure', including a fully staffed acupuncture clinic to be open 24-hours a day, a full service rehabilitation center and a 24-hour hotline." (pp. 207-208).

Other early trials of electroacupuncture included diverse and contradictory findings. MacQuarrie (1974) reported the work of L. K. Ding of the Discharge Prisoners Aid Society of Hong Kong. After several clinical trials Ding concluded that electroacupuncture by itself was often not sufficient to relieve withdrawal symptoms. He used it on a "voluntary basis" for some patients as well as making it part of his standard treatment in conjunction with methadone withdrawal. Sainsbury (1974) reported a detailed case study of an 18 year old Australian woman withdrawn successfully from heroin by electroacupuncture.

Patterson (1974, 1976), a British surgeon who worked with Wen in Hong Kong and returned to London, observed that electrical stimulation was of greater significance in the treatment than the needling of acupuncture points. She continues to work on the intensity and frequency of the electrical current in electrostimulation treatment (Patterson, 1991).

The use of electrostimulation has been studied more extensively than manual acupuncture, although the latter is more widely used clinically. Researchers using TENS apparatus for symptoms of withdrawal (Gomez & Mikhail, 1974; Patterson, 1991; Smith &

O'Neil, 1975) suggest that it is the electrical frequency used during stimulation rather than the specific acupuncture points stimulated that has greater medicinal effect (Katims et al, 1992). In Honolulu, Severson et al (1977) followed eight outpatient heroin addicts who were administered electrostimulation for four to seven days. Five of these clients were successfully detoxified on a short term basis but only one remained drug free at four-month follow-up.

In a landmark clinical trial, Wen (1977) treated 51 heroin addicts with the combined approach of Auricular-Electrostimulation (AES) plus naloxone. He used the naloxone to flush opiates from receptor sites in the brain, speeding the detoxification process to a few days rather than the three weeks to six months recommended in standard methadone detoxification (Anglin & McGlothlin, 1985). The AES successfully suppressed withdrawal symptoms. Forty-one of the 51 heroin addicts in the study were successfully detoxified. This surpassed AES alone and was more successful than detoxification with methadone. Small amounts of naloxone could suppress acupuncture analgesia. This suggested a similarity in the neurochemical sites of action of acupuncture and heroin, since the pain relief aspect of both could be blocked by naloxone. Wen hypothesized that the pain reducing capacity of acupuncture may be due to the brain releasing endorphins.

Lewenberg (1985) reported a clinical trial on 106 addicts using a combination of treatments. He used electrical stimulation, TENS and medication with small doses of antidepressant and Clonidine - a chemical compound used for treatment of high blood pressure and other medical problems, which was given only to severely addicted patients suffering from chills. Fifty-six attended more than four treatments; 35 of these were heroin users and 21 were methadone users; 33 of these stopped or "substantially reduced" their opiate use by the end of the third week of treatment. Long term recovery recommendations included psycho-social support and lifestyle changes. Although this study had no follow-up and no control group, it has been cited as a rationale against using acupuncture alone by those more supportive of using medications to accomplish detoxification.

In his article "Acupuncture and Addiction: An Overview" Lau (1976) described several addiction treatment programs in Canada which offered auricular electroacupuncture detoxification. Although he mentioned seven locations including several clinics in Toronto and single clinics in North York, Ontario, and Winnipeg, these were anecdotal reports of very few cases. Lau also described a film called "Acupuncture -A Technique for Treating Alcoholism" prepared by D. Kubitz, a psychiatrist, marketed by Faces West Productions, San Francisco.

Staplepuncture, a variation of auricular acupuncture which did not use electrostimulation, was described by Sachs (1975) and Tennant (1977) of Los Angeles. This technique involved the placing of surgical staples on the ears up to six months. Sachs treated 170 cases using the lung points. Eighteen patients were totally detoxified with no withdrawal symptoms, 97 patients were detoxified successfully with minimal remaining symptoms, and 67 patients were unaffected.

A clinical trial that changed the attitude of many Western scientists was conducted at the University of California, Los Angeles [UCLA] Medical School, Department of Anesthesiology Pain Clinic (Kroening & Oleson, 1985). Chronic pain inpatients who had become addicted to opioids were rapidly detoxified using both auricular electroacupuncture and naloxone, the treatment reported by Wen in 1977. Of the 14 subjects in the study, 12 of them (85%) were completely withdrawn from high doses of methadone within 2-7 days. These patients exhibited minimal or no withdrawal symptoms during the detoxification procedure and remained off narcotic medication for follow-up periods of over one year. Although there was no control group, this study showed a higher success rate than previous studies of methadone detoxification (Jaffe, 1985; Kleber, 1977). The authors themselves observed that the subjects studied were inpatient pain patients rather than street addicts which may have accounted for the very positive results.

When Lincoln Clinic was still using electroacupuncture, it reported a study on the largest number of subjects followed up the that time (Shakur & Smith, 1979). More than 3,000 outpatient heroin addicts had been treated by electrostimulation. In follow-up interviews with the first 200 clients, 80% reported that acupuncture relieved some withdrawal symptoms. Long term follow-up was not included.

Smith, Squires, Aponte, Rabinowitz and Bonilla-Rodriguez, (1982) and Smith and Kahn (1988) reported that auricular acupuncture without electrostimulation was successful in the treatment of all substances of abuse including heroin, cocaine, crack cocaine and alcohol.

Most reports of treatment at Lincoln Clinic have been primarily anecdotal, such as the following survey results reported in 1982 (Smith, et al, 1982): (a) 90% relief of symptoms in acute withdrawal clients following acupuncture according to symptom surveys; (b) 90% of all detoxification intake clients returned for further acupuncture treatment with no ancillary incentives such as other medications, welfare credit or probation merits; (c) an estimated 60% of all acupuncture clients receiving the full series of treatments remained drug and alcohol free for at least several months. Smith cited budgetary limitations and an ever-increasing patient load as the reasons no formal statistical studies had been undertaken up to that time. Similarly, Traditional Chinese Medicine [TCM] resists the investment in Western style research at the expense of treatment availability (Ford-Geiger, 1986). In 1990 a placebo control study was completed at Lincoln demonstrating the efficacy of this treatment modality for crack/cocaine addiction (Lipton, Brewington, & Smith, 1990).

The results of manual auricular acupuncture treatment at the Hooper Center in Portland Oregon, a county funded treatment center based on Lincoln Clinic which offers a full spectrum of inpatient and outpatient modalities were reported (Lane, 1988). Acupuncture was used as an adjunct in all phases of treatment. Inpatients receiving acupuncture had a higher detoxification program completion rate than those receiving traditional treatment. Clients interviewed were very positive about remaining substance free and about the role of acupuncture in their efforts. They generally reported great relief of withdrawal symptoms. Acupuncture was also found to be remarkably inexpensive at approximately $2.00 per treatment when added to the existing chemical dependency programs.

Acupuncture has been mentioned frequently in overviews of treatment interventions for addiction. As early as 1974 a letter had appeared in The Lancet describing auricular electroacupuncture as a possible treatment intervention for drug addiction (Tseung, 1974). Whitehead (1978) called for controlled studies and single blind studies which would allow easier evaluation of acupuncture treatment in terms of Western medicine. He criticized the acupuncture clinical trials described up to 1976 for their lack of clarity and follow-up. Lau (1976) in an overview, "Acupuncture and Addiction, " described possible mechanisms of acupuncture and encouraged continued research. Lipton and Maranda (1983) suggested acupuncture detoxification as an entry point to methadone maintenance. Other overviews of treatment which included acupuncture suggested further investigation. (Colvin, 1983; Katmins et al, 1992; Kleber & Riordan 1982; Resnick, 1983.

Auricular acupuncture detoxification has been recognized for its value in AIDS prevention (Konefal, 1989) and appears in a summary of available treatments (Citizens Commission on AIDS, 1989). The Family Therapy Networker featured acupuncture in an issue devoted to the crack epidemic (Morley, 1990).

Many feature stories on acupuncture treatment for chemical dependency have appeared in the lay press and on television. Most of the coverage has focused on Lincoln Clinic. Under the leadership of Michael Smith, M.D., current director of Lincoln Clinic, the program has become a large scale treatment provider and the model for other program throughout the United States and abroad (Lane, 1988; Smith, 1987).

Comparison Studies

Although eagerly examined by a treatment community desperate for a cure for opiate addiction, the shortcomings of the initial report by Wen and Chueng (1973) are representative of the conceptual flaws which continue to plague the literature on acupuncture detoxification. The first report was criticized as "an inadequate and inconclusive clinical trial that suggested a need for further research" (Whitehead, 1978, p. 9). Measured by Western scientific research standards, the following were lacking: (a) there was no control or alternate treatment group; (b) follow-up beyond discharge was unclear, (c) the difference between a "cure" as opposed to reduction of withdrawal symptoms was unclear,(d) severity of addiction (how much, how long), and (e) substances abused (opium vs heroin vs alcohol) were unclear, (f) placebo tests had not yet been done; and (g) there was no comparison of points used. The first and last two issues have been addressed in subsequent research on acupuncture detoxification. The other issues are the same as the methodological problems that need to be addressed in the field of chemical dependency research in general.

Wen and Teo (1974) provided the first comparison study of acupuncture and methadone. In a group of 70 male addicts, half were administered AES to the lung point and the remainder were treated with methadone. Fifty-one percent of the AES group, compared to 28.6% of the methadone group, remained abstinent for one year. They speculated that effectiveness of AES would be considerably higher with follow-up outpatient treatment.

Tennant (1977) observed that while all 18 patients in an auricular staplepuncture group he treated reported significant reduction of withdrawal scores on the first day of treatment, only three of these patients returned for at least five sessions; only one addict was successfully detoxified. Many patients in the methadone comparison group did complete their treatment and 13 were able to be withdrawn from narcotics.

Man and Chuang (1980) concluded that acupuncture was as effective as methadone for detoxification when three of 18 electroacupuncture compared to three of 17 methadone clients were detoxified and remained in treatment.

In the Netherlands, Geerlings, Bos, Schakin and Wouters (1985) compared electrostimulation to oral methadone with a group of 93 heroin addicts admitted to an inpatient drug detoxification unit. More drop-outs were found among electrostimulation patients than methadone detoxification patients. Logistic regression analysis found that electrostimulation was more successful with older, severely addicted female heroin addicts.

A large scale comparison study with an 18-month follow-up was reported by Newmeyer, et al (1984). This outpatient study, conducted at the Haight-Ashbury Free Medical Clinic in San Francisco, compared auricular electroacupuncture detoxification to the combination of auricular electroacupuncture plus medication and to medication only. Of the 460 clients in the initial research sample, only 72 chose auricular electroacupuncture alone. In 30-minute sessions electrostimulation was administered to the lung and *shen-men* ear points. Clients who chose acupuncture were more likely to be white, better educated and employed compared to the general opiate treatment population of San Francisco at the time. In comparison with methadone treatment generally, auricular electroacupuncture clients were more likely to drop out and on readmission were more likely to choose methadone as opposed to choosing acupuncture treatment again. However, auricular electroacupuncture clients exhibited a dramatic improvement compared to the methadone clients in symptomatology and mood states, particularly anxiety and depression. They tended to provide more negative urine tests and self reported less heroin use than the medications group. Cost benefit analysis found that acupuncture detoxification was much less expensive than the medication and counseling combination. The follow-up of successfully detoxified subjects suggested that less severely addicted heroin addicts were more amenable to the auricular electroacupuncture treatment compared to longer term addicts. However, findings at Lincoln Clinic suggest that severely addicted users benefit most from manual auricular acupuncture which helps to restore systemic balance (Smith, 1985).

Many confounding variables shade the outcome of the Haight-Ashbury Clinic study, although it received much attention at the time of its publication and has since been cited as demonstrating that the outcome of acupuncture treatment is questionable. Treatment consisted of electroacupuncture using only two ear points which produced an unexpectedly high level of pain for addicts. The Lincoln Clinic five-point manual acupuncture protocol now in use is relatively painless and has been found much more effective than electroacupuncture (Smith & Kahn, 1988). Acupuncture treatments at the Haight-Ashbury Clinic were also less convenient than medication treatments in terms of time and accessibility. In addition, a peer support component was missing. Clients were seen on an individual basis, missing the group support that was available to those receiving medication and counseling in the control section of the study. Territorial disputes among the staff also contributed to a non-supportive atmosphere. A class phenomenon seemed to exist whereby "middle class whites" responded to acupuncture on an intellectual level while "lower class minority" clients were ostensibly alienated by the approach. The appeal to diverse ethnic communities, particularly to those who are economically disadvantaged has since been substantiated, particularly for the Puerto Rican, African-American, Native American, and Latino communities (Chao, Smith & Davidson, 1990; Clark, 1990; Lane, 1989).

Promising results from a large comparison study have also been reported from Dade County Florida (Konefal, 1990). In an unpublished report of the first phase of a three year study in progress, auricular acupuncture was found to be more beneficial than urine testing alone in treatment of nonpregnant polydrug abusers in the criminal justice system.

Placebo Control Studies

Was the success of acupuncture treatment due to a placebo effect? Studies were needed to address this possibility. Leung (1977) conducted an early placebo study and found that narcotic addicts whose lung points were stimulated with electroacupuncture exhibited fewer withdrawal symptoms than subjects given placebo acupuncture. However, there was such a high dropout rate for both groups that statistical analysis was not possible.

A randomized single blind control study was conducted by researchers at the University of Minnesota (Bullock, Yumen,

Culliton & Olander, 1987). This rigorous placebo study used manual acupuncture detoxification treatment on chronic recidivistic male alcoholics on an inpatient treatment unit. Fifty-four severe alcoholics were randomly assigned to one of two groups. Group I received manual auricular acupuncture on points specific to the treatment of addiction (*shen-men*, lung, kidney or liver) and two wrist points (hoku and weiguan). Group II received sham manual auricular acupuncture on points known to have no relation to relief of withdrawal symptoms. Treatment was divided into three phases: Phase I -daily treatment for five days; Phase II -three treatments per week for 28 days; Phase III -treatment twice per week for 45 days. Thirty-seven percent of the treatment group (N=10) compared to 7.4% of the control group (N=2), completed all three phases of the study. There were highly significant differences between the two groups across all treatment phases on self assessment of desire to drink, number of drinking episodes and readmission for subsequent redetoxification. The study also confirmed earlier observations that acupuncture detoxification was cost effective: overhead costs were low, minimal equipment was needed, and many patients were treated simultaneously by one acupuncturist (Clark, 1990).

A second larger placebo study was conducted by Bullock, Culliton and Olander (1989) and reported in The Lancet. This study of 80 subjects employed a single blind random assignment design to compare sham and real manual auricular acupuncture in the treatment of recidivistic chronic male alcoholic inpatients. The treatment for this second trial was divided into slightly different phases: Phase I - five times a week for two weeks; Phase II - three times a week for four weeks; and Phase III -twice a week for two weeks. The completion rate was higher for this study than for the pilot: 21 (52.3%) of the 40 patients in the treatment group completed all phases of the program compared to one (2.5%) of the 40 controls. Only three (7.5%) treatment patients left the program during Phase I; 19 (47.5%) control patients terminated treatment during the first phase. This was a very high dropout rate among the control patients despite the promise of incentive payments. At six month follow-up, six of the 21 patients in the treatment group who had completed the program reported that they had not taken any alcohol in the interim. In addition, none had been readmitted to the detoxification center, whereas 39 control patients and all treatment patients who had failed to complete the program reported drinking episodes. Cost effectiveness was again found to be significant. The encouraging results in program retention with the acupuncture treatment group suggested a valuable treatment tool had been found for this difficult recidivistic population.

Another large control study of acupuncture treatment, this time comparing acupuncture and methadone in relation to heroin addiction, was reported August 15, 1990, from the MIRA Outpatient Clinic at Bayview Hunter's Point, San Francisco (Clark, 1990). This one and one half year study, commissioned by the California State Legislature has not yet been published but the results have been reported to the State Legislature. Newmeyer participated as one of the co-investigators on this study addressing many of the issues raised by Newmeyer et al (1984). The first phase of the study sought to assess the efficacy of manual auricular acupuncture, using a randomized single blind placebo design similar to the Bullock studies (1987; 1989). During the 21 day detoxification trial, 100 subjects were followed for withdrawal signs and symptoms, as well as attendance patterns and periodic urine testing. The treatment group, which received authentic auricular acupuncture, attended the clinic more days and stayed in treatment significantly longer than the control group, which received sham auricular acupuncture. Sixteen treatment as opposed to four control subjects remained in the study beyond 21 days. However, fewer than 25% of the treatment group remained in the study beyond two weeks and only 33% of this group produced negative urine tests at 15 days.

After this comparison was completed, another 50 addicts were recruited and treated using true acupuncture points for phase two of the study. This second phase compared clients choosing acupuncture detoxification to clients choosing methadone detoxification. Cross sectional comparison was made of demographic characteristics and treatment patterns of all detoxification clients choosing acupuncture treatment compared to all detoxification clients choosing methadone or other treatment modalities throughout San Francisco during the time of the study. Participants choosing acupuncture tended to be older. A higher proportion was African-American, as opposed to the earlier findings of Newmeyer et al (1984).

The study's third phase investigated the treatment outcome of acupuncture compared to methadone detoxification. Thirty-three acupuncture and 30 methadone clients were compared as to urine test results and self reports at the end of 30 days. Nine of the acupuncture clients, or 27%, and three of the methadone clients, or 10%, had negative urines. Of the acupuncture clients with positive urine tests, 54% were positive for heroin and 21% for cocaine. Similarly, for the methadone clients who tested positive, 62% tested positive for heroin although they were receiving methadone maintenance and 21% tested positive for cocaine. Only one subject, an acupuncture client, reported no use of drugs or alcohol in the 30 day period prior to follow-up. It was concluded that auricular acupuncture clients did at least as well as methadone clients at follow-up. Acupuncture clients were more likely to have negative urinalyses and report longer periods of abstinence with fewer problem days than their methadone controls. This was especially significant because methadone treatment has several drawbacks not found with acupuncture: methadone is an addictive drug, has side-effects and is teratogenic (Cregler & Mark, 1986).

Clients reported the following responses to acupuncture detoxification: they felt relaxed and comfortable during the 20 to 40 minutes of the procedure, treatment prevented withdrawal symptoms for about eight hours with effects lasting increasingly longer as days in treatment increased, and at one week they felt less irritable and their thinking was more clear. Clients with many previous detoxification experiences using other treatment modalities appreciated the simplicity of the acupuncture treatment. They felt they were not "just trading one addiction for another" as was the case with methadone maintenance (Washburn, Kennan &

Nazareno, 1990). Finally, clients reported that the group setting, where as many as 40 people were seen at one time, was their one consistently positive social interaction and found it a pleasant way to begin the day.

Crack/cocaine users were the focus of a placebo control experiment designed by Lipton et al (1990) following the protocol established by Bullock et al (1989). One hundred fifty subjects were randomly assigned to received experimental acupuncture or placebo acupuncture only in an outpatient setting for one month. Although it usually recommended that acupuncture treatment be administered in conjunction with counseling and other recovery services, for the purposes of research clarity these subjects received acupuncture only. Outcome measures included urinalysis profiles, self reports including the Addiction Severity Index (McLellan, Luborsky, O'Brien & Woody, 1980) and treatment retention. Urinalysis results indicated that after two weeks of treatment experimental subjects had significantly lower cocaine metabolite levels than the placebo controls subjects. The researchers noted that "no specific pharmacologic treatment for cocaine abuse is currently widely used or generally recognized as effective" (p. 27). They further observed that acupuncture seems to be the most widely used medical treatment for crack/cocaine abuse in New York City. Lincoln Clinic alone has treated more than 8,000 such patients.

Studies Regarding Pregnant Addicts.

Although no research has been published as yet specific to acupuncture detoxification of pregnant women, one recent pilot program demonstrated the success of acupuncture treatment with substance abusing pregnant women. Fifteen cocaine addicted women receiving treatment during pregnancy at a high risk prenatal clinic at Columbia Presbyterian Hospital in New York City were treated with acupuncture for chemical dependency. They all received at least five prenatal care visits as well as supportive counseling. When the birth weights of infants born to these women were compared to birth weights of fifteen infants born to women who received comparable care without the acupuncture treatment, the birth weights in the treatment group were found to be significantly higher than those who did not receive acupuncture, 3400 grams compared to 2800 grams. The women who did not originally receive acupuncture due to its unavailability at their particular clinic in the multilevel structure of clinics at this hospital chose to receive acupuncture after delivery (M. Smith, M.D. personal communication, October 23, 1992).

Another study of pregnant substance abusers receiving acupuncture treatment is currently underway at Saint Raphael's Hospital in New Haven, CT. More than 300 women have been treated, with only 50 having positive drug toxicologies at delivery. There have been no untoward effects from the acupuncture, no deaths, and no Intensive Care Unit [ICU] admissions (W. Rugero, personal communication, February 11, 1992).

In 1989 an outcome study on postpartum women was reported (Chao et al, 1989). The treatment of 290 postpartum substance abusing women whose babies had been held in the hospital because of positive cocaine toxicologies at delivery yielded positive results. Seventy percent of all postpartum referrals attended acupuncture treatment and counseling on the prescribed schedule for at least two consecutive weeks. Fifty percent of all referrals provided an average of ten or more negative daily urine tests. It was on this basis that more than half of the infants retained at the hospital after delivery due to the addiction of the mother -boarder-babies -were returned to the custody of their mothers. Women who were referred immediately postpartum had significantly fewer positive urine tests than women referred two months or more after delivery. The latter group had only a 37% return of infants as opposed to 58% in the entire sample. The savings in foster care expenses alone make this a compelling treatment consideration.

Two innovative perinatal substance abuse treatment programs incorporating acupuncture as a primary treatment component have been recognized for their clinical success.

The first, the Maternal Substance Abuse Acupuncture Services of Lincoln Hospital, an outpatient clinic established in 1986, treats primarily crack/cocaine dependent women. They have developed a six-week program and a six month protocol for the 80% of their clients who are referred by the Child Welfare Administration. According to director Nancy Small, the program recognizes that "women are busy people" (Ackerman, 1992), the program is organized so that clients need be in the clinic no longer than two hours per day. In depth counseling is provided after ten days of negative urine toxicologies. Counseling, 12-Step meetings, "Women's Rap Group" group education/discussion sessions and parenting classes are all mandatory treatment components. The success rate with court referred clients, defined as drug free for at least two months is greater than 50% (AHA, 1991).

The second program, the Ramsey County Maternal/Child Project, is located in St. Paul, MN. This unique program provides acupuncture treatment for its clients in their own home as well as in a group/clinic setting. Based on a family preservation model, treatment is provided for twelve weeks or more in the home by a team which includes the acupuncturist, child protection specialist, family therapist, chemical dependency counselor and a public health nurse. In this way all the members of the woman's immediate support environment can be addressed. The prevention impact of these services has been widely recognized and results in a reduction in emergency use of medical and social services not only for the identified client but also for the extended family. A program modeled on this protocol has recently been licensed as a institutional care provider, although all services are all home-based, and is contracting with private insurance companies as well as public social service agencies (K. Ganley, personal communication, October 3, 1992).

The literature regarding acupuncture detoxification has revealed many anecdotal clinical reports, comparison studies, and four recent placebo control studies. In the early studies, two auricular acupuncture points (lung and *shen-men*) were treated by electrostimulation. Electroacupuncture was found to be only moderately satisfactory. It was also expensive, since electroacupuncture involved costly equipment and was usually administered on an inpatient basis. In more recent studies, manual stimulation of three to five-points (*shen-men*, sympathetic, kidney, liver and lung) has been used with greater clinical and cost effectiveness. Reports on perinatal application of acupuncture treatment were also described, including two scientific control studies not yet published. Documentation of this ground swell/grass roots treatment phenomenon is clearly progressing

References:

Academy of Traditional Chinese Medicine. (1975). *An outline of acupuncture.* Peking: Foreign Language Press.

Ackerman, R. (1992)*. *Treating pregnant and postpartum substance abusing women with acupuncture for detoxification, preparation for counseling and relapse prevention.* (Video: available from 2417 Castillo St. Santa Barbara, CA 93105).

All-China Society of Acupuncture and Moxibustion. (1984). *The second national symposium on acupuncture and moxibustion and acupunctuure anesthesia.* Bejing, China: Author

American Hospital Association (1991). *Hospital and community partnerships: prenatal, infant care, and pediatric models for underserved women* (Available from The American Hospital Association. 840 North Lake Shore Drive, Chicago, IL. 60611).

Anglin, M. D. (1989). Alcohol use by heroin addicts: Evidence for an inverse relationship. *American Journal of Drug and Alcohol Abuse*, 15, 191-207.

Anglin, M.D., & McGlothlin, W. H. (1985). Methadone maintenance in California. In L. Brill & C. Winick (Eds.) *The Yearbook of Substance Use and Abuse*, 3 (pp. 219-280). New York: Human Science Press.

Barbor, T. F., Stephens R.S., & Marlatt, G.A. (1987). Verbal report methods in clinical research on alcoholism: Response bias and its minimization. *Journal of Studies on Alcohol*, 48, (5), 410-424.

Becke, H. (1988, October). Dangerous acupuncture points in pregnancy. *Deutsche Zeitschrift fur Akupunktur*, 5, 110-111.

Becker, R.O. & Selden, G. (1985). *The Body Electric*. New York: William Morrow.

Blum, K. (1990). *Alcohol and the addictive brain*. The New Free Press News.

Blum, K. (1990, September-October). The 'Alcoholic' Gene. *Professional Counselor*.

Bullock, M.L., Culliton, P.D., & Olander, R.T. (1989, June 24). Controlled trial of acupuncture for severe recidivistic alcoholism. *The Lancet*, 1435-439.

Bullock, M.L., Ymen, A.J., Culliton, P.D., & Olander, R.T. (1987, May-June). Acupuncture treatment of alcoholic recidivism: A pilot study. *Alcoholism: Clinical and Experimental Research*, 11(3), 292-295.

Chao, C.E., Smith, M.O., & Davidson, R. (1989). *Evaluation of the effectiveness of acupuncture on maternal substance abuse clients*. New York: New York City Department of Health, Health Research Training Program.

Chaudron, C., & Wilkinson, D. (Eds.) (1988). *Theories on Alcoholism*. Toronto: Addiction Research Foundation.

Cheng, R.S., & Pomeranz, B. (1979). Electroacupuncture analgesia could be mediated by at least two pain-relieving mechanisms: Endorphin and non-endorphin systems. *Life Sciences*, 2, 1957-1962.

Clark, W. (1990, August 15). Trial of acupuncture detoxification (TRIAD). Final report (Available from California State Legislature).

Clement-Jones, V., McLoughlin, L., Lowry, P.J., Bresser, G.M., Rees, L.H., & Wen, H.L. (1979). Acupuncture in heroin addicts: Changes in met-enkephalin and beta-endorphin in blood and cerebrospinal fluid. *Lancet* 2, 380-383.

Cocchi, R., Lorini, G., Fusari, A. & Carrossino, R. (1979). Experience with detoxification and weaning of heroin addicts by means of acupuncture, gabergic drugs and psychopharmalogic agents in low doses. *Minerva Med.* 70(24), 1735-1744.

Colvin, M. (1983, January - June). A counseling approach to outpatient benzodiazapine detoxification. *Journal of Psychoactive Drugs*, 15(1-2), 105-108.

Cosser, M.H., Brower, K.J., & Bersford, T.P. (1990, April). Treatment of alprazolam withdrawal with substitution and gradual reduction of chloridazepoxide. Paper presented at the annual meeting of the American Society for Addiction Medicine, Phoenix, AZ.

Cregler, L.L. & Mark, H. (1986). Medical complications of drug abuse. *New England Journal of Medicine*, 315, 1495-1500.

Dackis, C.A. & Gold, M.S. (1985). New concepts in cocaine addiction: The dopamine depletion hypothesis. *Neuroscience and Bio-Behavioral Reviews*, 9, 469-477.

Dackis, C.A., Gold, M.S., Sweeney, D.R., Byron, J.P., & Climko, R. (1987). Single dose bromacriptine reverses cocaine craving. *Psychiatric Research*, 20, 261-264.

Darras & De Vernejoul. (1986). *Visualization of acupuncture pathways*. World Research Foundation Congress of Bio-Energetic Medicine. Los Angeles. Video Tape.

Diamond, E. (1971). Acupuncture anesthesia. *Journal of American Medical Association*, 218, 1558-1563.

Donovan, D. & Marlatt, G. (1988). *Assessment of Addictive Behaviors*. NY: Guildford Press.

Donovan, D. (1988). Assessment of addictive behaviors: Implications of an emerging biopsychosocial model. In D. Donovan & G. Marlatt (Eds.) *Assessment of addictive behaviors* (pp. 3-50). New York: Guilford Press.

Dumitrescu, I., & Kenyon, J. (1983). *Electrographic imaging in medicine and biology*. Sudbury, Suffolk, Great Britain: Neville Spearman Limited.

Fetzer Foundation. (1989). *Energy fields in medicine: A study of device technology based on acupuncture meridians and chi energy.* Kalamazoo, MI: John E. Fetzer Foundation.

Fingarette, H. (1988). *Heavy drinking*. Berkeley: University of California Press.

Finnegan, L.P., Connaughton, J.F., Emich, J.P. & Wieland, W.F. (1972). Comprehensive care of the pregnancy addict and its effect on maternal and infant outcome. *Contemporary Drug Problems: I*, 794-81

Fitzgerald, K.W. (1988). *Alcoholism: The genetic inheritance*. NY: Doubleday.

Ford-Geiger, E. (1986). *The psychotherapeutic utilization of acupuncture* (Doctoral dissertation, University of Massachusetts).

Frances, R. (1989). *Concise Guide To Treatment of Alcoholism and Addictions*. Washington, D.C.: American Psychiatric Press.

Frawley, P.J. (1990, April 23). Private sector research studies on alcoholism treatment. Paper presented at the meeting of the American Society of Addiction Research Medicine Symposium, Phoenix, AZ.

Gawin, F. H. (1988). Chronic neuropharmacology of cocaine: Progress in pharmacotherapy. *Journal of Clinical Psychiatry*, 49, 11-16.

Gawin, F.H., & Ellinwood, E., Jr. (1989) Cocaine and other stimulates: Action, abuse and treatment. *New England Journal of Medicine*, 318, 1173-1182.

Gawin, F.H., & Kleber, H.D. (1986b). *Medical management of cocaine withdrawal*. New Haven, CT: APT Foundation.

Geerlings, P.J., Bos, T.W., Schakin, H.F., & Wouters, L.F. (1985). Detoxification of heroin addicts with electrostimulation or methadone. *Tijdschrift Voor Alcohol, Drugs, En Andere Psychotrope Stoffen*, 11(2), 80-85.

Gold, M.S., Washton, A., & Dackis, C.A. (1985). Cocaine abuse, neurochemistry, phenomenology and treatment. In N.J. Kozel & E.H. Adams (Eds.). *Cocaine use in America: Epidemiologic and clinical perspectives*. (NIDA Research Monograph No. 61.) U.S. Government Printing Office, Washington, D.C.

Goleman, D. (1990, July 7). Drug addiction linked to brain irregularities. *Santa Barbara News Press*, p. A15.

Gomez, E. & Mikhail, A. (1974). Treatment of methadone withdrawal with cerebral electrotherapy (electrosleep). Paper presented at the annual meeting of the American Psychiatric Association, Detroit, MI.

Han, J., Li, S., & Tang, J. (1981). Tolerance to electroacupuncture and its cross tolerance to morphine. *Neuropharmacology*, 6, 593-596.

Han, J., Tang, J., Huang, B., Liang, X. & Zhang, N. (1979). Acupuncture tolerance in rats: Antiopiate substrate implicated. *Chinese Medical Journal*, 9(9), 625-627.

Hayshiada, M., Alterman, A., McLellan, T., O'Brien, C., Purtill, J., Volpicelli, J., Raphaelson, A. & Hall, C. (1989, February 9). Comparative effectiveness and costs of in-patient and out-patient detoxification of patients with mild to moderate alcohol withdrawal syndrome. *New England Journal of Medicine*, 320(6), 358-365.

Heggenhougen, H.K. (1984). Traditional medicine and the treatment of drug addicts: three examples from Southeast Asia. *Medical Anthropology Quarterly*, 16(1), 3-7.

Jacobs, S., Anderson, G., Bailey, S., Ottaviano, J. & McCarthy, V. (1977). Neurophysiological correlates of acupuncture: Limbic and thalamic responses to analgesic studies in nonhuman primates. *Journal of Life Sciences*, 7(3), 37-42.

Jaffe, J.H. (1985). Drug addiction and drug abuse. In A. Goodman, L.S. Goodman, & Y. Gilman (Eds.) *The Pharmacological Basis of Therapeutics*, 7th ed. (pp.550-554). New York: MacMillan.

Kao, A. H. & Lu, L.Y.C. (1974). Acupuncture procedure for treating drug addiction. *American Journal of Acupuncture*, 2: 201-207.

Kaptchuk, T. (1983). *The web that has no weaver: Understanding Chinese medicine*. New York: Congdon and Weed.

Katims, J.J., Ng, L.K.Y., & Lowinson, J.H. (1992). Acupuncture and transcutaneous electrical nerve stimulation: Afferent nerve stimulation (ANS) in the treatment of addiction. In J. H. Lowinson, P. Ruiz, R.B. Millman & J. G. Langrod (Eds.), *Substance abuse: A comprehensive textbook* (pp. 574-583). Philadelphia: Williams & Wilkins.

Kaufman, E., & McNaul, I. P. (1992). Recent development in understanding and treating drug abuse and dependence. *Hospital and Community Psychiatry*, 43 (3), 223-236.

Keenan, P. (1990, February). Treatment of pregnant substance abusers. Paper presented at the National Acupuncture Detoxification Association Conference, Research Subsection, Miami, Florida.

Kenyon, J. (1983). *Modern techniques of acupuncture, volume 2: A practical scientific guide to electroacupuncture.* New York: Thorsons Publishers Limited.

Kleber, H. (1977). Detoxification from methadone maintenance: The state of the art. *International Journal of Addiction,* 12, 897-920.

Kleber, H.D. & Riordan, C.E. (1982, June). The treatment of narcotic withdrawal: Historical review. *Journal of Clinical Psychiatry* 43, 30-34.

Konefal, J. (1989, March 10). Drug abuse detoxification study for risk behavior of aids. Grant application to the Department of Health and Human Services, Public Health Service (Available from Dept. of Psychiatry, University of Miami, Miami, FL).

Konefal, J. (1990, September). Acupuncture program services: Mid-year progress report - 1990 (Available from University of Miami, School of Medicine, Dept. of Psychiatry, Miami, FL.).

Kosten, T. R. (1989, July). Pharmacotherapeutic interventions for cocaine abuse: Matching patients to treatment. *J. Of Nervous and Mental Disease,* 177 (7), 379-389.

Kosten, T.R., Kleber, H.D. & Morgan, C. (1989). Treatment of cocaine abuse with buprenorphine. *Biologic Psychiatry,* 26, 637-639.

Kroening, R.J., & Oleson, T.D. (1985). Rapid narcotic detoxification in chronic pain patients treated with auricular electroacupuncture and naloxone. *The International Journal of the Addictions,* 20,(9), 1347-1360.

Kroger, W.S. (1973). The scientific rationale for acupunctural analgesia. *Psychosomatics* 14(4), 191-194.

Lane, C.A. (1988). Final evaluation report: Acupuncture detoxification research demonstration project (Available from Alcohol and Drug Program, Multnomah County, Oregon).

Lau, M.P. (1976). Acupuncture and addiction: An overview. *Addictive Diseases,* 2, 449-463.

Lei, C. (1973). Neurological basis of pain and its possible relationship to acupuncture analgesia. *American Journal of Chinese Medicine,* 1, 61-72.

Leung, A.J.H. (1977). Acupuncture treatment and withdrawal symptoms. *American Journal of Acupuncture,* 5, 43-50.

Lewenberg, A. (1985). The utility of acupuncture in combination with antidepressants or clonidine in the treatment of opiate addiction. *Advances in Therapy,* 2(4), 143-149.

Liao, Y.Y., Seto, K., Saito, H., Fugita, M., & Kawakami, M. (1979). Effects of acupuncture on adrenocortical hormone production: I. Variation in the ability for adrenocortical production for the duration of acupuncture stimulation. *American Journal of Chinese Medicine,*(4), 362-371.

Lipton, D.S., & Miranda, M.J. (1983). Detoxification from heroin dependency: an overview of method and effectiveness. *Evaluation of Drug Treatment Programs.* (pp. 31-55). New York: The Haworth Press.

Lipton, D.S., Brewington, V. & Smith, M.O. (1990). Acupuncture and crack addicts: A single blind placebo test of efficacy. Paper presented at the National Institute on Drug Abuse (NIDA). Technical review meeting, Advances in Cocaine Treatment. National Institutes of Health Campus. Bethesda, MD.

Lorini, G., Fazio, L., Cocchi, R., Fusari, A. & Roccia, L. (1979). Acupuncture as a part of a program of detoxification and weaning from opiates: 25 cases. *Minerva Medica,* 70(56), 3831-3836.

Lowinson, J. H., Ruiz, P. Millman, R. B., & Langrod, J. G. (Eds.). (1992). *Substance abuse: A comprehensive textbook.* Philadelphia: Williams & Wilkins.

Macek, C. (1984, January 27). East meets west to balance immunologic yin and yang. *Journal of the American Medical Association,* 251(4), 433-439.

MacQuarrie, L. (1974). In Hong Kong, acupuncture: It still has a place. *J. of Addictions Research Foundation of Ontario,* 3 (11) 10.

Man, P.L., & Chuang, M.Y. (1980). Acupuncture in methadone withdrawal. *International Journal of Addiction,* 15, 921-926.

Mann, F. (1973). Acupuncture: *The ancient Chinese art of healing and how it works scientifically.* New York: Vintage Books.

Mayer, D.J., Price, D.D., & Raffi, A. (1977). Antagonism of acupuncture and analgesia in man by the narcotic antagonist naloxone. *Brain Research,* 121, 368-372.

McLellan, A., Luborsky, L., O'Brien, C., & Woody, G. (1980). An Improved Evaluation Instrument for Substance Abuse Patients: The Addiction Severity Index. *Journal of Nervous and Mental Diseases,* 1968. 26-33.

Morley, J. (1990, November-December). The War on Crack: Deescalating the War. *Family Therapy Networker,* 14 (6), 24-36.

Moyers, W. (1993). *Healing and the mind.* NY: Doubleday.

Navach, J. (1989). Thermodynamic, biochemical and electromagnetic views of chi. *Energy Fields in Medicine: A Device Technology Based on Acupuncture Meridians and Chi Energy,* 193-122. The John E. Fetzer Foundation, 929 West KL Avenue, Kalamazoo, Michigan 49009.

Newmeyer, J.A., Johnson, G., & Klot, S. (1984, July-September). Acupuncture as a detoxification modality. Journal of Psychoactive Drugs, 16(3), 241-261.

Ng, L.K.Y., Donthill, T.C., Thoa, N.B. & Albert, C.A. (1975a). Modification of morphine syndrome in rats following transauricular electrostimulation: An experimental paradigm for auricular electroacupuncture. *Biological Psychiatry,* 10, 575-580.

Ng, L.K.Y., Thoa, N.B,, Donthill, T.C., & Albert, C.A. (1975b). Experimental "auricular electroacupuncture" in morphine dependent rats: behavioral and biochemical observations. *American Journal of Chinese Medicine*, 3, 335-341.

Nogier, P.F.M. (1983). *From Auriculotherapy to Auriculomedicine*. Sainte-Ruffine, France: Maisonneuve.

Omura, Y. (1976). Patho-physiology of acupuncture effects, ACTH and brain morphine-like substances, pain, phantom sensations (phantom pain, itch and coldness), brain micro-circulation, and memory. *Acupuncture and Electrotherapeutics Res.*, International Journal, 2, 1-31.

Omura, Y. (1978). Pain threshold measurement before and after acupuncture. *Acupuncture and Electro Therapeutic Research*, 3, 1-22.

Patterson, M.A. (1974). Electroacupuncture and alcohol and drug addictions. *Clinical Medicine*, 81, 9-13.

Patterson, M.A. (1976). Effects of neuroelectric therapy (N.E.T.) in drug addiction: Interim report. *Bulletin of Narcotics*, 28, 55-62.

Patterson, M.A. (1991). Neuroelectric therapy: the new approach to drug treatment, and its scientific basis. Paper presented at the first annual meeting of the Subtle Energies and Energy Medicine Society. (pp.76-79) (Available from the International Society for the Study of Subtle Energies and Energy Medicine. First Annual Conference. June 21-25, 1991. Boulder, CO).

Peets, J.M. & Pomeranz, B. (1978). CXBK-mice deficient in opiate receptors show poor electro-acupuncture analgesia. *Nature*, 273, 675-676.

Peng, C.H., Yang, M.M., Kok, S.H., & Woo, Y.K. (1978). Endorphin release: A possible mechanism of acupuncture analgesia. *Comparative Medicine East and West*, 6(1), 57-60.

Pert, A., Dionne, R., Ng, L., Bragin, E., Moody, T.W. & Pert, C.B. (1981). Alterations in rat central nervous system endorphins following transauricular electroacupuncture. *Brain Research*, 224, 83-93.

Pittman, L. (1992). Acupuncture detoxification for homeless substance abusers. Report for the Department of Human Resources, Jersey City, NJ.

Pomeranz, B. & Chieu, D. (1976). Naloxone blockade of acupuncture analgesia: Endorphin implicated. *Life Sciences*, 19, 1757-1762.

Pomeranz, B. (1981). Neural mechanisms of acupuncture and analgesia. In S. Lipton & J. Miles (Eds.). *Persistent Pain, Modern Methods of Treatment*. (pp. 241-257). London: Academic Press.

Pomeranz, B. (1987). Acupuncture neurophysiology. In G. Adelman (Ed.) *Encyclopedia of Neuroscience, I* (pp. 6-7). Boston: Brikhauser.

Resnick, R. (1983). Methadone detoxification from illicit opiates and methadone maintenance. *New York College Division of Drug Abuse and*

Treatment, National Institute on Drug Abuse: Treatment and Research Monographs, (No. 83-1281), 160-167.

Sachs, L.L. (1975). Drug addiction, alcoholism, smoking, obesity treated by auricular staplepuncture. *American Journal of Acupuncture*, 3, (2), 147-150.

Sainsbury, M.J. (1974). Acupuncture in heroin withdrawal. *Medical Journal of Australia*, 3, 102-105.

"Scientists say enzyme could combat cocaine" (1993, March 26). *Santa Barbara News Press*.

Severson, L., Markoff, R.A. & Chun-Hoon, H. (1977). Heroin detoxification with acupuncture and electrical stimulation. *International Journal of Addiction*, 12, 911-922.

Shaffer, H. (1986). Conceptual crises and the addictions: Philosophy of science perspective. *Journal of Substance Abuse Treatment*, 3, 285-296.

Shaiub, M. (1976). Acupuncture treatment of drug dependence in Pakistan. *American Journal of Chinese Medicine*, 4, 403-407.

Shakur, M., & Smith, M. (1979). The use of acupuncture in the treatment of drug addiction. *American Journal of Acupuncture*, 7, 223-234.

Shanghai College of Traditional Medicine. (1981). *Acupuncture: A comprehensive text*. J. O'Connor & D. Bensky, (Eds.). Chicago: Eastland Press.

Shaowanasai, A. & Visuthima, H. (1975). Acupuncture and the treatment of heroin addiction. Paper presented at the 31st International Congress on Alcoholism and Drug Dependence: Bangkok, Thailand.

Shaowanasai, A. (1975). Report on acupuncture detoxification in Mauritius. In P. Bourne (Ed.). *Acupuncture and the Detoxification of Opiate Addicts*. Unpublished report. Washington, D.C.: Drug Abuse Council.

Smith, M. (1987). Acupuncture Treatment for Substance Abuse (Available from Lincoln Hospital Division of Substance Abuse, 349 East 140th Street, Bronx, NY 10454).

Smith, M. (1989a, November). The Challenge of Treating Maternal Substance Abuse. National Acupuncture Detoxification Association, 3115 Broadway #51, New York, New York 10027.

Smith, M. O. (1989b, July 5). The Lincoln Hospital Drug Abuse Program. Testimony Presented to the Select Committee on Narcotics of the House of Representatives of the United States. Washington, DC.

Smith, M. O., Alvarez, C. & Smalls, N. (1987, September 10). Criminal justice referrals to acupuncture detoxification: Pilot program shows encouraging results (Available from Substance Abuse Division, Lincoln Hospital, Bronx, NY).

Smith, M.O. (1979). Acupuncture and natural healing in drug detoxification. *American Journal of Acupuncture*, 7, 97-107.

Smith, M.O. (1985). Chinese theory of acupuncture detoxification. *American Journal of Acupuncture*, 13(4), 386-387.

Smith, M.O. (1988a, April 11). Acupuncture as a treatment for drug dependent mothers: Testimony presented to the New York City Council, New York, NY.

Smith, M.O. (1988b). Acupuncture treatment for crack: clinical survey of 1,500 patients. *American Journal of Acupuncture*, 16(3), 241-247.

Smith, M.O. (1988c). The pregnant substance abuser: Recognizing and treating the patient (Available from March of Dimes Birth Defect Foundation, Greater New York Chapter, 233 Park Avenue South, New York, New York 10003).

Smith, M.O. (1990a, September). NADA Newsletter, 1-3 (Available through Lincoln Hospital, Maternal Substance Abuse Services. 349 East 140th Street, Bronx, New York 10454).

Smith, M.O. (1990b, September). The Miami success story: Transforming the criminal justice system with an acupuncture based diversion program. National Acupuncture Detoxification Association Newsletter, 1-3 (Available from NADA, 3115 Broadway, #51, New York, New York 10027).

Smith, M.O. (1990c). Raising Healthy Babies for the 90's (Available through [Lincoln Hospital, Maternal Substance Abuse Services, 349 East 140th Street, Bronx, New York 10454).

Smith, M.O., & Khan, I. (1988). An acupuncture programme for the treatment of drug-addicted persons. *Bulletin on Narcotics*, XL(1), 35-41.

Smith, M.O., & Ra, K. (1985, July 22-26). Acupuncture and the treatment of chemical dependency and violence. Paper presented at the Caribbean Mental Health Conference, Nassau, Bahamas.

Smith, M.O., Squires, R., Aponte, J., Rabinowitz, N., & Bonilla-Rodriguez, R. (1982). Acupuncture treatment of drug addiction and alcohol abuse. *American Journal of Acupuncture*, 10(2), 161-163.

Smith, R. B., O'Neil, L.O. (1975). Electrosleep in the management of alcoholism. *Biological Psychiatry*, 10 (B), 675-680.

Spencer, C.P., Heggenhougen, H.K., & Navaratam, V. (1980). *American Journal of Chinese Medicine* 8(3), 230-238.

Summer, G.L. (1990, April). Cocaine treatment: The first twelve months (Available from Hanley-Hazelden Center, Saint Mary's Hospital, P. O. Box 4424, West Palm Beach FL 14302).

Tennant, F.S. (1977). Outpatient heroin detoxification with acupuncture and staplepuncture. *Western Journal of Medicine*, 125, 141-144.

Trachtenberg, M. and Blum, K. (1988). Improvements of cocaine induced neuromodulator deficits by the neuronutrient Tropamine. *Journal of Psychoactive Drugs*, 20(3), July-September.

Wallace, J. (1989,June). A biopsychosocial model of alcoholism. *Social Casework*, 70(6), 325-332.

Washburn, A.N., Keenan, P.A., & Nazareno, J.P. (1990). Preliminary findings: Study of acupuncture assisted detoxification. *MIRA Newsletter* (Available from Bay View Hunters Point Foundation for Community Improvement, U.C.S.F. Center for Aids Prevention Studies, P.O. Box 0886, University of California, San Francisco, CA 94143).

Wen, H.L. & Cheung, S.Y.C. (1973). Treatment of drug addiction by acupuncture and electrical stimulation. *Asian Journal of Medicine*, 9, 138-141.

Wen, H.L. (1977). Fast detoxification of heroin addicts by acupuncture and electrical stimulation (AES) in combination with naloxone. *Comp. Med. East-West*, 5, 257-263.

Wen, H.L. (1980, Winter). Clinical experience and mechanisms of acupuncture and electrical stimulation (AES) in the treatment of drug abuse. *American Journal of Chinese Medicine*, 8(4), 349-353.

Wen, H.L., & Teo, S.W. (1974). Experience in the treatment of drug addiction by electroacupuncture. *Modern Medicine of Asia*, 11, 23-24.

Wen, H.L., Ho, W.K., Wong, H.K., Mehal, Z.D., Ng, Y.H. & Ma, L. (1979). Changes in adrenocorticotropic hormone (ACTH) and cortisol levels in drug addicts treated by a new and rapid detoxification procedure during acupuncture and naloxone. *Comp. Med. East-West*, 6(3), 241-245.

Wen, H.L., Ho, W.K.K., Ling, N., Ma, L. & Choa, G.H. (1979). The influence of electroacupuncture on naloxone induced morphine withdrawal. II. Elevation of immunoassayable beta-endorphin activity in the brain but not in the blood. *American Journal of Chinese Medicine*, 7(3), 237-240.

Wen, H.L., Ho, W.K.K., Wong, H.K., Mehal, Z.D., Ng, W.H. & Ma, L. (1978). Reduction of adrenocorticotropic hormone (ACTH) and corticol and drug addicts treated by acupuncture and electrical stimulation. *Comp. Med. East-West*, 61-66.

Whitehead, D. (1978). Acupuncture and the treatment of addiction: A review and analysis. *International Journal of Addictions*, 13(1), 1-16.

Wu, C. & Hsu, C. (1979). Neurogenic regulation of lipid metabolism in the rabbit. *Atherosclerosis*, 33,153-164.

Zuckerman, B. & Alpert, J. (1988, March 9). Commentary: Alcohol and psychoactive drug use during pregnancy. *Pediatrics in Review*, 9 (9), 271.

Appendix X: **"So You Want to Start an Acupuncture Treatment Program for Detoxification, Relapse Prevention, and Preparation for Counseling" - A Case History of the Development of an Acupuncture Demonstration Program**

This paper was written by Ruth W. Ackerman, Ph.D., L.C.S.W., based upon her experience in starting Project Recovery, the author's program in Santa Barbara, California. It is reprinted with permission.

Developing an acupuncture-based chemical dependency program offers an opportunity to learn about the mysteries of program funding, policy development and strategic planning. The following is a brief sketch, using our experience in Santa Barbara, California as a case study, of elements to consider. Although specifics may vary from community to community, there are often common elements.

Project Recovery--A Case Study

Project Recovery provides low-cost outpatient alcohol and drug detoxification and relapse prevention treatment to Santa Barbara's homeless, low-income, and adolescent populations. Project Recovery started in 1988 with the cooperation of the Community Action Commission[279] which provided an administrative umbrella for the first nine months. An independent nonprofit agency, Alcohol and Drug Treatment, Inc., was incorporated to get the project off the ground, with a plan to find it a permanent home with an existing agency. It found a home at the Santa Barbara

Council on Alcoholism and Drug Abuse where it has been located since 1989.

The program is barrier-free: no appointments are necessary, and sobriety is not a prerequisite for treatment. As the effectiveness of acupuncture became clear, some county funding was made available after one year of operation. Now, five years later, Project Recovery provides services offsite at Casa Rosa (a residential facility for young, alcohol and/or drug-dependent mothers and their babies),[280] at Zona Chica (a state Medi-Cal funded day-treatment program for substance-abusing expectant mothers), as part of a demonstration project in the county jail, and as part of the free detoxification program offered at the Salvation Army's Hospitality House shelter where the Santa Barbara Council maintains six beds for Project Recovery clients. The Council pays the Salvation Army for the beds, meals, and laundry for these six clients, who are picked up at 7:00 a.m. for a Project Recovery day treatment program, and are returned to the Salvation Army residence at night. Initial results here and elsewhere indicate that acupuncture is the most effective treatment to date with the resistant population referred for treatment by the criminal justice system.

How To Start a Program - Removing Barriers to Treatment on the Community Level

After hearing about this unique treatment and then visiting Lincoln Clinic in the South Bronx, New York, it was apparent that this treatment worked and was a necessity in our community. We received generous consultation and encouragement from Michael Smith, M.D., Director of Lincoln Clinic, and other National Acupuncture Detoxification Association (NADA) members including Carol Taub, David Eisen, Pat Keenan and Janet Konefal. Information and technical support is available from NADA, 3115 Broadway #51, New York, NY, 10027.

We immediately approached the alcohol and drug office at the County Health Department. Although Dr. Smith came to Santa Barbara for our first presentation to the county medical director and his staff, they rejected our proposal for a demonstration project. We then developed an alternate strategy: to find an established nonprofit provider with whom to collaborate.

Dr. Smith suggested we target a population that was not currently receiving services, that presented a visible problem in the community, and that was not potential income for any existing programs. In short, we tried to avoid competing with anyone for a client population.

In the start-up phase we worked closely with one or two leaders in the acupuncture community. The director of the Santa Barbara College of Oriental Medicine, JoAnn Hickey, D.O.M., was particularly helpful.

We determined that our first target group should be the substance abusing homeless and those at high risk for homeless. The lack of services to this adult population had far-reaching effects. For example, in our community, if a parent is "under the influence" when a family appears at the homeless shelter, the family including the children cannot obtain shelter. Before Project Recovery, our county lacked resources for detoxification and treatment except for inpatient residential treatment which averaged $6,000 to $13,000 per month.

Detoxification services had been identified in our community as a critical need. Most communities have drafted a needs assessment for alcohol and drug Commissions, which should be available from your county Board of Supervisors, City Council, and the public library.

Before we could provide acupuncture based services, we had to identify and acquaint the key stakeholders in the community with our goals and our innovative method. First, we contacted the community we intended to serve. We met with The Homeless Coalition whose membership is drawn from the homeless community. The next stop was the Monday group, an informal gathering of community members interested the issue of homelessness. We also contacted leaders in the Native American, Latino and African-American Communities to learn about needs from their points of view and to familiarize them with this treatment modality.

Groups with special interest in human services such as the Medical Society Auxiliary, the Junior League, and several local private foundations were approached both to familiarize them with this new treatment concept and to ask them for direction, guidance and funding.

We knew that there was resistance to acupuncture in the medical community, which dominated existing treatment resources. Therefore, very early on, we contacted the physicians - individually, and in groups, by presenting at hospital grand rounds, and organizationally, by presenting our plan to the County Medical Society.

Our presentations included an acupuncture treatment and a video tape presentation of Lincoln Clinic. There are now several videos appropriate for that purpose available from the NADA Literature Clearinghouse, PO Box 1927, Vancouver, WA, 98668-1927; 206-254-0186. We received excellent advice from an African-American social worker in the community who saw the Lincoln Clinic tape. She suggested we make our own video as soon as we could to counter the resistance and denial in our community which insisted that we had no indigent addicts here and that addiction is a problem only in large urban areas.

Examples of groups we spoke to included the directors and staffs of the County Drug and Alcohol Services Department, Chief of Police, Sheriff, Jail Administrator, District Attorney, Public Defender, Association of Trial Lawyers, Chamber of Commerce, Down Town Merchants Association, the newspaper publishers, South Coast Coordinating Council on Social Services, City Council, County Board of Supervisors, County Alcohol Advisory Board, County Drug Advisory Board, Franklin Center staff (health and social services provider in the African American Community), Human Services Commission, Santa Barbara Council on Alcoholism and Drug Abuse, Transition House Homeless Services, Zona Seca (nonprofit substance abuse treatment provider for the Latino/a community), Community Health Clinics, Isla Vista

Health Services, Cottage Care (our local, private detox and 28-day program provider), Shick Hospital, The Care Unit (a 28-day treatment program which has since closed), Klein Bottle Services (our adolescent drug and alcohol treatment provider), and the methadone clinic.

We had direct access to all these groups by virtue of connections from working long years in the social service community. If you don't have them yourself, find connections who will provide linkage to these systems.

What to Tell an Audience

With enthusiasm and respect, tell them what you are going to tell them, tell it, then tell them what you told them and allow for questions.

What you tell them might include:

1. What and how you define the need for this substance abuse treatment based on local needs assessments.

2. Describe and demonstrate acupuncture detox treatment.

3. Refer to successful outcomes elsewhere.

4. Describe the program you are proposing locally.

5. Suggest how that particular audience might help (i.e. a letter of support, contributions, or linkage to key decision makers).

6. ALWAYS leave a copy of or reference to the EXCELLENT studies from Minneapolis, "Controlled Trial of Acupuncture for Severe Recidivistic Alcoholism" by Bullock, Culliton, and Olander, (*The Lancet,* June 24, 1989, pp. 1435-1439), or the original (pre-followup) report of the same study, "Acupuncture Treatment of Alcoholic Recidivism: A Pilot Study" by Bullock, Umen, Culliton, and Olander, (*Alcoholism: Clinical and Experimental Research, 11*(3), May-June, 1987, pp. 292-295).[281] The fact that these research reports had appeared in peer-reviewed journals was critical in gaining the support or at least tolerance from the medical and chemical dependency communities.

7. Show a video, selected according to your audience.

8. Give them contact names and numbers of people in successful programs. Call NADA if you need assistance identifying appropriate contacts.

9. Arrange for key decision makers to visit New York, or other communities which have established programs. Or arrange a visit *to* your site from someone from these programs.

Where to Locate the Program

Our vision was to simply add acupuncture treatment to existing chemical dependency programs. The intent was to establish a pilot program at an existing service agency located near the homeless shelter.

The dream is a long range plan, the reality takes time. After many months it became apparent that our efforts to be "adopted" by an existing agency were not going to be successful, EVEN THOUGH WE OFFERED TO RAISE ALL THE MONEY FOR THE PROJECT OURSELVES. The primary obstacles were skepticism regarding acupuncture as an effective treatment and fears of liability.

Liability

Trustees on boards of nonprofits were fearful of their liability exposure. Provision of acupuncture is considered a physical treatment and most providers were not covered for any treatment beyond counseling. Thus we obtained professional liability insurance for each acupuncturist. The agency advanced them the money for the premiums and they have paid it off over time. This worked for us, but may not work for you. We recommend professional consultation on this matter from your attorney.

Starting a Nonprofit

Because we could not get "adopted," we started a new (there are now 760 of these in Santa Barbara County alone) nonprofit corporation. The Legal Aid Foundation connected us with an attorney who donated $4,000 in professional services and obtained nonprofit status for us. This tax exempt 501(C)(3) status allowed us to receive contributions from individuals and charitable foundations. It is possible to establish your own nonprofit without incurring legal fees. A "How to" book with do-it-yourself tear-out forms is published by NOLO Press, Berkeley, California.

To create a nonprofit, you must have a board of trustees. Board members should be selected strategically. We included the following:

- an accountant.
- a prominent physician.
- an attorney (Our first choice accepted. She was a recovering alcoholic with five years of sobriety. She committed suicide by taking an overdose the day we were to meet for the first time. The disease of alcoholism is cunning and baffling. We require our staff to attend at least six Al Anon meetings as part of their orientation).
- the director of the most prominent adolescent substance abuse program in town.
- a Latina psychologist who is an international consultant on addiction.
- the director of a local charitable foundation with skills in community organizing and ties to private donors.
- a local realtor/counselor who became one of our most generous private donors.
- A professor of anthropology at our local university who is a well respected activist in the African-American community.

This board met twice a year. Members had no responsibilities in relation to fund raising or policy, but their names on the letter head was as good as gold. We purchased "errors and omissions" Board liability insurance and strongly recommend any nonprofit do so.

Our financial strategy was to raise enough money to sustain the project for three years. We did not want to disappear for lack of funding after a successful six-month demonstration project. Initially we obtained a small grant ($900) from a nonprofit foundation interested in supporting start-up progressive social change activities. That not only enabled us to cover mounting clerical expenses related to initial educational outreach, but also gave us credibility which made subsequent fund raising activities much easier. Similar groups may exist in your community. Contact the Funding Exchange, New York City for information regarding similar resources.

Some of our initial funding came from these sources:

$900--Start up funding from the Fund for Santa Barbara

$2000--City Human Services Commission

$2000--Equipment grant from the Santa Barbara Foundation

$2000--Private donor/family foundation

$5000 --Individual donor/board member

$5000--Exxon

$5000--Individual donor/family foundation

$7500--McKinney money/federal funds

$5000--Individual contributions from $5 to $250.

We were ready to start our program as a new nonprofit when our request for a sponsoring agency bore fruit: the Community Action Commission of Santa Barbara offered some funding and provided a part-time administrative assistant for our first year. It would be well worth checking on this potential resource if your community is in the United States.

After less than one year we were permanently adopted by the Santa Barbara Council on Alcoholism and Drug Abuse. We retained our nonprofit status for another year to be sure that the relationship with the Santa Barbara Council would be satisfactory. At the end of that time we dissolved our organization and terminated our nonprofit status.

Suggestions for Grantseekers

We wish we would have had "7 Steps to Secure a Grant for Your Project" by Keith Melville. Here is the essence of his comments.

Seven Steps to Secure a Grant for Your Project

Obtaining grant funding for a project is a research intensive task. Careful and focused research will greatly increase chances for getting funded and reduce time spent pursuing inappropriate funding sources. Don't expect shortcuts. The following seven steps outline the process.

1. Self/organizational assessment: Determine if your organization is structured to receive grant funding. If you seek funding within an organization in the United States, it must have a 501(c)(3) nonprofit tax exempt status. Most private sector funding goes to nonprofit organizations.

2. Define your project: What do you want to do? Be concrete. You may have only a vague idea of your goals; to solidify them you may want to do some background research and find out about other organizations and individuals who are doing similar projects. Contact NADA for information about programs nearest you. Before you even begin to research funding sources you should be able to describe:

   a. What your project is.

   b. The geographic location of your project.

   c. What problem/need your project addresses.

   d. What concrete steps you need to take to implement your project.

   e. Time frame for completion of your project.

   f. Total costs.

Any attempt to secure funding for a vague (even if brilliant) idea will fail. Many funding sources have very specific criteria for their giving; you have to know whether your project will meet these criteria before you apply. Grantmakers want to know that you have a clear plan and that you are qualified to carry it out.

3. Consult the list of Foundation Center Library affiliates and locate the one nearest you, as well as a convenient university library and/or public library. You will need to research funding sources extensively. Foundation Library affiliates and university libraries have most comprehensive resources.

4. Research funding sources and develop a list of potential funders. Familiarize yourself with all resources available. Directories to foundations based on geographic location and subject narrow your search quickly and can save time. Utilize periodicals for current information/spotlights on particular types of private giving.

5. Find out as much as possible about each of the funding sources on your list: request annual reports if available; find out about past giving through IRS records; request application guidelines if they have them; find out preferred approach of each fund source and grant cycle deadlines.

6. Prepare a proposal tailored to each funding source that show how your project fulfills its stated objectives. Send the proposal and appropriate attachments as required to potential funders before their deadlines for accepting proposals.

7. A few weeks after submitting the proposal, call to make sure the foundation/funding source has received your materials, and find out if they require any additional materials to process your application. Grant review procedures may take anywhere from a few weeks to six months, so be patient.

Here are some additional "do's and don'ts":

Do

- Do your HOMEWORK. Carefully and exhaustively research potential funders.
- Find out if funding sources prefer a letter of introduction or a phone call as a first step before you waste time and money writing and mailing a full length proposal.
- Respect deadlines. Your application may be disqualified on these grounds alone.

- Always address your cover letter to a specific individual at a foundation; verify the spelling of the name, title, and address. Contacts at funding sources do help, but are not substitutes for a well written proposal.
- Make each proposal unique, demonstrate your knowledge of the foundation, their interests, and how these relate to your project.
- If a foundation has application guidelines, follow them to the letter.
- Be a shameless self promoter to establish the validity of your organization or project. Use testimonial quotes.

Don't

- Don't use the mass mailing approach; it doesn't work and can damage your reputation with potential funders. Grantmakers will not be receptive to a generic application that does not address the concerns of their foundation.
- Don't focus all of your efforts on one ideal funder.
- Don't expect contacts at a particular funding source to guarantee success. Especially at larger foundations, demonstrating that your project is well designed and that your organization has a committed and experienced staff (or you have extensive knowledge of the field) will impress grant makers more than a personal contact.
- Don't use jargon or acronyms in you proposal when avoidable. You should write your proposal in concise, clear prose, in the active voice. Don't include unnecessary graphs or charts. Keep your proposal to the point and avoid emotional appeals.
- Don't make your proposal beautiful but unreadable. A well written proposal is more important than a fancy binding.
- Don't give up if your proposal is rejected. Most funders receive more proposals than they can fund in a given year. If you are unsure why your proposal was rejected, ask. Find out if that funder would consider your proposal in upcom-

ing grant cycles or if they have suggestions about other sources of funding.

Potential Funding Sources

There are many areas of potential funding for your work. Your local County Drug and Alcohol Services should be able to assist you in obtaining information in your own community. Call them, meet with their staff, let them educate you about funding process.

1.   Private Donors

Soliciting funds from individual donors is both an art and a science. Raising money for start-up and long established projects can range from holding rummage and bake sales to individual donor solicitation of the take-a-prospect-to-lunch variety. Accessing established donor networks is difficult but not impossible. However, there are fewer charity dollars to go around and much more competition for them.

We constantly ask those interested in our project for names of prospective donors. We then invite the potential donor (and the person who referred us to them) to see a demonstration of the treatment. We contact them with a personal follow-up and ask for a donation. One donor often leads us to the next.

Nonprofit board members often assume responsibility for funding. While the board of the Alcohol and Drug Treatment, Inc. never assumed that responsibility, the Santa Barbara Council certainly does!

2.   Foundations

Funding is often available, even for innovative, non-traditional programming, through private foundations as well as individual private donors. The research librarian at your local public library will be a great resource in showing you the directories on private and public giving. There are many popular books on accessing foundation funding, including how to identify the foundation most appropriate for your project and how to write a proposal.

There are several categories of foundations:

National foundations are large foundations that do not limit their giving on the basis of geographic location. For example, the Ford Foundation.

Special Interest Foundations only support specific fields of interest.

Family Foundations/Funds, range from large to small, make up the largest category of foundations, often limit their giving to a particular locality.

Community Foundations/ Funds, also called Public Charities, collect money from corporations, private donors, and the public. These collective funds make grants only within the community for which they are named. Community leaders often administer funds, and tend to focus on community development and enhancement.

Corporate Giving: (Distinct from corporate foundations). Some corporations make charitable donations, give gifts, and supply in-kind donations such as equipment. These corporations generally do not have application guidelines or professional grant reviewers. Total corporate giving is about 5% of all philanthropic giving and goes mostly to education and health and human services. Usually corporations give to programs that will affect their employees or enhance their image. This type of giving usually has geographic limitations.

We were able to engage many foundation donors with the notion of a "private/public" partnership. This meant balancing private funding with public funding over time.

An important selling point to all donors was the potential this treatment model had for becoming self sustaining on the basis of fees collected, including insurance and Medi-Cal. Although the process of obtaining Medi-Cal funding has taken much longer than we anticipated, we are still aiming at relative independence.

3. Federal Government

Applying for government funding is a complex process that may require more time and labor than the applications for private foundations. This should not be a deterrent. Keep in mind that federal agencies prefer projects that can serve as prototypes or models. Local government funders require strong evidence of community support.

Securing government funding requires perseverance. Government grants usually have stringent reporting requirements which require extremely careful record keeping; this means higher administrative costs.

The National Institutes of Health and the Department of Health and Human Services provide opportunities for funding. Check directly with National Institute on Drug Abuse, [NIDA] National Institute on Alcoholism and Alcohol Abuse, [NIAAA], Center for Substance Abuse Treatment (CSAT) Center for Substance Abuse Prevention (CSAP), and the office of Alternate Therapies. These are generally multi-year research-oriented or model program grants. They usually require collaborative work with a primary investigator from a university with a track-record in working with federal grants, or with a well established agency.

4. County Drug and Alcohol

These include federal block grant monies allocated to the state and filtered on to county levels. Some of these funds are mandated for AIDS, HIV, intravenous drug users or perinatal substance abuse.[282] The allocations are often retained by particular county's office of alcohol and drug services, particularly if it provides substance abuse treatment directly. Other counties such as ours do not provide direct service but contract-out to nonprofit providers. There is tremendous competition among established providers for these funds. Find out from your county drug and alcohol office if there is a funding cycle for new programs and when applications or Request for Proposals (RFP) are due (usually beginning in January or February). Also ask if there is a county Master Plan that you can review.

5. County Mental Health Services

In some locations this agency handles substance abuse treatment as well as mental health services. In California, it is almost an administrative impossibility to be both mentally ill and chemically dependent simultaneously.

6. County/City Human Services Commissions

offer services aimed at the economically and socially disenfranchised. Limited funding may be available.

7. AIDS

By collaborating with existing AIDS programs you may have a natural home for acupuncture services. AIDS funding, including Ryan White funds, may be available specifically for chemical dependency prevention.

8. Medi-Cal [California]

Becoming a Medi-Cal provider allows you to collect "stickers" as an optional treatment provider. Although there are only two available per month, they may be also used for counseling and other alternate health treatments. Medi-Cal does fund traditional treatment and efforts are being made to expand coverage to include outpatient acupuncture. Becoming a licensed treatment site will help allow you to access Medi-Cal funding. Contact your local Medi-Cal information officer at the Department of Health, or your local Alcohol and Drug Program Administrator.

9. Insurance

Most companies are reducing their coverage of inpatient substance abuse treatment. Be a pioneer and arrange directly with the insurer to bill insurance for outpatient acupuncture detoxification services.

10. Fee for Service

Many clinics operate on a sliding fee scale. Our charges range from $0 to $35 per treatment. Regular collection of fees reduces the ill effects of co-dependency, and dignifies the client. Often "in kind" work can be part of recovery for the client with limited financial resources.

11. Criminal Justice System

This source of funding has not traditionally included substance abuse treatment, but times are changing. Many jurisdictions have set aside money for jail over-crowding and these funds may be available for diversion funding based on just the kind of treatment you plan to offer. The appointment of Janet Reno as Attorney General is a good sign, as is President Clinton's recent decision to change the tactics of the war on drugs to emphasize treatment. Model programs exist in Dade County, Florida; Portland, Oregon; Santa Maria, California, and throughout Minnesota.

12. Probation and Parole.

Particularly with state parole, treatment can sometimes be purchased and program component requirements worked out with the referring agents. Some jurisdictions now mandate treatment during probation or parole and require payment as part of the suspended sentencing process. It may take a lot of political work and perseverance, but this treatment BELONGS in those programs.

13. Driving Under the Influence [DUI]

In many locations treatment is mandated for those arrested for a DUI. We have not yet been successful in becoming a mandated part of our local program, but other acupuncture-based programs have been able to do so.

14. Family Violence

Family violence treatment programs exist in most California counties and are often used by the courts as diversion sentencing in domestic violence cases. You can try to attach acupuncture to existing programs or develop a comprehensive program with acupuncture, counseling and education. Chemical dependency is highly associated with domestic violence.

15. Victim/Witness

Victim/witness funds may be available for victims of domestic and other violent crimes. This funding is available on the state level and is usually administered through the county District Attorney's office. Be creative and persistent.

Let Us Help You

If further information would be valuable to you, please let us know. You will find NADA members and others affiliated with clinics using the NADA protocol most generous with their time.

Section A: Eight Sample Program Proposals

Following are a sample of eight various acupuncture-related proposals from the author's program. They are reprinted by permission of the Santa Barbara Council on Alcoholism and Drug Abuse. Some are in the form of memorandum, some are one page summaries, and others are more developed in detail. All are proposals that were actually submitted, and they are presented as they were submitted, except that in some cases the names of persons and agencies have been deleted. Some were funded, some were not, and some are still pending.[283] They are included as a resource will help the reader in developing language for his or her own proposals.

Most proposals we submit are accompanied by the following brief history and description of our program:

Santa Barbara Council on Alcoholism and Drug Abuse
Project Recovery

History and Overview

Throughout 1987 and into the Spring of 1988 in Santa Barbara, a number of individuals in the community developed private and public funding for a one year outpatient demonstration of the efficacy of acupuncture in the treatment of symptoms of acute withdrawal from psychoactive drugs. Funding for this project became complete when our local Community Action Commission agreed to manage the project and to provide as partial funding a portion of their McKinney homeless money so that the program would target homeless alcoholics and drug addicts.

Project Recovery operated through the summer of 1989 at the Franklin Community center, a well utilized multi-service facility in a Latino residential area of Santa Barbara. With successful statistics and enthusiastic support from the treatment community at large, the Community Action Commission began seeking a "home" for the project with an agency whose primary expertise was in the chemical dependency field. In November of 1989, the administration of the program was transferred to the Santa Barbara Council on Alcoholism and Drug Abuse. The funding base of Project Recovery had by then expanded to include County Drug and Alcohol support.

As of this date, Project Recovery has provided treatment to over 2500 unduplicated clients. Due to increased community acceptance, the project has expanded its services to include education/counseling group support in both English and Spanish, case management, individual and referral counseling, and a sophisticated computer tracking system to maintain current attendance data for local probation, parole, and child protective services.

Acute Treatment Program

Project Recovery also operates a county-funded six bed six to 21 day acute care detoxification program in conjunction with the Salvation Army Hospitality House at 423 Chapala Street. Both male and female chemically dependent clients are under the custodial care of the Salvation Army. Day treatment is provided at our Haley Street clinic including twice-daily acupuncture, individual and group counseling, education, and Twelve Step meeting involvement.

Fees for this service are on a sliding scale, and intakes are from 1:00 to 4:00 P.M. daily at the Salvation Army. Call 963-3315 for information.

Acupuncture

Acupuncture is a foundation for psycho-social rehabilitation, and is most effective when used in conjunction with counseling, Twelve Step programs, and case management. Acupuncture not only controls withdrawal symptoms and craving, but it also reduces fears and hostilities that usually disturb drug abuse treatment settings. Acupuncture has a balancing effect on the autonomic and neurotransmitter systems as well as an apparently rejuvenating effect. REM rebound sleep dysfunction - including insomnia and "drug dreams" - typically accompany acute and post-acute withdrawal, and 92% of Project Recovery clients report that acupuncture provides relief from these symptoms. Clinical experience has also demonstrated that acupuncture is helpful in treating other post-acute withdrawal symptoms and the symptoms that forebode relapse.

At a very low cost compared with other treatment modalities, acupuncture provides the opportunity for multiple contacts between the client and the treatment system. Patients learn to have confidence in daily acupuncture visits and the relief that consistently occurs. This modality facilitates constructive, non-antagonistic counseling and breaks down the barriers that usually inhibit group process. The consistently calm atmosphere in the treatment area is a marked contrast to the tense mood of jail, of the streets, or even of the best conventional drug program.

Protocol

The acupuncture protocol used at Project Recovery was developed between 1972 and 1974 by Michael Smith, M.D., Director of Substance Abuse at the Lincoln Hospital in New York (349 East 140th Street, Bronx, N.Y. 10454 [212] 993-3100) and founder of the National Acupuncture Detoxification Association (NADA). The specific procedure was based on the initial findings of acupuncture researchers. Clinicians at Lincoln subsequently explored whether different acupuncture points or treatments would enhance the effects of the detoxification process. The points selected at Lincoln were thus based upon research and clinical experience. The procedure is simple, easy to apply, and does not require electrical stimulation. Reports have indicated that these points are equally effective in the treatment of heroin, cocaine, crack cocaine, alcohol, methamphetamines, and nicotine.

Five thin needles (0.25 mm diameter, 15 mm long) are inserted into the appropriate are of the ear cartilage ridge, located next to the outer rim of both ears. The five corresponding points are "*shen-men*," sympathetic, kidney, liver, and lung. The patient is required to sit and relax for 45 minutes with the needles in place. The needles are then removed. Before insertion, the auricular points are cleansed with a 75% alcohol prep pad.

Research

In a clinical evaluation at Lincoln during 1987-88 of 1,500 unscreened court-mandated outpatient "crack" cocaine abusers, more than 50% provided negative urine toxicologies for longer than two months.

Dr. Milton Bullock of the Hennepin County Medical Center in Minneapolis conducted a controlled placebo trial of the NADA acupuncture protocol. His study, published initially in the journal *Alcoholism* in June, 1987, and subsequently in the British medical journal *Lancet* in June of 1989, showed that 93% of chronic, late-stage male alcoholic standard treatment patients completed the eight week program, compared with two and a half percent of the control group. Six month follow-up statistics showed that men in the control group were re-admitted to detox more than twice as often and had more than twice the number of drinking episodes than men in the standard treatment group.

In 1987, a pilot program was established in the public detox unit in Portland, Oregon. The county of Multnomah voted to allot $90,000 of their federal Bureau of Justice Administration funds to create several acupuncture components in both outpatient and in-patient treatment and shelter settings. Before acupuncture was used, 34% completed the detoxification program; now 98% of the patients complete the program. The Oregon State Department of Corrections has helped establish a Criminal Bed Reduction Program using acupuncture in the correctional facility in Salem. A clinic for runaway youth and a community based program have been started. For information, contact David Eisen, M.A., Director of Acupuncture Services, Hooper Memorial Detox Program, 20 N.E. Union Street, Portland, OR 97232, (503) 238-2067.

The National Institute on Drug Abuse has funded a three year research grant to demonstrate reduction in the spread of AIDS by improving treatment for drug abuse in Dade County, which has incorporated acupuncture into all aspects of drug treatment. In this multi-phasic program, first and second cocaine offenders receive daily acupuncture in lieu of incarceration, and then move into a vocational rehabilitation and case management program. Of the first 1600 offenders to enter the program, only 2% had been rear-rested in the first eight months. The program also includes over 500 treatment beds in the Dade County Stockade, and an acupuncture treatment program for AIDS. For further information contact Janet Konefal, Ph.D., University of Miami School of Medicine, Department of Epidemiology, Graduate Programs in Public Health, P.O. Box 016069, Miami, FL 33101 (305) 547-6759.

Relapse

The disease of alcoholism and drug addiction is a chronic re-lapsing disorder. Transitional and early recovery periods, even among the most highly motivated clients, are characterized by in-termittent relapse. In traditional alcohol and drug treatment set-tings, relapse generally equates with program drop-out. One rea-son for the growing popularity of acupuncture-based programs with the criminal justice community is that these programs are able to hold clients in treatment during the early relapsing periods. Clients can return for daily acupuncture treatment regardless of use patterns and find physical support for the process of protracted withdrawal. The subjective benefits of acupuncture increase over time with daily treatments, and relapses tend to be shallow rather that catastrophic. The non-judgmental ambience of the acupunc-ture treatment setting generates trust with the clinical staff so that more productive relapse-prevention counseling and education can occur.

· · ·

Proposal 1:   **Six month jail demonstration project proposal**

$18,000 is needed to provide a six month treatment demon-stration project at the Santa Barbara County Jail. 50 individuals with a history of substance abuse who are incarcerated at the Honor Farm will volunteer for or, as a pre-sentencing condition due to a violation of probation, be required to complete the following:

- daily acupuncture 30 days prior to release.
- attendance at meetings of Alcoholics Anonymous, Narcotics Anonymous, or Cocaine Anonymous.
- pre-release assessment

These individuals will continue treatment in our outpatient program upon release.

Our goal for beginning this project is April 1, 1991.

Budget - Level I (6 month jail demonstration pilot)

Salaries:	Cost
Program Director	1,500
Adm. Asst.	1,000
Clinical Director	1,500
Acupuncturist	5,850
	9,850
Expenditures:	Cost
Needles, etc.	3,650
Printing	500
Start-up/adm.overhead	4,000
TOTAL	**18,000**

. . .

Proposal 2: **Letter requested by Director of Inmate Services at County Jail concerning possible resumption of funding for treatment for in-custody female clients**

This is a proposal to provide acupuncture treatment services for substance abuse and related problems to women incarcerated at the county Jail's minimum security facility.

As you are aware, a very substantial majority of all inmates incarcerated at La Mirada have a history of alcohol or other drug dependencies. The acupuncture treatment protocol we use was developed specifically for substance abuse at New York's Lincoln Hospital in the South Bronx and established by the National Acupuncture Detoxification Association. These treatments assist inmates in "post acute withdrawal" - a cycle of anxiety, depression, and drug craving often accompanied by sleep disturbance that is typical among drug dependent persons during the first year of abstinence.

By treating this condition in the incarcerated setting, we hope to prevent relapse among these inmates on their release. We also use this treatment as an opportunity to offer referral and recovery counseling in hopes that the clients can become involved in outpatient or other appropriate treatment or recovery programs upon release from custody.

We studied re-incarceration rates among a group of women who received this treatment at La Mirada during 1991-92, comparing their re-incarceration rates with a sample control population of the year prior.[284] We found that:

1. Women in the control group were twice as likely to be re-incarcerated during the first 120 days following release as women who received acupuncture.

2. Women receiving acupuncture had a 17% lower re-incarceration rate overall than the controls.

3. Women receiving 32 or more treatments while in custody had an overall re-incarceration rate 26% lower than the controls, and a rate 17% lower than those receiving fewer than 32 treatments.

We would be able to resume this program at a cost of $52 per 90 minute treatment session. That includes all medical supplies and "detox tea" for a maximum of 20 persons treated per session.

The minimum level of service that would still yield a benefit would be three treatment sessions per week (at a cost of approximately $675 monthly). The optimum service level is to provide the treatment daily, six days per week (at an approximate cost of $1350 monthly).

I would be pleased to provide any additional information or answer any questions, or to arrange a demonstration treatment and presentation, on request.

Sincerely,

Proposal 3: **This is a proposal requested by a private post-release services agency for State prisoners**

Proposal for a Daily Acupuncture Demonstration for Drug and Alcohol Sobriety Maintenance in a (agency) Setting

This is a proposal for a six month demonstration program to deliver daily acupuncture treatments for drug and alcohol sobriety maintenance to 12 (twelve) State Correction inmates in residence at the (agency) facility in Isla Vista.

Treatments will be performed by an acupuncturist on contract with the Santa Barbara Council on Alcoholism and Drug Abuse. The proposed protocol was developed by the National Acupuncture Detoxification Association and is currently in use in criminal justice settings in Miami, New York, Minnesota, and Salem, Oregon. An abstract of this treatment protocol and research is attached.

Treatment time is approximately one hour and would be performed at the convenience of the (agency) staff.

Six-month cost of the program with treatments seven days per week is $7,045.

Proposed Budget

Acupuncturist:+	4,550
Medical Supplies*	1,320
Administrative time#	1,175
TOTAL	**7,045**

+ 182 days @ $25

* 2200 treatments @ .60

includes [agency] staff training and start-up) @ 20%

. . .

Proposal 4:   **This is a proposal to provide substance abuse counseling/prevention/intervention services for persons and families residing at public housing complexes:**

Program Goals

1. To provide intensive alcohol and drug intervention and treatment program services on-site for residents of two housing authority locations to be determined by the (public housing agency).

2. To provide related but less intensive outreach, referral, and case management services on-site to residents of eight additional housing locations.

3. To provide acute treatment services at Project Recovery for identified (housing agency) residents.

Program Components

1. Prevention Alert Liaison (existing).

2. Acupuncture-based intervention, detoxification, and relapse prevention treatments.

3. In-patient detoxification.

4. Individual, group, family, crisis, and referral counseling on alcohol and other substance abuse.

5. Case management to provide networking and interface with other community health and social service providers such as (names of agencies).

6. Criminal Justice (police, municipal court, probation, and parole) liaison services.

7. Prevention/education services.

Program Description and Objectives

The Santa Barbara Council on Alcoholism and Drug Abuse will provide, through its Project Recovery Drug and Alcohol

Treatment Program, Community Services Coordinators, and Prevention Programs, the following services to a potential 175 unduplicated clients:

1. 1,872 acupuncture intervention, detoxification, and relapse prevention treatments, offered three times per week on-site at two Housing Authority locations to be designated by (housing agency). Services will be provided by state-licensed acupuncturists on contract with the Santa Barbara Council on Alcoholism and Drug Abuse and certified by the National Acupuncture Detoxification Association. Subjective outcomes anticipated are that clients receiving treatment will:

    a) experience reduced physiologic craving and other withdrawal symptoms associated with abstinence.

    b) become more accepting of the need to be drug free and to face their denial.

    c) become accepting of their potential to stop using drugs.

    d) develop willingness to engage in ancillary treatment and support services.

2. Two "slots" at the Project Recovery Acute Care Detox, an intensive day treatment program which includes residency at the Salvation Army Hospitality House at 433 Chapala. This program accommodates men and women for six to 21 days during acute alcohol or other drug withdrawal, and involves twice-daily acupuncture, gender-based and mixed group counseling/education, individual counseling, and intensive 12-Step group involvement (Alcoholics Anonymous and Narcotics Anonymous).

This program also includes outpatient aftercare including group and individual counseling, acupuncture, and case management.

3. Nine hours per week at each of the two designated sites (eighteen hours total) of culturally sensitive case management and individual, group, youth, and family counseling. Some hours will coincide with and follow established acupuncture hours, and others will be flexibly scheduled to meet needs, such as during the evenings to accommodate families and youth groups, etc.

4. Twelve hours per week of crisis and referral counseling, case management, and outreach at the eight non-intensive sites. (Clients at these sites may be referred to either of the targeted program sites or to Project Recovery for treatment).

5. MFCC supervision for all counseling program personnel.

6. Program interface with county probation and state parole to assure involvement of clients who are on probation/parole with their officers, and to maximize making program involvement a part of probation or parole requirements as appropriate.

7. Presentations throughout the year at all sites of culturally sensitive group education on the issues of alcoholism, family systems, recovery, relapse prevention, and nutrition and other health issues such as HIV/AIDS, Fetal Alcohol Syndrome, etc. Sessions will be scheduled at the convenience of those participating.

Budget

Salaries			
Position	**FTE**	**Rate**	**Cost**
Acupuncture		25	9,750
Counseling/Case Mgt.		11	6,864
Counseling*		22	6,864
Intensive Case Mgt.		17	5,304
Outreach Worker		11	3,432
Supervision		22	915
Subtotal Salaries			34,720
Expenditures:			
Administrative Overhead	12%		4,280
Supplies	0 .85/tx		1,591
Subtotal Expenditures			5,871
TOTAL			**39,000**

Proposal 5: **Following is a proposed treatment option for state parolees that was requested by the director of the local parole office**

OUTPATIENT SERVICES

Goal: To provide acupuncture-based outpatient drug-free alcohol and other drug treatment services.

The protocol for services contracted for is that established by the National Acupuncture Detoxification Association. Parameters under the contract would be for a standard 90 day treatment program providing

- 24   treatments for the first thirty day period.
- 12   treatments during the second thirty day period
- 8   treatments during the final thirty day period.

Up to eight aftercare treatments per month would be reimbursed for an additional six months following program completion.

Included in the Program protocol would be a ten week, weekly group counseling/education session. a half-hour individual counseling session per week.

The program would also monitor attendance at Narcotics Anonymous or Cocaine Anonymous meetings on request.

. . .

Proposal 6 **This is another state parole proposal to provide more intensive day treatment/case management services**

This program is to provide acupuncture and case-management-based drug-free alcohol/drug day treatment services and to assist parolees in networking and accessing community resources for sobriety maintenance and vocational and basic life skills.

- Parolees referred to this program on a week-to-week basis will receive:
- twice-daily acupuncture.
- supervised day treatment Monday thru Friday from
- 8:00 A.M. to 5:00 P.M. to include:
- intensive case management for issues of sobriety maintenance, vocation and educational issues, and
- basic living and life adjustment skills.
- individual and group counseling and education
- for substance abuse and relapse prevention.
- supervised attendance twice-daily at Narcotics, Alcoholics, or Cocaine Anonymous meetings.
- once-weekly men's or women's group counseling sessions.

This program is not confined to a single "locked-down" location, but moves under supervision between our clinic at 133 East Haley, the Haley Center, the Alano Club, other Twelve Step meeting locations, and other community agencies as appropriate to client need. Clients begin and end the treatment day at the Project Recovery clinic at 133 East Haley.

This program is under the supervision of (staff), and is billed to parole at a rate of $380 per week for a five-day week, and pro-rated at a rate of $76 per day.

. . .

Proposal 7:   **This letter reflects an collaborative effort between our program and a perinatal treatment provider**

Dear (agency director),

Our agency would like to express our support of (agency) in developing a day treatment program for perinatal alcohol clients.

We are willing to subcontract with (agency) for a nutritional counseling and education component of such a program, including acupuncture treatment for mothers as well as a modified acupuncture treatment protocol using herbal seeds that would extend to alcohol or drug exposed infants in the program.

All aspects of our treatment program could be accomplished for $12,500 per fiscal year, which would include acupuncture four times each week plus 1.5 hours three times per week for small group nutritional education and counseling. A budget breakdown for these services is as follows:

Acupuncturist +	5,200
Group Counseling/Education *	3,276
Medical supplies/tea	1,774
Educational Materials	1,000
Administrative Overhead/Start-up 9%	1,250
TOTAL	**12,500**

+ 208 hours @ $25
* 234 hours @ $14

. . .

Proposal 8: **Portions of a Proposal for a Collaborative Substance Abuse Intervention Program between Santa Barbara County Public Health and the Santa Barbara Council on Alcoholism and Drug Abuse.**

Rationale

The New York State Division of Substance Abuse Services has described acupuncture as "an entry service to assist individuals accessing substance abuse treatment programs and support services," and as a "threshold technology" most useful with clients who resist initial treatment due either to active drug use, the presence of withdrawal symptoms, or denial.

We are aware that a substantial number of individuals accessing public health services in Santa Barbara County have substance abuse as an underlying or attending disorder. This is a proposal to begin a collaborative effort between Santa Barbara County Public Health and the Santa Barbara Council on Alcoholism and Drug Abuse to develop strategies for implementing acupuncture as an intervention modality at the county's outpatient health clinic.

Acupuncture has been shown to alleviate classic alcohol and drug withdrawal symptoms. But our experience in the use of the standard five-point auricular protocol that has been developed for acute withdrawal has shown that this treatment has great efficacy as well in addressing issues of stress, anxiety, and pain. In a public health outpatient setting, people might be encouraged to access this treatment for these other symptoms and, in the course of treatment, a substance abuse assessment and referral could be achieved.

This treatment can be accomplished in any group setting where people are seated. Treatment benefit requires that needles remain inserted for at least 1/2 hour. One acupuncturist can comfortably treat as many as 20 individuals at a time.

Cost

Acupuncture could be provided on a trial basis four hours daily, four days per week. The monthly cost for this service, at a rate of $35.00 per hour, would be approximately $2500. This could be recouped through fee-for-service Medi-Cal (at 150 billable treatments per month). Or Santa Barbara Health Initiative (which administers Medi-Cal in the county) may be open to contracting for this service if a plan is developed.

Implementation

It is proposed that meetings be developed between the clinical staffs of both the county Outpatient Clinic and Project Recovery to study ways of implementing this service, and between the administrative staffs to develop an appropriate plan for Medi-Cal billing.

Public health -

The role of Public health delivery in homeless substance abuse is twofold.

First, the accessing of public health services on the part of homeless persons is a premier intervention opportunity. Therefore, intervention modalities need to be available on sight at the primary health care access point in south county. Besides an outpatient acupuncture clinic with case management back-up opportunity at the County Department of Public Health, funding is proposed for an "Acu-Van" - a mobile treatment unit to deliver acupuncture detoxification, public health, and case management services to areas where homeless substance abusers are known to sleep and congregate.

Second, linkage between public health and substance abuse is necessary so that non-substance abuse health problems that may be precipitating factors in the substance abuse or in substance abuse relapse may be identified and appropriate services provided in the same treatment setting. Such issues include but are not limited to:

- chronic pain
- traumatic injury
- mental health issues, including Post Traumatic Stress Syndrome
- HIV/AIDS

Social Services

Case Managers providing SSI Protective Payee services have been shown to be effective in addressing substance abuse issues among the homeless. Our agency currently provides this service to 20 SSI recipients, and this program will be expanded. The role of the case manager is to make appropriate assessments and subsequently:

1. To support the client in substance abuse recovery and assure that the client has access to appropriate treatment, health, and recovery resources.

2. To assist the client in accessing appropriate housing, social, vocational, educational, and legal resources.

3. To provide education, guidance, and oversight in the client's management of social security benefits.

Section B: Health and Safety Standards

Following is a sample needle safety protocol that complies with standards recommended by the California Office of Health and Safety.

Acupuncture Clinic and Counselor Safety Protocol and Exposure Control Plan

This acupuncture clinic protocol has been developed to protect at-risk workers and clients of (name of program) against blood-borne pathogens, including the hepatitis B virus (HBV) and the human immunodeficiency virus (HIV).

Employees at Risk

Workers at (program) with occupational exposure to blood and other infectious material include acupuncturists and counselors who work in or around the clinic site during clinic hours.

The (program), in order to provide a safe work environment at these sites, provides to at-risk workers the following:

1. Testing for Hepatitis B and tuberculoses and, when indicated, vaccine for Hepatitis B.

2. Rubber gloves, disinfectant cleaner, and medical waste containers.

3. Bleach-based disinfectant soap and hot running water.

4. Information and training on the procedures and protocols described in this document.

The (program) provides orientation and information to clients on the procedures and protocols described in this document.

Acupuncture Protocol

The acupuncture detoxification treatment protocol is designed to augment and support other aspects of a broader comprehensive approach to substance abuse treatment. The clients participate in their treatment in a variety of ways including:

1. The maintenance of the treatment room.

2. Respecting and reminding others to respect the quiet meditative milieu.

3. Signing in and out of the clinic.

4. Removing of their own auricular point needles

5. Wiping their ears after treatment

6. Asking for assistance when needed

7. Making sure the acupuncturist removes all body point needles.

8. Discarding of waste products appropriately.

The clients are instructed to wipe their ears with cotton after removing the needles. If one of the points should bleed, the client is instructed to hold the cotton on the point and call the acupuncturist to handle the bleeding.

Acupuncture Detoxification

Treatment Orientation

Clients are oriented to acupuncture treatment and safety precautions during the intake session. Safety precautions are included in the client "Welcome" document distributed to each client and are posted in the clinic.

Procedures Followed by Client

1. When entering the clinic, all clients report to the client reception area, which is staffed by the (program) Clinic Coordinator. Here they:

a) sign the client roster.

b) receive their treatment cards.

c) clean the cartilage area of both ears with cotton with an alcohol solution.

d) select packages of ten disposable acupuncture needles.

2. Clients select a seat and check to be sure there are no loose needles on or around the chair area. If loose needles are found, they are reported to the acupuncturist.

3. Clients open their packs of needles by peeling back paper and exposing the handle end of the needles, and await the acupuncturist to insert the needles.

4. After the acupuncturist inserts the needles according to the acupuncture detoxification treatment protocol, the client remains seated with the inserted needles for 45 minutes. If a needle falls out prior to the completion of treatment, the client notifies the acupuncturist who appropriately disposes of the loose needle.

5. The client removes and counts their own auricular needles after 45 minutes and drops them in the medical waste dispenser. If one of the points should bleed, the client holds a cotton ball on the point that has bled, and calls the acupuncturist to handle the bleeding and assure that any blood-exposed cotton is properly disposed of. If the client contaminates their hands with their own blood, the client washes them with soap and water. If one or more needle is missing, the client assists the acupuncturist in locating the lost needle(s).

Procedures Followed by Acupuncturists and/or At-Risk Workers

All acupuncturists and other at-risk workers:

1. Wash hands with soap and water before entering the clinic.

2. Wear rubber gloves as appropriate to handle dirty or bloody cotton and, at the discretion of the acupuncturist, when needling. When handling something bloody, the acupuncturist or at-risk worker should put gloves on both hands and appropriately dispose of gloves following any such exposure.

3. Wash hands with soap and water following each exposure to blood or tissue or to blood- or tissue-exposed cotton.

Acupuncturist:

4. Treats additional body points for side effects of drug withdrawal depending upon the discretion of the acupuncturist with the consent or at the request of the client.
   a) Selects points appropriate to the presenting problem
   b) Inserts and removes all body needles
   c) Records additional treatment on the client's treatment card.

5. Inserts needles following sterile procedure - i.e., needle is grasped by the handle so that the tip and shaft are not touched and do not touch anything prior to insertion.

6. Washes hands after contact with a client who presents an obvious skin infection, severe acne, or if client has bled.

7. At their own discretion re-needles auricular point using a sterile needle should a needle fall out after initial insertion.

8. Removes all body point needles using cotton balls.

9. Removes auricular point needles on request using cotton balls.

10. Asks client to assist in locating missing needles following needle count.

11. Discards needles into biohazard disposal container.

Needle Safety Rules

1. Each new client is to read these needle safety precautions and to be given these precautions in writing.

2. In case you are stuck with a non-sterile/previously used needle, notify the acupuncturist immediately.

3. Do not leave the treatment area for any reason with needles inserted. PLEASE USE THE RESTROOM BEFORE RECEIVING TREATMENT.

4. Please do not walk around (including going to the bathroom or getting tea) with needles inserted unless you are going to the needle removal area to remove your needles.

5. Check area around your chair before and after treatment to be sure there are no stray or loose needles; count your needles as you take them out to be sure that none fell out during treatment; if any are missing, notify the acupuncturist immediately and assist in locating the missing needle(s).

Needle Stick Protocol

The following guidelines are to be followed toward preventing the possibility of a double stick (a used acupuncture needle piercing the skin of a second person):

1. Once needles are inserted, the client is to stay seated during treatment. The Clinic Coordinator will assist in serving tea.

2. Clients are instructed to check area on and around their chair before and after treatment to be sure there are no stray or loose needles.

3. Clients are instructed to count ear needles upon removal to be sure that none fell out during treatment; if any are missing, they will notify the acupuncturist immediately and assist in locating the missing needle(s). Only the acupuncturist should remove body needles.

4. In the event of a double stick, the acupuncturist will immediately bring the client to the Program Director or, if he/she is unavailable, the Program assistant to assist in assessing whether testing for communicable disease is indicated. In any event, the client will be advised of client rights to be tested for a communicable disease. The acupuncturist shall file an incident report with the Program Director. One copy of the report will be kept in the client's file, and another copy will be given to the Executive Director.

A document similar to the following should be explained and given to each client upon intake, and posted in the clinic:

Needle Safety and What to do in Case of Bleeding

To avoid contagious disease or injury, please observe the following simple rules regarding needles:

1. Do not leave the treatment area for any reason with needles inserted. **PLEASE USE THE RESTROOM BEFORE RECEIVING TREATMENT AND GETTING YOUR TEA.**

2. Clean the cartilage area of both ears with an alcohol swab.

3. Select two packages of disposable acupuncture needles (5 needles per pack).

4. Before you sit down, check to be sure there are no loose needles on or around the chair area. If loose needles are found, please report it to the acupuncturist or other (program) staff member.

5. Open your packs of needles by peeling back the paper and exposing the handle end of the needles, and wait for the acupuncturist to insert the needles. The acupuncturist will tell you how many needles he or she inserted.

6. After the acupuncturist inserts the needles, remain seated with the inserted needles for 45 minutes. If a needle falls out, notify the acupuncturist or a staff member who will appropriately disposes of the loose needle.

To Remove Needles

1. If you have needles in your arms, hands, or legs, wait for the acupuncturist to remove them. DO NOT WALK WITH NEEDLES IN.

2. After body points are removed, use the mirror and pull your ear needles out in the direction from which they were inserted. Have a cotton ball ready in case blood appears after a needle is removed. Remove one needle at a time. Drop them in the red plastic medical waste container. COUNT YOUR NEEDLES as you take them out to be sure that you have the same number as were put in. If you are missing any, notify a staff person immediately.

3. Using a clean piece of dry cotton, check both ears for any spots that have bled. PRESS THE COTTON ONTO ANY POINTS THAT ARE BLEEDING. DISCARD THE COTTON ONLY IN RED PLASTIC MEDICAL WASTE CONTAINER.

4. If you have any questions or need help, ask a staff person.

5. If you accidentally get blood on your hands, wash them with soap and water.

6.. In case you are accidentally stuck with a non-sterile or previously used needle, notify the acupuncturist immediately.

Safety Inspection and Maintenance

It is the policy of the (program) that all client treatment program areas and buildings shall be inspected on a bi-monthly basis for any condition which poses a potential hazard to client health and safety. This inspection shall include but not be limited to flooring, window areas, door and door perimeters, and electrical and mechanical fixtures.

It is a further policy of the (program) that a "SAFETY INSPECTION AND MAINTENANCE LOG" shall be maintained at a designated location in the Agency. The Log shall contain the report of the findings and maintenance recommendations for each bi-monthly inspection. The log shall contain a description of any condition found which represents a potential hazard to client health and safety, and a copy of such finding shall be filed with the Executive Director within twenty-four hours, and the Executive Director shall effect the necessary repairs or correction prior to further client use of the area. If no such condition is found during the inspection, the staff person conducting the inspection shall make verification to that effect in the "SAFETY INSPECTION AND MAINTENANCE LOG."

Section C: Sample Client Intake Materials and Client Confidentiality

These procedures and materials have been developed from a variety of NADA programs.

1) "Welcome" document:

2) Client Rights and Grievance Procedures

3) Intake Form: (The funding agency may require special Client Intake forms. Most programs start out asking the client for more information than is necessary, and end up shortening the intake requirements. The form provided contains most of the information required by various state and federal agencies.)

4) Sliding Fee Scale

5) Referral forms: Standard "Treatment Plan" referral forms may be used by criminal justice or other referring agencies who have mandated clients to attend. Clients are instructed to bring these signed forms with them when they come to the clinic. Includes instructions to the client and hours, days and location of the clinic.

6) Sliding Fee Scale for Special Programs

. . . .

(Name of Program, address, phone #)

WELCOME

Acupuncture is an ancient form of healing. We use acupuncture and herbal tea as an aid in detoxification and in maintaining sobriety. Acupuncture is not a miracle, but it will reduce craving and much of the discomfort of "kicking" while it helps restore the body's own energy.

CLINIC HOURS AND LOCATIONS

(Clinic treatment days, hours, and locations. Clinic hours should reflect the fact that the treatment takes 45 minutes.)

ADMISSION TO (PROGRAM)

You are welcome here and there are no special requirements to enter our program. Whether you are coming voluntarily or have been referred by the courts, parole or probation, simply come to the clinic during clinic hours and see a counselor for an intake. No appointment is necessary. During this interview, you will have an opportunity to ask questions about the treatments and discuss the best treatment plan for you. The interview will take about 20 minutes.

DAILY PROCEDURE

Each day you come for treatment (describe procedure for recording attendance or participation. This should involve a client treatment card, on which are recorded daily treatments and symptoms.) Clean your ears with alcohol and cotton, select your needles, pulling the wrapper open to expose the needle handles. Find a place to sit and wait for the acupuncturist. Hair hanging over the ears must be pulled back during treatment.

ABOUT TREATMENTS

Allow 45 minutes to an hour for treatment. Following treatment, sit at the mirror in the clinic and remove the needles from your ears. If you do not feel comfortable doing this, ask the acupuncturist to do it for you. For needle safety reasons, the following rules must be followed:

1. Check area around your chair before and after treatment to be sure there are no stray or loose needles; count your needles when you remove them to be sure that none fall out during treatment; if any are missing, notify the acupuncturist immediately and assist in locating the missing needle(s).

2. In case you are stuck with a non-sterile/previously used needle, notify the acupuncturist immediately.

3. No client may leave the treatment area for any reason with needles inserted. If one of your needles falls within reach hold it and give it to the acupuncturist to discard. If you want more tea ask a staff person to get it for you.

4. Clients may not walk around (including going to the bathroom or getting tea) with needles inserted.

5. If you see a random needle, tell a staff person, but do not pick it up yourself.

Come as clean and sober as you can. For best results, you should come at least daily for the first two weeks, but you are welcome to come as often as you like.

You will get the most out of your treatment if you relax quietly in your chair, sitting quietly with arms and legs uncrossed. Talking, reading, eating, smoking, and gum chewing interfere with the effectiveness of the treatment. People sometimes use the treatment time to meditate or doze.

ABOUT COUNSELING AND MEETINGS

We have (describe any education/counseling or recovery group activities on site. Ideally, an opportunity should be provided for clients to stay after treatment or to come back during the day and talk to a staff member about acupuncture, drugs, sobriety, recovery, Twelve Step programs, or any other issues with which they might need assistance or information.).

Acupuncture is effective with other recovery activities and support. A.A., N.A., and C.A. schedules are available in the clinic. Ask (staff) for additional information.

ABOUT THE TEA

The tea is not a narcotic or sedative, but it will relax you. Following treatment, drink as much as you like. The tea is available for sale at cost or may be purchased in bulk at (local outlet is available). It contains chamomile, peppermint, hops, valerian root, yarrow, and scullcap.

FEES

(Depends upon policy) No one is turned away for lack of funds. You are encouraged to be self-supporting in sobriety, so, if you are not working, please pay what you are able for your treatments. If you are employed, treatment fees are charged on a sliding scale based on income.

RULES

No weapons, violence, or threat of violence.

No smoking, eating or talking in the clinic.

Please respect the treatment time of others.

For issues concerning client confidentiality, see *Confidentiality: A Guide to Federal Laws and Regulations*, published by and available from the Legal Action Center, 153 Waverly Place, New York, NY 10014. If the program receives public funding, forms which place the program in compliance with these laws are usually provided by the local administering agency.

Laws require that clients sign an Informed Consent and statement of Client Rights. Concerning acupuncture, the following Informed Consent may be used:

(Name of Program)
INFORMED CONSENT

1.   I, the undersigned client/participant, hereby authorize the clinical staff of (Program) to perform treatment including acupuncture procedures induced by the insertion of special needles into the underlying tissues at certain points on the surface of the body.

2.   Acupuncture detoxification has shown through experience to be helpful in relieving acute symptoms of withdrawal from alcohol and other drugs. I realize, however, that no guarantees have been given me regarding cure or improvement.

3.   The confidentiality of all client records maintained by this Program is protected by federal law. The Program Staff may not say to a person outside the Program that a client attends the Program or disclose any information identifying a client as an alcohol or drug user unless:

   a)   The client consents in writing.
   b)   The disclosure is allowed by a court order.
   c)   The disclosure is made to medical personnel in a medical emergency, or to qualified personnel for research, audit, or Program evaluation.
   d)   The Program Staff believes the client to be in danger to self or to another person or to the property of another person.
   e)   The appropriate state or local authorities when child, dependent adult, or elder abuse is observed or suspected (11161.5 State Penal Code; 15600 et. seq. and 9387 et. seq. Welfare and Institutions Code; 42 U.S.C. 290ee-3;42 C.F.R. Part 2).

4.   Federal law and regulations do not protect any information about crime committed by a client either at the Program or against any person who works for the Program or about any threat to commit such a crime.

5.   If my attendance here is mandated or required by a government agency, I realize that the referring agency may impose adverse consequences as a result of my failure to comply with treatment plans.

6.   I understand that I am free to withdraw my consent at any time.

_____   ___/___/___

Signature of Client/Participant

_____   ___/___/___

Signature of Staff

(Name of Program)

Client Rights, Nondiscrimination Policy, and Grievance Procedures

Admission to the (Name of Program) is based upon expressed willingness to attempt recovery from alcohol and/or other drugs, and upon a willingness to abide by the (Name of Program) rules as stated below.

No client will be denied admission to the program based upon race, ethnicity, national origin, gender, religious belief, or sexual preference.

Clients may be declined admission or may be discharged based upon medical screening if, in the opinion of a physician, it is inadvisable for them to undergo or continue the program.

Clients have the right to examine their client records upon petition to the Program Director.

If any grievances arise regarding admission, discharge, or relationship with supervising (program) staff, the following procedure should be followed:

1. Attempt to resolve the dispute with the responsible staff member.
2. If unsuccessful, contact the (program) Director in writing (mailing address), or in person (address) or by telephone (number).
3. If the problem or issue remains unresolved, submit a statement of the problem in writing to the Executive Director, (agency, address).
4. If the problem remains unresolved, an appeal may be filed in writing to the Secretary of the Board of Directors (or ultimate authority, agency, address).

Further appeal may be made (if public funding) to the Drug and Alcohol Administrator (county or local jurisdiction).

(Name of Program)

INTAKE FORM

Date:___/___/___   Social Security #:____-___-_____
Name:_____
Homeless? __   Address: _____
City: _____   Zip Code:_____   Phone#:_____
Birth Date:_____Age:_____   Gender:_____
Ethnicity: White; African American; American Indian; Asian; Filipino
          Pacific Islander; Latino.
Employment   Employed F T, Employed P T, Unemployed (Looking
Status: for work), Not in the work force (not seeking work).
Highest School Grade Completed? _____
Referring Agency: _____ Mandated: Y/N
_____Number of entries into Project Recovery.
_____Number of entries into all detox/recovery program.
_____Are you on (public insurance)?
_____Number of dependent children at home.
Please describe your drug use:

Choice	Drug	Route*	Freq#	Age of First Use	Date of Last Use
First					
Second					
Third					

*   Routes of Administration: oral, smoke, inhale, injection
#   Frequency of use in last month: daily, 4-6 times a week, 1-3 times a week, 2-3
    times a month, one time a month, no use
Any IV (needle) drug use in past year above? Y/N
Medical History : (circle condition for which you have recently been treated):

Liver Disease	Hepatitis	Asthma	Heart Disease
Kidney Disease	Diabetes	Lung Disease	Hemophilia

Physician_____ Date last seen_____
Current medication:_____
Are you being treated for any psychiatric disorder? _____
Women: *Are you pregnant Now? Y/N Month:*_____
Family history of alcohol or drug addiction: father, mother, aunt, uncle,
other: _____
Describe any treatment program, drug or alcohol rehab, or detox program
you   have   gone   through   in   the   past   six   months.
_____
comments:_____

(Name of Program)

Weekly Fee Schedule for Acupuncture Treatments

Gross Monthly Income	Per Treatment	Unlimited Treatments
Less than 738	2	5
738 - 1037	4	10
1038 - 1338	12	32
1339 - 1638	24	65
1639 - 1938	32	90
1939 - 2538	40	125
2539 - 3138	48	150
Over 3138	55	200

* Deduct 20% of fee for each person other than yourself who depends upon this income

I agree to pay $_____for each week of treatment.

_____   ___/___/___

Signature of Client/Participant

Probation Referral Form
(Parole, Child Protective Services, etc.)
To (program):_____   Date: ___/___/___
_____ is being referred to Project Recovery for the following
treatment services:

Instructions to Client
To begin your treatment program, bring this completed form with you
Project Recovery at any of the times listed. You do not need an appointment.
Give this form to the acupuncturist or counselor and they will set a time for your
intake, usually right after your first acupuncture treatment. During the intake,
your intake counselor will explain the program to you and answer any questions.

Acupuncture Times and Location
(Name of Program)
(phone #)
(address)
(clinic days and hours)

To be completed by the Referring Officer

___**Treatment Plan A (30 days):**
Acupuncture 5 x per week for 30 days.
Weekly drug/alcohol counseling/education group:
Daily N.A./C.A./A.A. meetings for 30 days.

___**Treatment Plan B (60 days):**
Acupuncture:
5 x per week for 30 days.
then 3 x per week for 30 days.
Weekly drug/alcohol counseling/education group:
N.A./C.A./A.A. meetings 3 x per week for 60 days.

___**Treatment Plan C (90 days):**
Acupuncture:
5 x per week for 30 days.
then 3 x per week for 30 days.
then 2 x per week for 30 days.
Weekly drug/alcohol counseling/education group:
N.A./C.A./A.A. meetings 3 x per week for 90 days.

___Other treatment plan or recommended services (please describe):
_____

Referring Officer: _____   Phone #: _____

(Name of Program)

Fee schedule for 30 day, 60 day, 90 day, and six month tracking programs:

Total Program Fee: $_____

Gross Monthly Income	30	60	90	180
Less than 738:	25	38	55	104
738 - 1037:	120	180	325	465
1038 - 1338:	160	240	432	618
1339 - 1638:	212	320	575	822
1639 - 1938:	282	425	765	1093
1939 - 2538:	375	565	1017	1454
2538 - 3138:	499	751	1352	1933
Over 3138:	663	999	1798	2572

Deduct 20% of fee for each person other than yourself who depends upon this income.

I agree to pay to the total amount of $ _____ with an initial payment of _____ on ___/___/___ and subsequent payments of _____ on every ____/____.

_____   ___/___/___
Client

_____   ___/___/___
Staff

Individual client "Treatment Cards" or daily private client log sheets are useful. One side of the card or log may give the client an opportunity to "rate" the severity of their symptoms that day on a scale of one to four. Common withdrawal symptoms from a variety of drugs might be listed, such as shakes, sweating, insomnia, anxiety, cravings, "drug dreams," depression, headaches, loss of appetite, nausea, diarrhea, and constipation. This allows the client to see progress during detoxification, and allows the acupuncturist to track persistent symptoms. A "Before treatment" and "After treatment" comparison is good, in which the client rates, on a scale, the degree of relief from the symptoms they were experiencing before treatment. Options can be checked in general response to the treatment such as "worse, no effect, slight relief, great relief." This will provide a helpful research tool to the program as well as validation of treatment effectiveness for the client. The card may also provide space for other information such as "date of last use" or any significant changes since the client's last treatment (employment, change in housing, etc.). And it is good to provide a place for the client to make subjective comments, "journal" or "diary" type entries as a way of marking their own progress.

This card or log should also have a place for the acupuncturist to sign or initial dates of treatment, and a place to list any special protocols or points used, especially if more than one acupuncturist is working in the clinic.

Section D: Sample Job Descriptions

Following are some sample descriptions of typical positions in an acupuncture-based program. The degree of specialization of positions depends, of course, on the size of the program, so duties may be consolidated or rearranged depending on need for the following:

- Program Director

- Administrative Assistant

- Coordinator of Clinical Services

- Program Assistant

- Acupuncturist

- Counselor

TITLE: Program Director
REPORTS TO: Agency Executive Director (or Board)
QUALIFICATIONS:

- If recovering, a minimum of five years continuous sobriety.
- College degree in helping profession (Counseling, Psychology, Sociology, etc.) and / or degree / certificate in Oriental Medicine or acupuncture preferred, equivalent experience acceptable. National Acupuncture Detoxification Association (NADA) certification or equivalent required. Minimum two years direct experience in the field of alcoholism / drug abuse required. Certificate in Alcohol/Drug Counseling or equivalent required.
- Specific knowledge of the principles of NADA protocol, of individual and group chemical dependency counseling techniques, of relapse prevention, and of basic pharmacology and specific withdrawal symptoms from all major categories of psychoactive drugs.
- Ability to write appropriate professional letters and reports, to communicate verbally with judges, attorneys, physicians, employers, and other professionals as well as clients from a wide range of socio-economic backgrounds.
- Public speaking skills for purposes of in-service training, press conferences, orientations, and other speaking engagements.
- Administrative and supervisory skills.
- Ability to recognize own professional limitations so that proper referrals can be made.
- High standard of professional ethics.

RESPONSIBILITIES:

Provides for all outpatient detoxification, counseling, and other treatment and case management services and assures that all such services are provided under the direct supervision of properly certified and insured practitioners employed by or under contract with (Agency/Program).

- Supervises and provides professional evaluations for (list of all subordinate staff positions).
- Assures proper case and staff meetings between case managers, probation, and community resources staff.
- Assists in the coordination of services with probation and community resource agencies.
- Insures delivery of client services at satellite locations including (list).
- Processes applicable paperwork, maintains accurate client records and computer files, and submits monthly statistics and other records as required by funding sources.
- Prepares reports to funding sources and assists in preparation of related grant proposals.

- Conducts grant research to remain aware of potential new funding for expansion and enhancement of services.
- Assures the provision of information and referral services to all clients as indicated by client need.
- Keeps abreast of all current alcohol and drug resources in the community.
- Recruits, trains, orients, motivates, and rewards an extensive corp of volunteers to assist with appropriate program activities.
- Coordinates with the (local college of Oriental medicine) the placement of acupuncture interns to provide (Name of Program) program services.
- Keeps abreast of the current literature and research in the field of alcoholism and drug abuse.
- Upholds a professional image of the (Agency/Program) at all times.
- Performs other related duties as assigned by the (Supervisor).

TITLE: Administrative Assistant
REPORTS TO: Program Director
QUALIFICATIONS:

- A minimum of two years of administrative and computer operation responsibility.
- Administrative, organizational, reception, and general office skills.
- Ability to write appropriate professional letters and reports, to communicate verbally with judges, attorneys, physicians, employers, and other professionals as well as clients from a wide range of socio-economic backgrounds.
- Computer data entry and program development skills.
- Ability to work on complex tasks under pressure.

RESPONSIBILITIES:

- To maintain all (Program) client intake and attendance records.
- To design and generate reports concerning client program activity for law enforcement and funding agencies and to assure that all records required by these agencies are properly maintained.
- To answer phones and provide information and program referral information.
- To assist the Program Director and his assistant in maintaining an appointment calendar and developing materials for public speaking, in-service and outreach presentations and trainings, press conferences, orientations, and other speaking and public relations engagements.
- To assist in maintaining all administrative program files.
- To manage the Program office including the ordering of all office supplies, and the maintenance of telephone, computer, and other office equipment.
- To assist in program correspondence.
- To assure that a client master roster is maintained concerning the status of each client.
- To assure the proper billing for all (public insurance) eligible treatment services.
- To uphold a professional image of the (Agency/Program) at all times.
- To maintain plants, empty trash, and clean clinic and office space between cleaning service visits.
- To perform other related duties as assigned by the Program Director.

TITLE: Program Assistant
REPORTS TO: Program Director
QUALIFICATIONS:

- If recovering, three years of continuous sobriety.
- College degree in helping profession (Counseling, Psychology, Sociology, etc.) and/or degree/ certificate in Oriental Medicine or acupuncture preferred, equivalent educational experience acceptable. National Acupuncture Detoxification Association (NADA) certification or equivalent required. Minimum one year direct experience in the field of chemical dependency required.
- Specific knowledge of the principles of NADA protocol, of individual and group chemical dependency counseling techniques, and of basic pharmacology and specific withdrawal symptoms from all major categories of psychoactive drugs.
- Ability to write appropriate professional letters, funding applications, and reports, to communicate verbally with judges, attorneys, physicians, employers, and other professionals as well as clients from a wide range of socio-economic backgrounds.
- Public speaking skills for purposes of in-service training, press conferences, orientations, and other speaking engagements.
- Ability to recognize own professional limitations so that proper referrals can be made.
- High standard of professional ethics.

RESPONSIBILITIES:

- The Project Recovery Program Assistant, working under the supervision of the Program Director, assists in the overall supervisory responsibility for all (program services and activities), and, in carrying out this responsibility:
- Insures a sterile field for acupuncture needles and their disposal, and manages clinic inventory of needles, cotton balls, alcohol, tea, dispensers, and other clinic accouterments.
- Carries out and supervises outpatient client intakes including appropriate assessment and the collection of client fees.
- Assists in the supervision of client intakes.
- Conducts referral counseling with clients and facilitates counseling/education groups.
- Assures that all records required by funding sources are properly maintained.
- Assures that all reports to funding sources are prepared and submitted in a timely manner.

- Maintains current schedules for acupuncturists and counselors on contract with the program, assuring for the accurate billing for these services.
- Assists in the research and development of program grant and funding proposals for maintaining and expanding services.
- Assures the availability of information and referral services to all clients as indicated by client need.
- Assures the availability of current program literature, including brochures, referral information, and intake forms.
- Assists in the proper and timely reporting of appropriate attendance data to all referring agencies.
- Keeps abreast of all current alcohol and drug resources in the community.
- Assists in the development and implementation of a comprehensive outreach program as appropriate to inform the community of (Program) services, and maintains an awareness of client and community needs.
- Assists in the recruitment and training of an extensive corp of volunteers and interns to assist with appropriate program activities and maintains intern records.
- Keeps abreast of the current literature and research in the field of alcoholism and drug abuse.
- Upholds a professional image of the (Agency/Program) at all times.
- Performs other related duties as assigned by the Program Director.

TITLE: Coordinator of Clinical Services
REPORTS TO: Program Director
QUALIFICATIONS:
- If recovering, a minimum of two years continuous sobriety.
- Written and spoken fluency in Spanish required; bi-cultural ethnicity preferred but not required.
- Certified acupuncturist preferred; college course work in chemical dependency or helping professions (psychology, sociology, etc.) preferred. NADA (National Acupuncture Detoxification Association) certification or equivalent required.
- Ability to write appropriate professional letters and reports, to communicate verbally with judges, attorneys, physicians, employers, and other professionals as well as clients from a wide range of socio-economic backgrounds.
- Public speaking skills for purposes of in-service training, press conferences, orientations, and other speaking engagements.
- Administrative and supervisory skills.
- Ability to recognize own professional limitations so that proper referrals can be made.
- High standard of professional ethics.

RESPONSIBILITIES:
- Provides all client services, written or spoken, in Spanish.
- Travels to and provides for all necessary supplies and for acupuncture treatment at assigned treatment sites.
- Acts as liaison between (Program) and the treatment satellite location staff persons.
- Provides for herbal tea at assigned acupuncture treatment sites.
- Insures a sterile field for acupuncture needles and their disposal, and manages clinic inventory of needles, cotton balls, alcohol, tea, dispensers, and other clinic supplies.
- Provides for therapeutic urinalysis on site, operates urine testing equipment, and manages clinic inventory of urinalysis equipment and supplies, and assures for proper maintenance and cleaning of urinalysis equipment.
- Collects client fees for services as appropriate.
- Maintains computer records and client files at assigned treatment sites, assuring for the proper computer entry of all urinalysis test results and treatment attendance.
- Provides other related duties as assigned by the Program Director.

TITLE: Acupuncturist
REPORTS TO: Program Assistant
QUALIFICATIONS:

- State Acupuncture license (or equivalent).
- National Acupuncture Detoxification Association (NADA) certification.
- $1,000,000 professional liability insurance policy in force listing the (Agency/Program) as additionally insured.

RESPONSIBILITIES:

- Performs NADA protocol auricular acupuncture on (Program) clients and potential clients and provides additional triage medical case management as appropriate.
- Assures that all clients receiving treatment have completed required consent forms and treatment cards.
- Documents treatments on appropriate treatment cards.
- Assists in maintaining clinic needles, supplies, and tea, and assures a sterile field for the performance of acupuncture treatment under the health and safety standards established by the clinic and by state and federal laws.
- Upholds a professional image of the (Program/Agency) at all times.
- Performs additional duties as assigned by the Program Assistant or Director.

TITLE: Counselor
REPORTS TO: Program Assistant
QUALIFICATIONS:

- Spanish/English bi-lingual, bi-cultural (as appropriate).
- College degree in helping profession (Counseling, Psychology, Sociology, etc.) and MFCC or CAC preferred. Equivalent experience acceptable. Minimum two years experience in the field of alcohol/drug counseling required. NADA Certification or equivalent required.
- Specific knowledge of individual and group counseling principles and techniques, and of substance abuse assessment and case planning.
- Ability to write appropriate professional letters and reports, to communicate verbally with professionals and with clients from diverse socio-economic and ethnic backgrounds.
- Ability to recognize own professional limitations so that appropriate referrals can be made.
- High standards of professional ethics.

RESPONSIBILITIES:

- Develops and implements outreach strategies in the Latino community.
- Conducts individual and group substance abuse counseling and education sessions.
- Conducts substance abuse severity assessments and produces appropriate treatment plans.
- Performs case management including maintaining files properly documented with client's progress and attendance.
- Keeps abreast of the current literature and research in the field of alcoholism and drug addiction/abuse.
- Upholds a professional image of the (Agency/Program) at all times.
- Performs additional duties as assigned by the Project Recovery Director.

Appendix XII: Treatment Resources

Section A: HIV/AIDS and Other Infectious Diseases

Increasingly, primary health issues are correlative factors that need to be addressed in a sustained way by the capable treatment provider. "There is a plenitude of anecdotal support for implementing or enhancing primary care as an avenue to increased compliance and (drug treatment) program retention." [285] Substance abuse is indeed profoundly linked, through high-risk behaviors and the physical vulnerability associated with chronic substance abuse, to human immunodeficiency virus (HIV), acquired immune deficiency syndrome (AIDS), tuberculosis (TB), sexually transmitted diseases (STDs), as well as diseases of the liver, brain, pancreas, and respiratory system. Therefore, an effective continuum of substance abuse treatment needs to have a sustained interactive relationship with primary health care and with health care case management services. Research indicates that infectious diseases such as AIDS, hepatitis B infection, STDs, and TB are increasing among drug users, and approaches to these diseases needs to be integrated with drug treatment and a public health approach if we are to reverse or at least stabilize the trends of those diseases. Drug abuse treatment settings are an ideal site to identify these infections and initiate and maintain appropriate medical management.[286]

The epidemic of HIV is one of the most serious current public health challenges, and injecting drug users are at increased risk for HIV infection because they often share contaminated injection equipment.[287] This drug-related HIV epidemic is having a disproportionate impact upon ethnic minorities such as African Americans and Hispanics,[288] African Americans comprising 51%, and Latinos 29%, of the HIV cases in which drug injection is the primary risk factor. Injecting needle users also place two other groups at risk for developing AIDS: their sexual partners and their children. Nationally, nearly 60% of pediatric AIDS patients contracted HIV through perinatal transmission from an injecting drug abusing mother or a mother who was having sex with an injecting drug abusers.[289]

Besides drug treatment itself, prevention campaigns promoting risk reduction measures (non-sharing of needles, monogamous relationships, sexual abstinence, and the use of latex condoms) are currently the primary means available for moderating the HIV epidemic's impact, and such campaign efforts should be a sustained and fully integrated feature of a comprehensive drug treatment program, indicating the desirability of making basic AIDS and AIDS prevention training mandatory for all treatment staff.[290] HIV testing on site has also been found to have a positive correlation with HIV risk behavior.[291]

Substance abuse and TB are also linked,[292] especially among those with AIDS.[293] Part of TB resurgence is co-occurrence with AIDS, and, according to a New York study,[294] TB/AIDS patients compared to AIDS patients without TB are more likely to be non-white and to be IV drug users. Jails and prisons are ideal environments for the spread of TB, and TB also touches the communities into which prisoners are released, indicating the need for supervision and case management of TB cases and community health surveillance.[295]

Here again, acupuncture can help to fill the operational gaps that generally exist between HIV and AIDS services and treatment and the chemical dependency treatment setting.[296]

HIV and AIDS recovery issues are also linked to the process of recovery from chemical dependency. The following paper is reprinted with permission of the author.

Thinking about HIV, AIDS, and Recovery (1993)
by Carol Crump, M.A.

AIDS is a bio-psycho-social disease, just as alcoholism is. It's influenced by physical, psychological, behavioral, and environmental conditions. It affects the mind, the body, and the emotions. Just as with alcoholism, there is no single, simple, magical cure.

The Program of Alcoholics Anonymous helps people learn when they need to ask for help, and how to discover within themselves the strength and courage to change. This is the same sort of learning required to avoid the risk of infection with HIV, and to slow progression of the disease if infection has already occurred.

Most AIDS patients have histories of past or present alcoholism or addiction. If you work in the area of chemical dependency, then you will be working with HIV+ people. That's a simple truth. If you work in recovery, you know that information and hope are some of our most powerful tools. These are the same tools we use in facing HIV and AIDS.

The Center for Disease Control (CDC), which records all reports of AIDS on a day-to-day basis, estimates that more than 1.5 million Americans have been exposed to HIV as of 1988. By the mid-1990s the tally may be as high as ten million. Remember that CDC counts only full-blown cases of AIDS in their statistics. Some people with HIV related diseases become so ill that they die without ever having met the specific criteria for AIDS diagnosis. The diagnostic classifications are only somewhat useful for us as counselors -- what's important for us to realize is that most people with HIV infection don't realize they are HIV+, and that most people with HIV infection have so far not become ill.

AIDS is not an illness of high-risk people. It is an illness of high-risk behaviors. It's easier to engage in high-risk behaviors when you're using alcohol or drugs.

Staff need not only learn about AIDS, but to integrate that knowledge into their work. That means talking about two subjects that have traditionally been hidden in our society: death and sexuality.

Feelings to be aware of:

The attitude that anyone with a positive HIV test is going to 'get it' (AIDS), and will soon die. Connected with this may be a feeling that it's not really worth it for the HIV+ person to stay clean and sober, because they're just going to die soon, anyway. These ideas aren't uncommon -- the question is whether you, as an addictions counselor, are holding these ideas anywhere in your mind, and how these may impact the way you treat a person with HIV.

Your own fears and attitudes may come up in thoughts like, 'Well, if I thought I was going to get AIDS, I'd probably drink, too...' Whether or not you ever say this out loud, the person you are counseling will, at some level, be aware that you feel that way. Can you find feelings like this in yourself? How would you deal with an HIV+ person who has just relapsed?

A.A. has a long history of providing real support for people with life-threatening illnesses of any kind. A friend of mine in the program, faced with leukemia, once said, "A.A. isn't just a great way to live -- it seems to be giving me a good way to die, too." If you find yourself with a lot of fear and negative thinking about serious illnesses, seek out the people in the program who are dealing with these: there are lots of them, and they can offer real support and inspiration to you and the clients you work with.

Some people carry feelings of blame towards HIV+ persons -- there's sometimes the sense that they were 'asking for it', or 'deserve it'. Many cancer or heart-disease patients may also carry some degree of responsibility for their illness, but, as we know in A.A., to hold responsibility is not the same as blaming a person for their disease. Ask yourself if you're treating the HIV+ person in the same way as you would a person struggling with cancer. If you feel differently about the person with HIV, then take some time to look at that.

If you are in recovery yourself, you are probably very aware that many physicians and health-care professionals are not well-educated about addiction, and that this lack of education can lead to over-medication or inappropriate prescribing of medication for alcoholics and addicts. The same thing is true of HIV infection and AIDS. Physicians may carry the same fears and beliefs about AIDS that were mentioned before: a fatalistic idea that being HIV+ means an inevitable and horrible death, the idea that an HIV+ alcoholic may just as well keep drinking because they'll die soon. More commonly, if an HIV+ alcoholic or addict is trying to get clean and sober, it's not at all unusual for physicians to prescribe addictive medications like Valium and Ativan to 'help' the addict 'cope'. Those of us with a solid recovery program know very well that there's a big difference between medications like those and medications properly prescribed and appropriately used. A.A.'s guidelines for the use of painkilling or mind-altering medications apply just as much to the HIV+ alcoholic as they do to any other addict. As a counselor, you will be an important source of information and support for the HIV+ addict who is trying to find a way to live with HIV infection while staying sober, and who may be faced with professionals offering unnecessary types or amounts of medication.

Like alcoholism, AIDS isn't just going to disappear from our world. Whether you yourself ever have the virus or not, AIDS will be part of your life in sobriety. By 1995, it is very likely that every A.A. or N.A. group in the United States will have lost a member to the disease.

Alcoholics were stigmatized and despised for far too long. As people in recovery, we hold the tools to ensure that the same tragedy doesn't have to happen to those with HIV and AIDS in our midst. As people who, in our disease, probably engaged in unsafe behaviors, the saying "There but for the grace of God go I" applies now more than ever before.

Alcoholism used to be considered a moral deficiency. Now some people look at persons with AIDS in the same way. We in recovery don't have to let that happen. People in recovery know what it is like to feel hopeless and then to receive help. Knowing that, the doors of A.A. and N.A. cannot be shut to anyone, no matter how ill they may be.

Our recovery program will sustain us in the face of AIDS only as long as we give it away.

"When anyone, anywhere, reaches out for help, I want the hand of A.A. always to be there. And for that: I am responsible."[297]

Other helpful papers on this subject include Neil R. Schram, M.D.'s "Refining Safer Sex," *FOCUS*,[298] June, 1990, p. 3; "Rebecca Cole and Sally Cooper's "Lesbian Exclusion from

HIV/AIDS Education: Ten Years of Low-Risk Identity and High Risk Behavior," SIECUS Report, December 1990/January 1991, pp 18-23, and Jose Pares-Avila and Nicolas Parkhurst Carballeira's "Providing Culturally Competent HIV Counseling Services to Latinos: A Training Module for Community Mental Health Service Providers" (draft), available from the National Institutes of Mental Health, Public Inquiries Branch, Room 15C-05, 5600 Fishers Lane, Rockville, MD 20857.

Section B: Dual Diagnosis

A correlative factor that needs to be addressed in comprehensive drug and alcohol treatment is dual diagnosis. According to the National Institute on Drug Abuse (NIDA), drug dependence frequently occurs in conjunction with, or secondary to, other psychiatric disorders such as depression, organic impairment, or schizophrenia.[299] Some researchers[300] have found that as many as 78% of individuals seeking assistance for alcohol and other drug abuse problems showed evidence of an additional psychiatric disorder at some point in their lives, and other studies[301] have found that over a third of admitted general psychiatry patients have been found to have problems that are significantly influenced or precipitated by their drug abuse. According to Rosenthal,[302] the problems that plague conventional treatment providers around the issues of dual diagnosis clients "arise out of the historical bifurcation of psychiatric and substance abuse services into separate, independently administered treatment domains, in which different physical locations, staffing patterns, and treatment philosophies reflect the frequently mistaken assumption that patients fall neatly into one category or the other." Acupuncture, because of its effectiveness in treating many mental health disorders,[303] can help in filling this operational "gap" between conventional mental health and chemical dependency treatment services, in which many clients become lost. Here, as with the relationship between the criminal justice system and the substance abuse treatment provider, a historical rift exists which must be bridged if the complex needs of the dual diagnosed population are to be addressed. While there is some controversy in the literature about whether dual diagnosis treatment should go on in more than one setting or under a single roof, there is evidence that successful treatment, as measured by abstinence rates and decreased hospitalization, can be accomplished in a primary substance abuse treatment setting for the dual diagnosed with concurrent treatment by other providers.[304] (See pp. 183-184 for a discussion of dual diagnosis and strategies for addressing it in the acupuncture-based setting; see also *n.* #208)

Dual Diagnosis is difficult if not impossible to assess when an individual is chronically using psychoactive drugs, because some symptoms of both intoxication and acute withdrawal are parallel to symptoms of mental disorders. It is only following the detoxification phase that an accurate diagnosis can begin to be made. Even then, post acute withdrawal syndrome, which lasts for months, can manifest some symptoms that resemble those common to mood disorders and personality disorders.[305] Acupuncture is helpful here as well, because the basic NADA protocol has efficacy in addressing many of these symptoms regardless.

It is Anne Wilson Schaef's opinion that all so-called psychiatric disorders (to which, of course, the conventional Western response is usually drug therapy), are "abnormalities" of the imposed Cartesian mind/body dualism, and therefore exist on the addictive continuum. They are, in this sense, like chronic drug use, "normal" and understandable survival-based reactions to the internalized oppression of the addictive system. Alice is herself not crazy! Many of these disorders do, indeed, respond to Twelve Step program involvement, and a special dual diagnosis Twelve Step meeting format ("Double Trudgers") has been developed in many regions.

Complete Western clinical definitions of all psychiatric disorders may be found in the *Diagnostic and Statistical Manual of the American Psychiatric Association* (APA), *third edition revised* (DSMIII-R) which, as a clinic resource guide, should be accompanied of course in our setting by a comprehensive diagnostic Chinese medical reference.

For dealing with countertransference issues with Post Traumatic Stress clients, see K. McCann and L. A. Pearlman's "Vicarious Traumatization: A Framework for Understanding the Psychological Effects of Working with Victims," *Journal of Traumatic Stress*, Vol. 3(1), 1990.

Other resources specific to Post Traumatic Stress include George S. Everly Jr., *A Clinical Guide to the Treatment of the Human Stress Response*, available from Chevron Publishing Corporation, 5018 Dorsey Hall Drive, Suite 104, Ellicott City, MD 21042, 410/740-0065, and J. Wilson and B. Raphael (editors), International Handbook for Traumatic Stress Syndromes, New York: Plenum (1992).

For other related resources, query:

Phoenix Springs Group
3345 Bee Caves Road, Suite 205
Austin, Texas 78746
512 / 327-3388

Mental Health Resources:
National Alliance for the Mentally Ill
1901 N. Fort Myer Drive, Suite 500
Arlington, VA 22209
703 / 524-7600

National Depressive and Manic Depressive Association
Merchandise Mart
Box 3395
Chicago, IL 60654
312 / 993-0066

National Institute of Mental Health
Public Inquiries Branch
Room 15C-05
5600 Fishers Lane
Rockville, MD 20857

National Mental Health Association
1021 Prince Street
Alexandria, VA 22314-722
703 / 684-7722

National Mental Health Consumer's Association
311 South Juniper Street, Room 902
Philadelphia, PA 19107

Phobic Society of America
P.O. Box 42514
Washington, DC 20015
301 / 231-9350

Section C: Gender, Age, Ethnicity, Race, and Sexual Preference:

Working Between Cultures

Harriet Beinfield and Efrem Korngold, *Between Heaven and Earth: A Guide to Chinese Medicine*, write (p. 381.) "By choosing between mutually exclusive either-or options, we splinter our world into winners and losers, masters and slaves, superiors and inferiors, haves and have-nots. Such hierarchical divisions are reinforced by a self-serving morality. We choose between what's good for my mind *or* body, me *or* you, my business or the environment, my national security or yours, means and ends, swaggering and sweating to defend what we arbitrarily decree as a righteous side of this tissue-paper wall. Rather than honoring our gender and ethnic differences with mutual respect, we confuse equal opportunity with homogeneity, crushing our diversity and imposing upon ourselves the banality of a mass monoculture."

The hope for the economic survival and spiritual flourishing of the nation and indeed of the human race is to acknowledge, honor, and embody the vast hidden treasures of cultural diversity that characterize modernity. In this, the challenges to the addiction treatment system are great indeed. It needs to serve as a haven of last resort to the most disenfranchised and wounded victims of the exclusionary, hierarchical, addictive society. It needs to become a safe harbor, a sanctuary for diversity, a place where healing begins, and an embarkation point for reentry into the larger emerging communities that it serves and that are being created out of the inclusionary principles of recovery.

There has been a great deal of research on cross-cultural training and counseling in the fields of psychiatry and anthropology, but the field of chemical dependency has lagged behind. Some of this is due to the influence of Alcoholics Anonymous, in which denying uniqueness has been seen as therapeutically desirable. Rather than uniqueness or differences, A.A. has emphasized the bond of alcoholism/addiction which makes everyone equal in the group. This "we are not unique" philosophy has helped thousands recover, and in fact is a philosophy that has been consistent with fundamental goals of the Civil Rights movement which has stressed equality (rather than differences) for African Americans, Latino/as, Native Americans, and others. This tendency toward "color-blindness" and "cultural-blindness" in which everyone is treated the same has been in conflict with an increasingly popular philosophy which emphasizes the need for people of color to appreciate their cultural differences and to identify with original (pre-migration) cultural values. Since addiction recovery, as we have been describing it in this book, is a process of a new emerging self, a transformation of ones consciousness of self, and since addiction, as we have described it, has resulted in part from the imposition of the White dominant values of Western culture, the identification of women with women, men with men, African Americans with African Americans, Native Americans with Native Americans, and so on, is an inevitable and necessary step in the recovery process. The validation of cultural experience and of cultural referents that are endogenous are vital.

Ethnicity and race, as well as gender and gender preference, are traditional "barriers" to drug and alcohol treatment in that conventional treatment, as well as research, is dominated by middle class White cultural values. This, in addition to racist attitudes among members of Twelve Step groups, have conveyed the tacit message that sobriety and "anglicization" are somehow parallel. Treatment needs to convey the strong message that *recovery is about becoming who you are.*

There are a number of things that a treatment program can do to address these barriers and to achieve cultural competence. The first and obvious goal is to recruit staff members who represent the ethnic, cultural, gender, and language characteristics of whatever client groups the program is targeting or expects to serve. If people of color are to be served, they will be heartened if the first staff people they meet in the program are also people of color. It is not enough to have "token" ethnic members on the Board of Directors or in administrative positions, although this is desirable. There must be a conscientious effort to recruit these individuals into front line staff positions. Unfortunately, while acupuncture itself transcends cultural differences, and can in fact be seen as a "global medicine" consistent with the folk medicine traditions of many ethnic minorities, acupuncturists themselves in this country tend to be Asian or White and middle class. There is a concerted effort within NADA to recruit and provide scholarships for people of color besides Asians who are interested in becoming acupuncturists.

As numbers warrant, ethnic- and language- and gender- specific groups should be available on the treatment site or, through linkages with other agencies, by referral.

All staff people working with clients, regardless of their own backgrounds, can also do a great deal to increase their own sensitivity to cultural differences so that they are able to honor all of the individuals who come to the clinic. Cross-cultural training should be accessed for all staff that will help the staff re-evaluate their own prejudices, giving them better insight into their own value system, and which will provide staff with the tools to assess clients more effectively and give them information which will help clients remain in treatment.

Treatment, therefore, needs to be able to speak different languages; it needs to transcend all boundaries in terms of accessibility and delivery of services; it needs to itself find "sponsorship" from within the communities it serves so that genuine bridges to those communities can be created, and it needs the capacity to integrate, in a therapeutic way, the cultural and gender issues that will become unmasked following detoxification - to become, inotherwords, itself a container for processing cultural and political issues.

Latino/a Culture:

Mexican, Puerto Rican, Cuban, and South American populations in the United States, particularly in inner cities, have grown dramatically in the past decade, as have drug and alcohol problems in this culture. The family values and extended family values of many in these cultures make seeking help from people outside the family extremely difficult, and families in these cultures are often very enabling of substance abusers who are members of the family, protecting them from the consequences of their addictions. Most acute drug and alcohol problems for members of these cultures, particularly among females, arise following the second and third generation in this country.

One valuable resource is "Quetzacoatl, Cortez, Y La Malinche: Counseling Latinos," a packet of resources collected by Jorge Cherbosque, PhD at the University of California, Los Angeles from the EAPA Western District Conference, April 18-21, 1993. This and other resources are available from the UCLA Latino American Center (213) 825-4571, and the UCLA Chicano Studies Research Center (213) 825-2363. Also of general value is Jose Pares-Avila and Nicolas Parkhurst Carballeira's "Providing Culturally Competent HIV Counseling Services to Latinos: A Training Module for Community Mental Health Service Providers" (draft), available from the National Institutes of Mental Health, Public Inquiries Branch, Room 15C-05, 5600 Fishers Lane, Rockville, MD 20857.

Adolescents:

The LifeBack Adult and Adolescent Substance Abuse Program in Michigan City, Indiana, has implemented an acupuncture component in their adolescent treatment program. See Richard Karrel's "Acupuncture In an Adolescent Treatment Setting, *Addiction and Recovery*, December, 1990, pp. 24-27.

Gays and Lesbians

While it is generally estimated that 10% of the general population have alcoholism or other drug dependency, a disproportionate percentage of the gay and lesbian adult population are thought to be afflicted. An extremely valuable, though somewhat regional, periodical is the *Gay and Lesbian Resource Center (GLRC) Bulletin*, 126 East Haley Street, Suite A-17, Santa Barbara, California, 93101. 805 / 963-3636. Monthly. $12/yr

The following is reprinted with permission from the author.

"Do You Work with Gay or Lesbian Clients? ...Some Things to Consider..."
by Carol Crump, M.A.

Homophobia is a harsh word, and painful to apply to ourselves or to other people. Try thinking of homophobia as the things we do, in our professional and personal lives, that make gay and lesbian people invisible. The ways in which we make a client invisible to ourselves represent lost opportunities to create connections, understanding, and the space for our clients and ourselves to find clarity and growth.

In counseling situations, all of the following are subtle (and not so subtle!) ways of being homophobic -- of erasing part of the reality of our clients lives:

Assuming that because you are a woman, you understand much of what it is to be a lesbian. Being quick to tell a lesbian that you "understand" her feelings, her circumstances, her life.

Finding yourself not wanting to really hear how a gay man or lesbian feels, acts with, lives with, their lover -- being a bit uncomfortable every tome a lesbian, for example, uses the word 'she' in place of 'he'. Be aware of whether you are aiming your questions or in just the right way to discourage her from speaking too directly of her relationship.

Assuming that to be gay or lesbian is a bedroom issue only. Demonstrating this with comments like, '...what somebody does in their own bedroom is nobody else's business'. Statements like this may be true in and of themselves, but fail to recognize the complex social, emotional, and political realities of the lives of gay men and lesbians.

Counseling a lesbian or gay man without having an extensive understanding of the gay and lesbian community where you live prevents your clients from accessing the resources that may be vital. Is the gay and lesbian community a large one? What kind of support and resources are available? What's the political climate within the community? Is it united and active or closeted and fearful? Is there little contact or interaction between gay men and lesbians, or are there some common projects, interests, and concerns? Is it a heavily bar-centered community? Is there active support for recovery from alcoholism and addiction, with gay and lesbian Twelve Step meetings? Are there support groups or 'safe houses' for battered lesbians or gay men? Do you know where to find this information?

Are there gay and lesbian therapists available? Are you willing to consult with them, refer clients to them, or ask them for supervision?

Do you believe that gay and lesbian relationships are basically 'just like' heterosexual relationships, except that the couple 'just happens' to be same-sex?

Have you had training in counseling gay, lesbian, and bisexual people? Training doesn't consist of one or two lectures in a course on human sexuality. It doesn't mean being an observer when a gay or lesbian speaks in a classroom situation: while this is certainly helpful, you're still in the role of passive observer -- a relatively 'safe' role which doesn't take you outside of your familiar comfort zone or invite you to look very deeply at yourself. Training means a combination of reading, study, supervision, and person-to-person experience with gay and lesbian people. Are you willing to seek out this kind of training?

Do you hold the belief that you 'don't have any problems' with people being gay or lesbian? Do you believe that only 'other people' are homophobic? Do you find yourself responding with statements starting with '...some of my best friends are...? ' Are you feeling a little angry at being asked this question? Feel into that. Wonder about it.

If you identify as gay or lesbian, to what extent have you examined your own internalized homophobia? What aspects of life in our community make you uneasy or uncomfortable? How might this discomfort play itself out in a counseling situation? Do you have a place to take these questions and work them out, not only in a personal sense, but in a clinical one as well?

Are you able to stay open to the idea of working through your own homophobia? Even for those of us who have been gay- or lesbian-identified for many years, the struggle with our internalized homophobia is something that goes on for a lifetime. As gay and lesbian counselors, if we aren't willing to see ourselves clearly, the messages we have internalized about ourselves can easily prevent us from being fully available to our clients. As heterosexual counselors working with gay and lesbian clients, you're faced not only with learning about what is essentially a different culture and community, but also with the painful task of acknowledging and reassessing some of the ideas you may hold. This is difficult work. Be gentle with yourself, but do it. One way of beginning this work is, when you are alone with yourself, ask how you really feel in your heart of hearts about gay and lesbian people. Don't judge your response, or worry about what 'other people' might think of you. Just notice it. Notice what your body is doing. Be with the images and pictures that come up in your mind. Let the words of your thoughts simply flow through your awareness. Take your time and let yourself feel your response clearly. Lean into it. Ask yourself about the ways in which your response may impact the way you are able to work with gay and lesbian clients. Honor your strengths. Give yourself permission to wonder about the parts of yourself that feel fear or a touch of disgust or impatience. Find a safe place to bring these out and to talk about them.

Section D: Counseling and Acupuncture

It is common for acupuncture-based programs to have difficulties in developing the proper balance between the acupuncture and the chemical dependency counseling portions of the program, as each staff learns about the other, and the as the best relationship is discovered. Our Santa Barbara program has gone through a long evolutionary process in the area, and following is a description of this counseling role in the acupuncture-based treatment setting, written by a a licensed counselor working adjunctively with the program. It is reprinted with permission from the author.

Detox, Counseling, and Acupuncture
by Faith Cavalier, MA., MFCC.

The Santa Barbara Council on Alcoholism and Drug Abuse's Project Recovery Detox and Acupuncture Program offers two forms of psychiatric intervention - individual counseling and group therapy. Each modality is offered twice a day, five days a week.

The first group generally takes place after the morning acupuncture clinic. On any given scheduled day the group may be male or female only, mixed, SSI, or [residential] Detox group only. The groups are held by Project Recovery staff and a Community Service Coordinator who is also available for case management purposes. A licensed Marriage Family and Child Counselor is also available and provides ongoing training and clinical supervision for staff, as well as counseling services for clients.

The second group held each day of the week is primarily for the [residential] Detox clients and graduates of this program. These groups are held by Community Service Coordinators or Interns. Case management services are also available if the need arises.

The groups may be educational, process, or relapse prevention in nature, depending on the needs of the group and the skill of the counselor. The groups are generally a mixture of alcoholics and drug addicts.

The individual counseling is 'drop-in' in nature, and is available during acupuncture clinic hours. A client may sign up for counseling at the same time as they sign in for acupuncture. The session will last anywhere from five to 30 minutes depending on available time and the length of the [counseling] waiting list. The counseling may take place in a private office if one is available, or out in the open nestled amongst the others [in the acupuncture clinic]. It is not unusual to find a client and a counselor both receiving acupuncture, sipping the herbal detox tea, as they work together on a particular issue or problem, but we avoid doing active counseling while the client is having treatment so that maximum benefit from the treatment can be achieved. If there is a crisis, this may not be possible.

For a population not generally having access to counselors or the willingness to utilize such services, this is a nice system as it tends to normalize and demystify the counseling process. Seeing a counselor becomes an acceptable part of the treatment as 'everyone' is seen doing it.

It is of value having counselors who are in Twelve Step recovery and who are able to model clean and sober living and the benefits of such a life. By the very nature of this persons existence, hope is offered to the chronic and severe relapser.

It is also desirable to have counselors who are sensitive and aware of cultural, gender, and age issues. It is a real advantage having counselors who are bilingual.

Counselors who understand dual diagnosis and feel confident working with the mentally ill substance abuser on psychotropic medications are an additional asset to the program.

Approximately 50% of people suffering from mental and emotional disorders such as schizophrenia, severe depression, or bipolar disorders have an alcohol or other drug dependence problem. When the counselor is trained in this area they are able to assess the situation and respond appropriately such as drawing up a 'no suicide' contract for a severely depressed person who is having suicide ideation. Or the counselor may call the psychiatric assessment team in the event the person is in imminent danger to self or another or is gravely disabled. It behooves the program and the client if the counselor has established a good working relationship with the case managers of the County Mental Health system.

It is recommended that counselors inform the client what the limits of confidentiality are and obtain a written release of information when consulting and networking with additional support systems (For a sample Release of Information form and statement of Federal confidentiality requirements, see Appendix XI, Section C). This contributes to the building of trust between client and counselor.

Since the sessions may be very brief with no guarantees that the sessions will be ongoing, it helps for the counselor to have developed strong listening skills and to be able to establish rapport in a very short period of time.

Having a strong referral base with available resources to connect the client with is conducive to their ability to maintain their sobriety. The following are resources we have found helpful: recovery homes; A.A., N.A. meetings; Double Trudgers (A.A. for the mentally ill); culturally relevant A.A. meetings for specific cultural populations such as Native Americans of African Americans or Spanish-speaking A.A.; employment services; therapists; [Western] medical services; HIV/AIDS testing sites and counseling services; gay and lesbian programs; general relief and SSI workers; petty cash (for client emergencies).

I recommend also that counselors be required to attend weekly clinical supervision meetings and be encouraged to take extra special care of themselves. Supervision is an ideal place to explore their countertransference issues, especially where it concerns wanting to fix or change the client in any way.

Finally, the clients seen at the clinic generally suffer from serious low self-esteem and traumatic, trust destroying situations in their far and recent past. This is an ideal place for the therapist along with the acupuncturist and other staff to begin developing and creating a safe, non-judgmental, respectful and honorable environment for the client to rest, collect themselves, and decide what direction they want to move in.

It's clear from this description that more than one counselor will need to be involved in our ideal program, especially given the number of hours our acupuncture clinic services will be operating.

In addition to our full time MFCC or LCSW, let's schedule an additional 40 hours per week of counseling. Any interns we are able to recruit will be a bonus.

A Counselor's Guide to Acupuncture in the Treatment of Addiction

by Cally Haber and Charles Singer
Reprinted by permission
P.O. Box 3115
Santa Cruz, CA 95063
(408)458-0809

What is Acupuncture?

Acupuncture is a therapy which was developed in China over 3000 years ago and has been used successfully to treat a variety of illnesses. It is now used world wide.

Acupuncture works by stimulating designated points on the body via the insertion of very fine acupuncture needles. These points correspond with the functions of internal organs and other bodily processes as defined by the principles of Chinese medicine.

How Does it Work as a Detoxification Method?

Acupuncture reduces symptoms of withdrawal as well as aiding in long term recovery. Substances that respond well to acupuncture include alcohol, heroin, crack, methamphetamine, methadone, and nicotine as well as other drugs. Acupuncture does not cure alcoholism or drug addiction. It alleviates withdrawal symptoms so that mental and physical stability are achieved as soon as possible, allowing involvement in counseling, Twelve Step programs, and other support systems as necessary for maintaining sobriety.

Specifically, acupuncture:

- lessens depression, anxiety, and insomnia;
- reduces or eliminates withdrawal symptoms such as drug craving, body aches, headache, nausea, sweating, muscle cramping, etc.;
- is useful in stress reduction and relapse prevention;

Treatment is performed by a licensed acupuncturist. Five new, sterilized, disposable, solid (that is, no hollow core) needles are inserted into specific points in each ear. Each point stimulates an internal body organ or function of the central nervous system, kidney, liver, and lungs that in turn assists in reducing the craving for alcohol or drugs. Needles remain in the ear for 45 minutes. Inserting the needles in the ear causes no to minimal discomfort.

Daily treatment for the first few weeks is most beneficial. The frequency of treatments can then be decreased over several months. More frequent treatment is also encouraged at any time when cravings return, when there is increased stress, or should relapse occur. Some clients like "tune-ups" once they have passed through the acute phase.

Traditional Chinese Medicine

Traditional Chinese Medicine (TCM) is a three thousand year old system of medicine. It is a comprehensive system of health care that offers patients treatment for illness and promotes optimum health and quality of life. There are many modalities of treatment in TCM, acupuncture and herbal therapy being the two most familiar to westerners.

Chinese understanding of human beings sees no separation between body, mind, and spirit; they are perceived as a whole. Each organ is believed to have an expression on the physical, emotional, and spiritual level. When doctors of Chinese medicine use the word "liver" they are referring to the physical liver with all its physiological functioning but additionally to the mental abilities of planning and implementing, the emotional capabilities of anger and determination, and the spiritual activity of hope.

The concept of *qi* (pronounced chi) is very important in TCM. *Qi* is considered to be the life force, the energy that powers the body, mind, and spirit. *Qi* circulates in the body through fourteen major pathways, or meridians, each of which has an internal branch to the organs. There are specific points along these meridians where the body's energy can be contacted through the insertion of acupuncture needles. Each point has its own function and effect on the *qi*.

Acupuncture's goal is to help the patient achieve balance. Symptoms are seen as the body/mind trying to get some attention and help. Illness is perceived as a loss of harmony or balance in the body, and may come from a hyper or hypo functioning of an organ(s). Symptoms may appear on the mental, emotional or physical levels (i.e. inability to concentrate, rage, headaches). Acupuncture is used to redirect the qi and restore function. Treatment is best when we pay attention to the small, initial symptoms, before they get too big. After a course of treatment (ten to twelve visits) has been completed, treatments can be done seasonally to keep a person well.

The points used in the ear treatment for the addicted person are the liver, kidney, lung, *shen-men*, and sympathetic. The first three are the major organs of detoxification at the physical level. Spiritually these points relate to the sense of hope/despair (liver), will power/hiding (kidney), and emptiness/inspiration (lung). Emotionally these three organs refer to anger/determination (liver), fear/courage(kidney), and self-esteem/self-loathing (lung). *Shen-men* means spirit gate. It is used to calm the patient. Sympathetic refers to the autonomic nervous system. This point balances the sympathetic and parasympathetic nervous systems, allowing the body/mind to come into a state of equilibrium. This treatment also functions to strengthen the adrenal glands, commonly in a state of depletion from stress and substance abuse. Treating this combination of points provides a comprehensive and effective medical approach.

Because people need to heal from addiction on many levels (physiological, psychological, spiritual), we believe that Chinese Medicine has an extremely useful role to play in assisting a person in their process of recovery.

Chinese Medicine is regulated in the United States by both national and state licensing boards. The National Commission of Certified Acupuncturists (NCCA) is an examination board that oversees testing at the national level. Most states require passage of this test to practice. California conducts its own test for licensure, and the Acupuncture Committee is under the auspices of the California Medical Board. Acupuncturists in California are primary health care providers. Acupuncture schools now provide a four year course of study with a Master's degree upon completion.

Acupuncture and Treatment of Addiction

Acupuncture is rapidly emerging as an important adjunctive therapy in the field of alcohol and other drug addiction. Since 1974, a successful program involving recovering drug users and alcoholics at Lincoln Hospital Substance Abuse Program in the South Bronx, New York City, has demonstrated that acupuncture has a remarkably positive effect on the recovery process. This program, directed by Dr. Michael Smith, documents the rehabilitative effects of acupuncture as well as the behavior modifications that ensue from the course of treatment he pioneered. Since then, more than 80 clinics in the U.S. and another 25 world wide have utilized an acupuncture component based upon the Lincoln Hospital model.

In 1989, the National Association of Criminal Justice Planners (NACJP) and the National Acupuncture Detoxification Association (NADA) released a suggested protocol that has been widely implemented with great success. They proposed a three tiered program that tapers the number of treatments to the length of sobriety. Realizing that relapse is part of recovery, this tiered program allows clients to progress at their own rate. If the patient fails in his/her second stage, they simply go back to the first stage which provides more frequent acupuncture treatment. In this way a patient is supported instead of punished for relapsing.

Acupuncture is an excellent modality because it treats in spite of denial. Acupuncture provides a non-confrontational approach in early recovery. It alleviates withdrawal symptoms and calms the patient, thus preparing the soil for further counseling and group work. This makes the initial days of detox much more manageable for both the client and counseling staff.

In 1985, the National Acupuncture Detoxification Association (NADA) was founded by clinicians who wanted to extend the example of the Lincoln Hospital experience into other treatment settings. NADA sets standards of certification for acupuncture detoxification specialists that are widely accepted in the field of chemical dependency. The group of acupuncturists that you work with are all NADA certified.

Chemical dependency professionals in both the private sector and the criminal justice system have taken a keen interest in the work done at Lincoln Hospital and other NADA affiliated programs. The introduction of an acupuncture component to an existing program provides a cost-efficient method for providing non-residential treatment to large numbers of drug dependent people, while increasing the effectiveness of existing services. Acupuncture also works well within the context of a residential treatment setting.

Regardless of the setting, and the substance abused, acupuncture treatment aids in patient detoxification. It does so by supporting the main organs of elimination in the body, speeding the body's ability to rid itself of toxins. Treatment improves mental clarity and the ability to focus. It also provides the patient with a sense of calmness and serenity. This creates a greater receptivity to the counseling process and decreased instances of clients' "acting out".

Treatment consists of the placement of five sterile needles just under the skin of both ears. The clients then sit quietly for 45 minutes. Treatment is more effective when done in a large group.

Approximately 30-35 people can be treated in one and a half hours, by one acupuncturist.

Dr. Smith says "acupuncture teaches the patient to relax from the inside out." This increased sense of calm and the quieting of symptoms that occurs as a result of the acupuncture treatment stimulates patients' own *qi* (one's inner energy) and brings them back into a more balanced state. As patients become calmer inside, they become much more aware of themselves and others. From this quieter, inner place, the patient can then make more careful choices in their reactions to life situations. This calmness seems to greatly enhance the effects of other treatment modalities for both the client and the provider.

The Hooper Center for Alcohol and Drug Intervention is a county-funded regional detoxification facility in Portland Oregon. Acupuncture is used in a subacute inpatient medical facility and in their four outpatient programs. In 1987 they instituted acupuncture as part of their total program and within six months saw some important clinical developments: their seizure rate decreased from 5-10 a month to 0-1 seizure a month; their need to medicate at all for alcohol withdrawal reduced by 40%; their monthly recidivist rate decreased from 27% to 5-7%; their nursing staff found that their own personal stress levels decreased. The only medical intervention they now use for cocaine and crack patients is acupuncture, with 90% of these patients now completing the program. People who are traditionally binge users use less drugs and come back into treatment much more quickly than before acupuncture intervention. People who receive treatment in their outpatient setting are twice as likely to stay sober over a 4-6 month period as those who don't use acupuncture.

Many new programs have opened in the last several years. Prison programs began in Florida, Oregon, New York, Minnesota, Maryland , California and Puerto Rico. Four new clinics opened in the San Francisco area in 1991 alone. In New York City, $2,700,000 was designated for acupuncture-based programs to be instituted in six more hospitals. It was the only budget increase for health care approved by the New York City government in 1991.

Why Acupuncture?

(extracted from: "Acupuncture Detoxification and Relapse Service: A Concept Paper," New York State Division of Substance Abuse Services, Arthur Webb, Director, October 1, 1991)

While acupuncture can assist most clients seeking treatment, it has a special application in helping addicted clients who resist initial treatment.

Typical beneficiaries are those who:

- need an immediate intervention for their substance abuse problem;
- may not be initially receptive to verbal, interpersonal intervention or counseling due to active drug use or presence of withdrawal symptoms;
- are in denial;
- are distressed and suffering from anxiety, depression, and other withdrawal symptoms;
- require a simple, non threatening and structured opportunity to begin to cope with their substance abuse problem in order to later engage in more formal treatment;
- need help in dealing with their cravings to use;
- are experiencing sleep disorders and drug dreams.

Commonly Asked Questions

1) Does it hurt?
Most often people barely feel the needle go in. Sometimes a point will be sensitive, but this small sting or pinch only lasts for a second. Tell the acupuncturist if a needle hurts during the treatment and they will adjust the needle for you. There should be no pain or discomfort during the treatment itself.

2) Any danger of AIDS?

Virtually none. The needles are sterile and have never been used on anyone else before. The needles are used only once and then thrown away.

3) Is the treatment itself dangerous?

No. Ear acupuncture is very safe. It is a treatment for balancing the body and gently engaging and enhancing the body's ability to heal itself.

4) Is it safe during and after pregnancy?

Yes! Acupuncture helps the health of both the mom and the developing baby. It is important that you tell the acupuncturist you are pregnant; they will do special points to help you.

5) What will it do for me?

Physically: relaxes and reduces stress, decreases pain, increases energy and immunity, helps withdrawal, normalizes sleep.

Mentally/Emotionally: helps you feel more clear, alert, calm, and focused.

6) How does it work?

The acupuncture needles connect to the body's energy or life-force, called "*qi*." This powers our body's organs and allows them to function. The treatments help increase the circulation of *qi* so the body's organs work more efficiently, therefore you feel better. It is like when your car needs a tune-up. After the car has the tune-up it runs much better, with more ease. You are much more important than your car, so we encourage frequent "tuneups."

7) *How often should I come?*

As often as you can. During the first four weeks of sobriety, it is best to come five days a week. The next month you should come three to four days a week. Continue to come at least once a week until you are six months sober. Remember to come in more often if you are experiencing a lot of stress or depression. These treatments are here for you to use to heal yourself and help yourself, for a better overall quality of life.

Why People Stop or Never Start Taking Treatment (reactions/reservations)

1) *I don't like needles.*

Acupuncture needles are very different from regular hypodermic needles. They are not hollow and are much thinner. It usually doesn't hurt going in, especially if you concentrate on your breathing. Most people barely feel the needles going in. At worst there is a very brief sting or pinching sensation.

2) *I don't want to become dependent on anything.*

This treatment is completely non-addicting, and there is a natural tendency to want or need less treatment as your recovery progresses.

3) *It gave me a headache.*

Occasionally people react like that. It may be your body detoxifying, or that you are very sensitive to the needles and the treatment brought too much blood and energy (qi) flow to the head. After the treatment, be sure you tell the acupuncturists that you got a headache, and they will adjust the treatment.

4) *The treatment made me too tired.*
Your body is detoxing and healing. This usually doesn't last more than one or two treatments. If it does, tell the acupuncturists and they will adjust the treatment.

5) *I had too much energy after the treatment and I couldn't go to sleep.*
Your body is detoxing and healing. This reaction should not last longer than one or two treatments. If it does, please tell the acupuncturists and they will adjust the treatment for you.

6) *I tried it and didn't feel anything.*
Some people feel something right away; others may take a week or two. Stick with it! It is like planting a seed and expecting a tomato harvest in one or two days. Anything worth having in your life takes time.

7) *My ears were hurting after treatment.*
Massage your ears after treatments. Tell the acupuncturist and they can do fewer needles for a few days.

8) *The points in my ears got too painful.*
If the needles hurt you a lot and you are afraid of them, there is something you can do. Concentrate on your breathing, especially remembering to breath through your mouth while you concentrate on exhaling the air. Put your mind on your breath, not on your ear! Relax rather than tensing your face, neck and shoulders. This will decrease the amount of pain you feel when the needle goes in.

Treatment Frequency Guidelines

Time Sober	*Treatments per Week*
First month	five
Second month	three to four
Third through Sixth month	one to two

We suggest more frequent treatment any time there is an increased tension level in your life, whether it is physical, mental or emotional. This applies no matter how long you have been sober. Sobriety includes finding a way to live with more comfort and ease even through hard times. Therefore, self care is an necessary thing to learn. The acupuncture treatments are a great way to care for yourself in a healthy way.

Things to Tell Clients

Acupuncture:

- is an effective treatment for any substance used.

- helps: headaches, body aches, sweats, sleep disturbances, tremors, anxiety, depression, mental clarity, decreases anger, reduces cravings for alcohol and other drugs.

- helps stabilize you physically and emotionally and increases your ability to focus.

- will help you stay clean and sober.

- relaxes you from the inside. So sit quietly during treatment.

- treatments stimulate your own body to heal itself. The treatments are not to sedate you but rather treatments that rebuild your physical and emotional self.

Come for treatment as often as you can. It works best when treatments are frequent and on going. These treatments will have a cumulative effect. If you are still using, or relapse, keep coming to treatment! The acupuncture will help you stop.

Avoid coffee, cigarettes, heavy meals, or being overly hungry before treatment. Sit quietly during the treatment with arms and legs uncrossed. Please respect the people near you who may be silently enjoying the benefit of their treatment.

Use the herbal tea formula as often as you like. It will help you relax throughout the day and may help normalize your sleep. The tea is safe, non narcotic and non-addictive. It is for sale here at the clinic for your later use at home.

Procedures for Clients to Follow

1. . Use the bathroom before starting your treatment.
   . Quietly enter the room.
   . Clean the inside of both ears with an alcohol swab
   . Don't touch your ears after you have cleaned them.
   . Get a cup of tea and take a seat.
   . Tell the acupuncturist each time if you are pregnant, or have a history of a bleeding disorder.
   . Give the acupuncturist your medical card when it is your turn for treatment.

2. Five sterile needles will be placed in each ear. These needles have never been used before and there is virtually no possibility of disease transmission.

3. Sit quietly for 45 minutes. Relax, meditate, visualize, or sleep.

4. Do not walk around after the needles are in your ear except to take them out. If you want more tea, raise your hand and an acupuncturist will be happy to get you some.

5. Sometimes an acupuncturist will needle other points that are not in the ear but on other parts of the body. These are to help conditions that are better treated with points other than those on the ear. Only the acupuncturist should take out the needles in these points.

6. If the needles fall out of your ear, just hold onto them. The points have already been stimulated and will not have to be re-needled.

7. Do not touch any needles but your own.

8. After 45 minutes, walk up to the mirror and take your needles out. Count them and make sure that you have all ten needles. If you don't have ten, please go back to your seat and find the lost needles. When you have all ten needles, dispose of them in the red container.

9. Check your ears in the mirror for blood after you have taken out the needles. If there is any bleeding, press a piece of cotton to the point for 30 seconds. Discard the cotton ball into the red container.

10. Consent for acupuncture treatment must have been read and signed before treatment is started.

Afterward: A Note to the TCM Community

Chinese Medicine and Chemical Dependency:
Some Pertinent Questions

The increased public interest in the use of acupuncture in the treatment of chemical dependency has raised some important questions for the Chinese medical community in the United States. It would have been serendipitous, from an idealistic perspective, had the addiction crisis in America waited to peak until Chinese medicine had achieved a foothold of acceptance in general health care in this culture, so that the chemical dependency treatment establishment could have found us professionally secure in our medicine and philosophy. But the reality has been otherwise. Chinese medicine is an infant in a foreign land, lacking the sort of strong legal, political, and social foundations that would make us strong, clear, and deliberate in our response to this keen and growing demand for our assistance; instead, unfortunately, we are found in something of a state of disarray, divided in a degree of controversy around a number of key issues precipitated by the adaptations required of Chinese medicine in the unique setting of substance abuse treatment and recovery in Western culture.

Some of the issues that divide the community are clinical in nature. Traditional Chinese medical texts (like their Western counterparts) are silent on the subject of alcoholism and drug addiction. So we are on a clinical frontier. With the complexities of the pathologies inherent in chronic drug addiction, generally tangled up as they are with a host of *attending* pathologies, we must acquiesce to the fact that final resolution of the many clinical questions that arise from a continuum of substance abuse treatment will result from thoughtful debate, research, and clinical experience over a substantial period of time.

Other dividing issues are, not surprisingly, economic in nature. The mounting interest of the federal government in acupuncture as a treatment specific to crack cocaine addiction has resulted in part from the successful Dade County, Florida drug court program which is rapidly becoming, in the administration's view, a prototype. Where federal interest is piqued in this manner, funding is generally soon to follow. Who will do the work? Who will certify that the work is done properly? And, of course, who will profit?

Five complex and related questions face the acupuncture profession in the area of educational and certification standards involving work with chemical dependency clients. These questions can be stated as follows:

1. What general educational standards, if any, concerning alcoholism, drug addiction, and substance abuse should be developed and adopted for the certification of *all individuals* who practice traditional Chinese medicine or acupuncture in the United States? How should such standards be developed, and by whom? What political priority should be given to implementing these standards, especially in "new" States who will be in the process of enacting acupuncture certification laws in the next several years?

2. What clinical training and supervision ought to be established for individuals administering acupuncture protocols in public chemical dependency treatment settings? How should these standards be developed, and by whom? In developing these standards, should any concessions be made in regions of the country where the numbers of licensed acupuncturists is not adequate to delivering services What legislative approaches should be urged to encourage an increase in licensed acupuncturists in these regions in order to meet the new demands for services?

3. Are there optimum, generic acupuncture protocols that should be used in first-phase recovery in a chemical dependency setting? What sort of research has already been accomplished, and what additional research is required in order to make this determination? How and by whom should such determinations be made? If such generic protocols are found to be appropriate, what is the proper relationship of expanded traditional Chinese medical protocols in these treatment settings to the generic protocol?

4. What process for resolution of these issues is indicated in the current political and funding environment? Might these issues be prioritized in a manner that would require that some of them are

deserving of more rapid resolution than others? What is the appropriate interface of the Chinese medical community with the chemical dependency treatment community in the resolution of these issues? Is there justification for the formation of a special and representative Commission charged with resolving these issues? If so, how should such a Commission be comprised, and what existing organizations or groups ought it to represent? What sources of funding are possible to finance the work of such a Commission?

5. What various impacts might the resolution of these issues, and the manner in which they are resolved, have upon the overall level of acceptance of Chinese medicine and acupuncture in the delivery of general health care in the United States? How might these influences be weighed?

Few would question the general need for an increased awareness of substance addiction and abuse on the part of practitioners of Chinese medicine and acupuncture in the United States. In spite of the enlightened work of many Western physicians in the field of alcoholism and substance abuse, Western medicine in general has made the error of operating in the vacuum of substantial denial of addiction. So, too, has the Western counseling/psychotherapy community. Both of these groups, in their tendency to address the attending or underlying syndromes that frequently accompany substance issues, have often in fact served to enable alcoholics and addicts to continue chronic use, even often complicating the condition through the prescription of other psychoactive drugs.

It would be a tragic loss to those who suffer from drug addiction if Chinese medicine, with its substantial arsenal of protocols that are relevant to addiction disorders, made the same mistake that Western medicine and psychology have made, proceeding in relative ignorance of the issues that make substance abuse such an endemic malaise in Western culture.

Since traditional Chinese texts, and the curriculum of colleges of Oriental medicine, do not address the issue of addiction, practitioners must educate themselves, or else develop meaningful networks with chemical dependency treatment and recovery resources in the communities they serve. The National Acupuncture

Detoxification Association (NADA) has been providing abbreviated trainings for acupuncturists in chemical dependency since 1985, but this training has been focused on specialized acupuncture protocols in the public detoxification setting, and does not emphasize the assessment, referral, or clinical skills that prepare individuals in private practice for the successful treatment of chemical dependency.

It is, of course, in large measure the result of the successful work of NADA in developing public, acupuncture-based chemical dependency treatment programs in Miami, Minneapolis, New York, Portland, Oregon, and elsewhere, and in the research that has resulted, that the concerns we have expressed above have taken on current significance. Funding of acupuncture-based chemical dependency treatment is likely to increase, perhaps dramatically, in the near future, and it behooves the Chinese medical community to address the issues listed above in anticipation of this potential entry into general health care in the United States.

Footnotes:

1   Acupuncture's primary clinical effectiveness is in (1) the relief of withdrawal symptoms, with the need for sedative drugs reduced or eliminated, (2) improved patient well-being and manageability, (3) lowered relapse rates, and (4) improved program completion rates (Jay Renaud, "Acupuncture," *Addiction and Recovery*, August, 1990).

2   Hillary Rodham Clinton makes specific reference to acupuncture's effectiveness in treating crack cocaine in the Miami drug court program in an interview in *Mirabella* magazine (August, 1993). For an overview of the drug court program, see "Miami's Drug Court: A Different Approach," National Institute of Justice, U.S. Department of Justice, Office of Justice Programs, NIJ: NCJ 142412 (June, 1993). Also see p. 192-194.

3   As Harriet Beinfield and Efrem Korngold write, "Medicine not only defines health and disease, but also makes implicit assumptions about what life is and what it is to be human. As such, it occupies a position of great power. In our view, Chinese medicine is not a replacement for Western medicine, but another window through which we can view ourselves, take stock of our personal and global situations, and use its insights to prompt a revolution in priorities, strategies, and choices." (*Between Heaven and Earth: A Guide to Chinese Medicine*, New York: Ballantine Books, 1991, p. 382).

4   We beg the forbearance of the more consummate traditional Chinese medical (TCM) practitioner. For while we shall, in this book, criticize the West in its tendency toward compartmentalization and reductionism in both its science and its medicine, we may ourselves, in our earnest zeal toward gaining acceptance of acupuncture as a treatment modality in and of itself, be found guilty of seeming to isolate acupuncture from the main body of TCM.

This is a criticism that seems reasonable. To disembody acupuncture as a method or technique in a highly localized setting seems in one sense an anathema to the sensibilities of the practitioner of TCM. However, note that acupuncture in the detoxification setting is not being accomplished in an isolated vacuum; rather, it is being performed in the striking context of transformational recovery from systemic addiction, and this recovery system has deep and profound resonances with TCM itself, resonances which we will investigate in this book.

Here, in this urgent context of recovery, there is less danger than one may think of acupuncture becoming lost, and there is little danger of the larger body of TCM being disparaged, for the philosophical organizing principles of TCM and those of recovery are the same: balance, integrity, and honor of the process of life. It is possible that what we are witnessing in this deceptively simple setting is the organic adaptation of TCM to the unique needs of Western culture. As Mark Seem writes, "In America ... we have the opportunity to participate in the reformulation of Oriental medicine to meet our own specific intellectual and healthcare needs. What emerges as American acupuncture will necessarily be different from what is being practiced elsewhere, and it will reflect the plurality of traditions and schools of thought that inform American practices and teachings." (*Acupuncture Imaging: Perceiving the Energy Pathways of the Body,* Rochester, VT: Healing Arts Press, 1990, p. 7)

There are many questions and many points of view that are currently being expressed by professional associations in the Chinese medical and acupuncture communities in the United States concerning acupuncture, Chinese medicine, and their use in chemical dependency. There is a degree of political and clinical controversy (see Afterword, p 427). While some of these issues will be touched upon in this book, it is not our primary purpose to explore these areas of controversy. It is our bias that this controversy will pass as acupuncture gains acceptance in the chemical dependency treatment arena and begins to secure a foothold in Western primary care. It is the bias of this book that the imperative of bringing the principles of Chinese medicine to the addiction crisis in America needs to overshadow current disagreements.

5   Americans are seeking alternative or non-conventional health care in increasing numbers. According to David Eisenberg, *et.al.,* "unconventional medicine has an enormous presence in the U. S. health care system. An estimated one in three persons in the U. S. adult population used unconventional therapy in 1990. The estimated number of visits made in 1990 to providers of unconventional therapy was greater than the number of visits to all primary care medical doctors nationwide, and the amount spent out of pocket on unconventional therapy was comperable to the amount spent out of pocket by Americans for all hospitalizations. Roughly 1 in 4 Americans who see their medical doctors for a serious health problem may be using unconventional therapy in addition to conventional medicine for that problem, and 7 of 10 such encounters take place without the patients' telling their medical doctors that they use unconventional therapy. Furthermore, use is distributed widely across all socio-demographic groups." ("Unconventional Medicine in the United States: Prevalence, Costs, and Patterns of Use," *The New England Journal of Medicine,* Vol. 328(4), January 28, 1993, pp. 246-250).

6   See G. DeLeon and S Holland, "Phoenix House: Criminal Activity of Dropouts," *Journal of the American Medical Association,* Vol. 222, 686-689 (1972); R. L. Hubbard, *et.al., Drug Abuse Treatment: A National Study of Effectiveness,* Chapel Hill, NC: University of North Carolina Press, p. 52, (1989); C. Leukefeld and F. Tims, "The Challenge of Drug Abuse Treatment in Prisons and Jails," in *Drug Abuse Treatment in Prisons and Jails,* Carl G. Leukefeld and Frank M. Tims, eds., NIDA, (1992); W. R. Miller, "The Effectiveness of Substance Abuse Treatment: Reasons for Optimism," *Journal of Substance Abuse Treatment,* Vol. 9, pp. 93-102 (1992); The U.S. Department of Justice Office of Justice Programs Bureau of Justice Statistics, *A National Report: Drugs, Crime, and the Justice*

System, December, 1992, NCJ-133652, U.S. Government Printing Office, Washington DC., p. 111 (1992), and H. K. Wexler, *et.al., A Criminal Justice System Strategy for Treating Cocaine-Heroin Abusing Offenders in Custody*, NIJ: NCJ-113915, U.S. Government Printing Office, Washington DC. *(1988)*.

7   See, for example, M. Burt, *et.al.*, "A Follow-up Study of 360 Former Participants in Narcotics Treatment," *International Journal of the Addictions*, V 15, N 3, p. 391-408 (1980).

8   See James Corrington, Jr., "Spirituality and Recovery: Relationships Between Levels of Spirituality, Contentment, and Stress During Recovery From Alcoholism in AA," *Alcoholism Treatment Quarterly*, 6(3/4), 1989, pp. 151-165. For a review of the research on AA effectiveness, see also Chad Emrick's "Alcoholics Anonymous: Affiliation Process and Effectiveness as Treatment," *Alcoholism: Clinical and Experimental Research*, 11(5), 1987, pp. 416-423.

9   We define "endemic" as something that lives within the culture, attacking those at risk. This is distinguished from "epidemic," which refers to a disease attacking, from the outside, many in a community simultaneously but which is not continuously present.

10   Herbert L. Gravitz is a California pioneer in the Adult Children of Trauma's (ACoT) clinical movement, and the quote is from a 1988 workshop. His published work includes, with Julie D. Bowden, *Guide to Recovery: A Book For Adult Children of Alcoholics* (Holmes Beach, FL: Learning Publications, Inc., 1986), and *Genesis* (Pompano Beach, FL: Health Communication, Inc. 1988).

11   *Alcoholics Anonymous*, 3rd ed. (New York: Alcoholics Anonymous World Services, Inc., 1976; orig. publ. 1939), pp. 58-9. Called *"The Big Book"* by AA members, the first 164 pages of this anonymously written AA handbook was substantially authored by AA co-founder Bill Wilson, a New York stock broker. The AA fellowship took its name from the book. In its three major revisions since 1939, the primary text of *Alcoholics Anonymous* has remained unchanged, but personal stories have been added.

12   Joe Califano, President of the Center on Addiction and Substance Abuse at Columbia University has taken on the task of finding a new word for the study of addiction, and recently solicited ideas. Terms reportedly under consideration are *addictionology*; *pharmacosiology* (from pharmaco-, "drug," and -osis, "disease;" *deditology* (from the Latin deditus, "addicted to;" and *etheology* (from the Greek ethos, "habit."

13   One of the peculiarities in this regard - in both social attitudes and public policy - has been the segregation of alcohol and nicotine from "other drugs." Until 1992, The National Drug Control Strategy was focused solely on illicit drugs such as cocaine, heroin, and marijuana, even though far more health problems and deaths can be attributed to alcohol and nicotine than to all illicit drugs combined.

Alcohol and nicotine have now been included in national drug policy and funding.

From a clinical point of view, there are of course differences among all drugs and drug classes, which we will describe in a later section. In general, however, we will use the terms *addiction, drug addiction, alcoholism, drug dependence*, and *substance abuse* somewhat interchangeably, except where noted.

14   See Appendix I, Section A for a review of drug legislation in the United States.

15   The attempts at defining drug addiction are complicated further by its variances with *non-addictive* patterns of psychoactive drug use, an area which has its own points of controversy. A scale is often used to differentiate among types of non-addictive, non-medical psychoactive drug use, such as "experimentation," "recreational" or "situational" use, and "habituation" (as distinct from the more extreme "abuse"). Using this frame, a way of differentiating *addiction* is that it is *progressive*: it gets worse if untreated. The non-addictive use categories are, by implication, static.

16   One of the salient features of the philosophy of Rationalism is the assumption of a fundamental dualism between ones inner life and the external world. The problems posed by this self/other division lie at the crux of addiction. According to the psychiatrist Stanislav Grof, "In the broadest sense, addiction can be defined as dependence on various aspects of the external world as exclusive sources of satisfaction. Addiction, understood this way, represents a prominent feature of the entire Western civilization, which has lost connection with the inner life and shows fascination with material pursuits. The great Eastern philosophies and the mystical traditions of all ages have emphasized that happiness is primarily an inner organismic condition and a state of consciousness. In contrast, the predominant life strategy in the West has been to expect satisfaction from material fetishes." ("Spirituality, Alcoholism, and Drug Abuse: Transpersonal Aspects of Addiction," editorial, *ReVision: The Journal of Consciousness and Change*, Fall, 1987, p. 3).

17   The theory of yin and yang, originating in ancient Taoism, provides the basis not only for Chinese medicine, but for the universe itself. David Eisenberg, M.D., quoting his teacher "Dr. Fang" in *Encounters with Qi: Exploring Chinese Medicine* (New York: W. W. Norton, 1985), writes "It is the principle of everything in Creation. It is the source of life and death...Yin and Yang represent opposing yet complementary aspects of the universe. For example, that which is cold is Yin, that which is hot is Yang. Night is Yin, day is Yang, and so on. Every object, every action, every aspect of time and space, can be thought of as a preponderance of either Yin or Yang. And within Yang there is something of Yin. For example, the roof of a house is Yang (up) relative to the ground, but Yin (down) relative to the stars. Nothing exists that is neither Yin nor Yang, and all

natural events are influenced by the constantly changing relationships of these two formless aspects of all things." (p. 37).

The use of the term "opposing" in the above description is worthy of comment. It is typical for Westerners interpreting yin-yang theory to ascribe to yin and yang the quality of opposition. The emphasis, however, in yin-yang philosophy is one of paired relationship rather than opposition. According to Nathan Sivin (*Traditional Medicine in Contemporary China*, Ann Arbor: Center for Chinese Studies, University of Michigan, 1987, pp. 204-205), "Traditional physicians believe that 'yin is born of yang, and yang of yin,' and that 'yin alone cannot be born; yang alone cannot mature.' That is to say, each depends on the other for is sustenance, and without one, the other cannot be. It is also said that 'when yin and yang are surrendered the vital energies expire.'"

Yin and yang, therefore, are not contradictory opposites in the Western linear or dialectical sense, but are totally bound in the context of one another with the emphasis upon *relationship*. They are never static, always in dynamic balance, in constant alternating cycles, and within one is always the seed of the other. Yin-yang philosophy does not deny differences; however, the significance is that yin and yang each complete and complement and ultimately culminate in one another.

Manfred Porkert and Christian Ullman, in *Chinese Medicine - Its History, Philosophy and Practice*, translated and adapted by Mark Howson (New York: William Morrow and Co., 1988), provide the following classifications:

YIN	YANG
constructive force	active force (determining principle)
completion	beginning
front	back
repose	transitional states
stasis	moving
consolidation	coming into being
concreteness	being moved
concentration	changing
solidity	developing
contraction	diffusing
extinction	dissolving
determinate	indeterminate
determined	dispersing
earth	sun
moon	heavens
fall	spring
winter	summer
water	fire

feminine	masculine
night	daylight
cold	hot
internal	external
dark	light
small	big
weak	strong
still	animated
on the bottom	on top
on the right	on the left
hours from noon to midnight	hours from midnight to noon
anything that acts on or is moving toward the interior	anything on or moving toward the surface
the trunk below the diaphragm	trunk above the diaphragm
the inner function meridians (in Chinese medicine)	the outer function meridians (in Chinese medicine)
transformational phase	stabilization phase
murky/opaque	clear
soft	hard
savory	tasteless
even numbered	odd numbered

Intuitive thought is yin, and rational thought is yang. Fritjof Capra, in *The Turning Point: Science, Society, and the Rising Culture* (New York: Bantam Doubleday, 1982, p. 38), writes: "The rational and the intuitive are complementary modes of functioning of the human mind. Rational thinking is linear, focused, and analytic. It belongs to the realm of the intellect, whose function it is to discriminate, measure, and categorize. Thus rational knowledge tends to be fragmented. Intuitive knowledge, on the other hand, in based on a direct, nonintellectual experience of reality arising in an expanded state of awareness. It tends to be synthesizing, holistic (from the Greek *holos* ["whole"]), and nonlinear. From this it is apparent that rational knowledge is likely to generate self-centered, or yang, activity, whereas intuitive wisdom is the basis of ecological, or yin, activity." Besides intuitive/rational, the useful associations of yin and yang for Capra are:

YIN	YANG
feminine	masculine
contractive	expansive
conservative	demanding
responsive	aggressive
cooperative	competitive

synthesizing   analytic

Another interesting grouping is offered by Sukie Colegrave, "Cosmic Masculine and Feminine," in John Welwood's *Challenge of the Heart: Love, Sex, and Intimacy in Changing Times* (edited work), Boston: Shambhala, 1985, p. 93

YIN	YANG
relationship	individualization
space	time
community	hierarchy/order
not-judging	judging
purposeless	purpose
nourisher	fertilizer
unity	polarity
acausal	causal
spontaneous	planned
oneness	differentiation

18   For an excellent historical and clinical overview of addiction, see Edward M. Brecher, *Licit and Illicit Drugs* (Boston: Little, Brown and Company, 1972).

19   Historically, heavy drinking has often been perceived as an acceptable stereotypical masculine trait, but never as a feminine one. The repulsion toward inebriation in women, a repulsion shared by men and women alike, has resulted in a deeply institutionalized stigma against and hence denial of alcoholism in women. See Florence V. Ridlon, *A Fallen Angel* (Associated University Press, 1988). For an analysis of this gender stigma as it applies to drugs besides alcohol, see L. and E. Peluso's *Women and Drugs* (Minnesota: CompCare Publishers, 1988), and E. M. Belle Muschinske's *A Description of the Personality Characteristics of Cocaine-Abusing Females* (available from the University of Microfilms Inc. in Ann Arbor, MI. (1990).

20   *Alcoholics Anonymous*, pp. xxiii-xxx, and 571-2. William Silkworth, M.D., who was instrumental in the formation of Alcoholics Anonymous, theorized that it was on the order of an allergy.

21   The "real" alcoholic, as AA describes, "at some stage of his drinking career begins to lose all control of his liquor consumption once he starts to drink." (*Ibid.*, p. 21).

22   In AA, there is a paradox in terms of responsibility on the part of the alcoholic for his or her alcoholism. Responsibility is assumed, but has an internal rather than an external locus. In its form, AA is hence non-authoritarian and non-directive. Its twelve steps are "suggested as a program of recovery" (*Alcoholics Anonymous*, p. 59). The responsibility for recovery is ultimately with the recoverer and his or her "higher power." This is not to say that there is not

leadership and direction in AA as it is practiced. The primary form this takes is "sponsorship." Sponsorship is the practice of the newcomer choosing an individual who has been sober and involved with the program for a substantial period of time to be a "mentor" or "advisor" on program issues. There is no established blueprint for sponsorship, but generally a sponsor is a member of the same gender (except for gays and lesbians) and provides emotional and social support to the sponsee, as well as advice on the Steps, meeting attendance, and other issues relative to sobriety and recovery.

23   *The U.S. Journal of Drug and Alcohol Dependence* - Vol. 12 #9 (Sept. 1988).

24   The Twelve Steps and Twelve Traditions of Alcoholics Anonymous are reprinted in their entirety in Appendix VI. The Twelve Steps are reprinted with permission of Alcoholics Anonymous World Services, Inc. Permission to reprint the Twelve Steps does not mean that AA has reviewed or approved the content of this publication, not that AA agrees with the views expressed herein. AA is a program of recovery from alcoholism - use of the Twelve Steps in connection with programs and activities which are patterned after AA, but which address other problems, does not imply otherwise.

25   *Ibid.*, p. 45.

26   Herbert Fingarette, *Heavy Drinking: The Myth of Alcoholism* (Berkeley: University of California Press, 1988). The research which led Fingarette to his thesis in this controversial book is challenged by anthropologist William Madsen in *Defending the Disease of Alcoholism: From Facts to Fingarette* (Akron, OH: Wilson, Brown and Co., 1989).

27   Stanton Peele, *The Meaning of Addiction* (Lexington: D.C. Heath and Co., 1985) and *Diseasing of America: Addiction Treatment Out of Control* (1989). Peele has also written "Why and by Whom the American Alcoholism Treatment Industry is Under Siege (*Journal of Psychoactive Drugs*, Vol. 22[1]: 1990, 1-13); "Ain't Misbehavin': Addiction has become an All Purpose Excuse" (*The Sciences*, July/August: 1989, 14-21); "Can Alcoholism and Other Drug Addiction Problems be Treated Away or is the Current Treatment Binge doing more Harm than Good?" (*Journal of Psychoactive Drugs*, Vol. 20[4]: 1988, 375-383), and "Through a Glass Darkly: Can Some Alcoholics Learn to Drink in Moderation? (*Psychology Today*, April: 1983, 38-42). In counterpoint of Peele's assertions, see John Wallace's "Controlled Drinking, Treatment Effectiveness, and the Disease Model of Addiction: A Commentary on the Ideological Wishes of Stanton Peele" (*Journal of Psychoactive Drugs*, Vol. 22[3], Jul.-Sep., 1990, 261-283). Wallace opens his commentary by saying that "Debating Stanton Peele reminds me of Marshall McLuhan's hypothetical mosquito in a nudist colony: there is so much to do, one does not know quite where to begin."

28   Peele, *Diseasing ...*, pp. 57-83.

29   See, for example, J. F. Maddux and D. P. Desmond's *Careers of Opiate Users* (New York: Praeger (1981); D. N. Nurco, et. al., "Addict Careers III: Trends Across Time, *International Journal of the Addictions*, 16:1353-1372 (1981), and D. Waldorf's *Careers in Dope* (Englewood Cliffs: Prentice Hall, 1973).

30   Kurtz, Ernest, *Not-God - A History of Alcoholics Anonymous* (Center City, MN: Hazelden Press, 1979).

31   "*Cogito ergo sum*," is the mantra of consecration by which rational thought is defined as the exclusive manner in which reality can be known. It forms the philosophical basis of what we will be calling the "theology" of Exclusionary Rationalism. It is, in essence, "nonparticipatory," in that the "body" (as distinct from "mind") is viewed as separate from the process of knowing. According to science historian Morris Berman in *The Reenchantment of the World* (Ithaca, New York: Cornell U. Press, 1981, p. 180), the weakness of science, and the fraud of the Cartesian paradigm, is that "there is no such thing as purely discursive knowing, and the sickness of our time is not the absence of participation but the stubborn denial that it exists - the denial of the body and its role in our cognition of reality."

Like the addict, it *thinks it is God.*

Kurtz (p. 169) remarks ominously that "Cartesian *cogito* with its futile quest for absolute objectivity was the final wedge that split man and his world irrevocably asunder."

32   Kurtz, p. 171.

33   Dualism, as we have suggested, is at the core of Rene Descartes' philosophy of rationalism. "I thence concluded," he wrote, "that I was a substance whose whole essence consists only in thinking, and which, that it may exist, has need of no place, nor is dependent on any material thing: so that 'I,' that is to say, the mind by which I am what I am, is wholly distinct from the body..." (*Discourse on Method and Selected Writings*, translated by John Veitch, New York: Dutton and Company, 1951, p. xx.)

Note also that the tacit assumption of choice in the designation "psychological dependence" reveals the Western rationalist (and Freudian) bias that *control* is tantamount to mental health.

34   Kurtz (p. 171) suggests that the inside/outside dilemma as it concerns the source of meaning of personal existence is a fundamental paradox of Twentieth-century America (for example, see note 22).

35   It is important from a political perspective to note that public insurance (Federal Medicaid and its State-level equivalents) have created a class system of health care delivery in general.

36   At present, more tranquilizers are sold in the U.S. than barbiturate sleeping pills, amphetamines, and opiate narcotics combined, and the majority of them are sold to women. According to Weldon Witters and Peter Venturelli (*Drugs and Society*, 2nd. Edition (Boston: Jones and Bartlett, 1988), there were an estimated 5 billion doses sold in 1979, with Valium representing one third of this. There have been more that 40 million Valium prescriptions written per year from the late 1970s through 1987, when there were an estimated 700 Valium imitations or substitutes on the market.

37   A major cause of Western doctors having their licenses suspended is the non-therapeutic prescription of drugs.

38   Early AA was a male dominated society (see note 182).

39   See Appendix VII for the full text of AA's twelve steps. Al-Anon's first step is the same as that of AA: "We admitted we were powerless over alcohol - that our lives had become unmanageable." The Codependents Anonymous (CoDA) first step replaces "alcohol" with the word "others."

40   Timmen Cermak (*Diagnosing and Treating Co-Dependence: A Guide for Professionals Who Work with Chemical Dependents, Their Spouses and Children*, Johnson Institute, 1986), is a pioneer in clinical codependence. Other significant works in this field are Melody Beattie's *Codependent No More: How to Stop Controlling Others and Start Caring for Yourself* (Minneapolis: Harper/Hazelden, 1987), and *Codependents' Guide to the Twelve Steps* (New York: Prentice Hall/Parkside, 1990); Susan Ricketson's *The Dilemma of Love: Healing Co-Dependent Relationships at Different Stages of Life* (Pompano Beach, FL: Health Communications, Inc., 1989), and Pia Mellody, Andrea Miller, and J. Keith Miller's *Facing Codependence: What It Is, Where It Comes From, How It Sabotages Our Lives* (San Francisco: Harper & Row, 1989).

41   This is a medical diagnostic, and hence insurance billable, criteria for codependence.

42   Anne Wilson Schaef, *Co-Dependence: Misunderstood, Mistreated* (San Francisco: Harper & Row, 1986).

43   Charlotte Kasl, *Many Roads, One Journey: Moving Beyond the Twelve Steps* (New York: Harper Collins, 1992), p. xv.

44   From the rational point of view, there is apparent paradox, or at least irony, in ascribing stress as a cause of psychoactive drug use. Psychoactive drug use and stress are indeed neurochemically linked. Before the end of LSD research in the 1970s, some psychologists, including Julian Silverman at Agnew State Hospital in California, hypothesized that LSD, like schizophrenia, simulated a high-stress state in the CNS. The sympathomimetic stimulants such as cocaine and the amphetamines could be said to do so as well, activating the "fight or flight"

neurochemical systems. Further, there is some evidence that prolonged stress itself, whether drug-induced or not, overworks the endorphin production system, and some research indicating that if addictive drinking or other psychoactive drug use begins, the endorphin is impaired (Kenneth Blum and Michael Trachtenberg, "Neurochemistry and Alcohol Craving," *California Society for the Treatment of Alcoholism and Other Drug Dependencies News*, Vol.13, No.2, Sept., 1986, p. 4).

One could therefore define the addictive cycle as the importing of an artificial stress-inducing chemical in order to deal with a stressful social environment.

45 See Appendix XII, Section B for resources concerning PTSD.

46 Among the failures of the Vietnam war is that because it lacked any degree of broad and genuine social support, the mechanisms by which soldiers generally develop comradeship and systemic validation for the trauma of their experiences were dysfunctional.

47 Lincoln Hospital has now, under Fullilove's direction, developed an ancillary women's treatment program specifically for trauma, with a facilitator's manual available from The Community Research Group, The New York State Psychiatric Institute, Unit 29, 722 West 168th Street, New York, NY 10032 (212-740-7292).

It is appropriate here to point out again that a singular virtue of Chinese medicine in the chemical dependency treatment setting is that it provides a drug-free arsenal of treatment responses for syndromes that become unmasked during the detoxification stage, and clinical protocols can be conveniently "transitioned" in the same treatment setting from detoxification to these subclinical issues as they arise.

48 It is not, therefore, a coincidence that virtually all chronic drug use is attended by ritual. Gloria Steinem, in her book *Revolution from Within: A Book of Self-Esteem* (Boston: Little, Brown, & Co., 1992, p. 313), writes: "In moments of sorrow or joy, too many of us are forced to turn to ceremonies that falsely elevate some and demean others, that separate us from nature, that make us feel ashamed of sacred parts of ourselves. It will take courage, creativity, and community to replace them with inclusive ceremonies that mark life passages; rituals that externalize universal myths and nature's symbols of old and continuing mysteries - and exclude no one."

Among the less obvious features of the organization of acupuncture-based drug treatment is the existence of ritual surrounding and attending the clinical process. Some clinics, such as Bayview Hunters Point in San Francisco, and El Rio in the South Bronx, have consciously incorporated and expanded ritual and celebration in the life of the clinic.

49 Genetic research is based on several models, including (1) animal models, (2) twin studies, (3) adoption studies, (4) family studies of alcoholics, and (5) studies

of persons assumed to be at high risk for developing alcoholism (Kenneth Blum and Michael Trachtenberg, "Neurochemistry and Alcohol Craving," p. 2). The classic twin studies carried out in Scandinavian countries demonstrating increased risk and based upon alcoholism in biological parents include those reported by D. W. Goodwin, F. Schulsinger, et.al.: "Alcohol Problems in Adoptees Raised Apart from Alcoholic Biological Parents," *Archives of General Psychiatry*, 1973; 28: 238-243) and M. Bohman: "Some Genetic Aspects of Alcoholism and Criminality: A Population of Adoptees," *Archives of General Psychiatry*, 1978; 35: 269-276. Brain wave amplitude differences were demonstrated in non-alcoholic children by a current leader in genetic research H. Begleiter, and reported (with B. Porjesz) in "Evoked Brain Potentials in Abstinent Alcoholics and Boys at Risk for Alcoholism," *Alcohol and Alcoholism*, V21(2), 1986, p. 64. Begleiter published numerous subsequent researches on the subject.

Animal researchers include Begleiter as well as G. E. McClearn ("Genetics and the Pharmacology of Alcohol," *Proceedings of the Sixth International Congress on Pharmacology*, 1975: 3: 59-66); K. Blum, A. H. Briggs, et.al. ("Evidence for the 'Genotype Theory' of Alcohol Seeking Behavior," *Alcohol and Drug Research*, 1986), and Dorothy Moore ("Laboratory Research in Advance of Clinical Trials," Alcohol, Health and Research World, Vol. 12(3), 1988, pp. 229-233).

For nutritional (and potential acupuncture) treatment implications, see also K. Blum and M. Trachtenberg's "Neurogenetic Deficits Caused by Alcoholism: Restoration by SAAVE, a Neuronutrient Intervention Adjunct," *Journal of Psychoactive Drugs*, Vol. 20(3), July-September, 1988, 297-313, and "Enkephalinase Inhibition and Precursor Amino Acid Loading Improves Inpatient Treatment of Alcohol and Polydrug Abusers: Double-Bind Placebo-Controlled Study of the Nutritional Adjunct SAAVE," *Alcohol*, Vol.5, 1989, pp. 481-493. (For information about SAAVE polynutritional supplements, see Appendix II.)

50   For a discussion of linked addictive and genetic effects, see Deborah Barnes, "The Biological Tangle of Drug Addiction," *Science*, Vol. 241(4864), July, 1988, pp. 415-417.

51   In 1973, three independent research groups identified a binding site in brain membranes for radiolabeled naloxone, a potent opiate antagonist. This discovery of opioid receptors was the precursor to the discovery of the natural or endogenous opiates met- and leu-enkephalin, and the endorphins (Richard Scheller and Zach Hall, "Chemical Messengers at Synapses," in Zach Hall's *An Introduction to Molecular Neurobiology*, Synderland, Massachusetts: Sinauer Associates, Inc., 1992, p. 129). One of these primary early researchers was Candace Pert, formerly of the National Institute for Mental Health. See her

"Opiate Receptor Demonstration in Nervous Tissue (with S. Snyder, *Science*, 1973, 179:1011).

52   For discussions of the gate theory of pain, particularly as it applies to acupuncture, see P.D. Wall's "The Gate Control Theory of Pain Mechanisms; A Re-examination and Restatement," *Brain* 101 (1978), 1-18; J. R. Melzack's "How Acupuncture Can Block Pain," *Impact of Science on Society* (UNESCO) 23 (1) (1973), 65; "Acupuncture Analgesia: A Psychophysiological Explanation, *Minnesota Medicine* 57 (1974), 161-166, and Chen Man's "Mechanisms of Acupunctural Anesthesia: the Two Gate Control Theory," *Diseases of the Nervous System* 33 (1972), 730-735, and "Acupuncture 'Anesthesia': A New Theory and Clinical Study, *Current Therapeutic Research* 14 (7) (1972), 390-394. For a general review of all of this literature, see Alan Bensoussan's *The Vital Meridian (*Edinburgh: Churchill Livingstone, 1990).

53   Pituitary peptides are one class of peptides released in the brain. These peptides include the adrenocorticotropic hormone (ACTH). The hypothalmus is involved in the release of peptides as well, and is also in the mediation of endorphin release. (Hall, p. 127).

54   K. Blum, *Alcohol and the Addictive Brain: New Hope for Alcoholics from Biogenetic Research* (New York: Free Press) 1991; F. George, and S Goldberg, "Genetic Differences in Responses to Cocaine," in *Mechanisms of Cocaine Abuse and Toxicity*, NIDA Research Monograph Series #88, 239-249; A. Oliverio, and C. Castellano, "Genotype Dependent Sensitivity to Morphine and Heroin: Dissociation between Opiate-induced Running and Analgesia in the Mouse." *Psychopharmacologia* 39:13-22, 1974; Ralph Tarter and Arthur Alterman, "Neuropsychological Deficits in Alcoholics: Etiological Considerations," *Journal of Studies on Alcohol*, Vol. 45(1), January, 1984, pp. 1-9; Arun Rawat, "Genetic Aspects of Ethanol Disposition and Dependence," *Neurobehavioral Toxicology and Teratology*, Vol. 5(2), March-April, 1983, pp. 193-199; Rachel Tyndale, "Genetically Polymorphic P450IID1 (Sparteine/Debrisoquine - Type CYP2D6): Neuronal Characterization and Structural Variants (Cytochrome P450IID1)," Volume 53/12-B of Dissertation Abstracts International, p. 6243, and John Murray, "Alcoholism: Etiologies Proposed and Therapeutic Approaches Tried," *Genetic, Social, and General Psychology Monographs*, Vol. 115(1), February, 1989, pp. 81-121.

55   Belle Muschinske (personal interviews) calls this theory the "Moths of Mt. St. Helens Theory of Alcoholism." It seems that before the 1980 volcanic eruption of Mt. St. Helens in Western Washington, the mountain was populated by white moths. Their color protected them from bird predators because the mountain was snow-covered year round. Before it erupted, however, black moths began to appear among the moth population. They were, of course, quickly preyed upon, and did not survive, but the genetic strain persisted, and, when the volcano

erupted, covering the snow with ash, it was the black population who survived on the new landscape. By analogy, Muschinske's theory is that alcoholism may not be a disease, but an genetic adaptation of sensitive people. The twelve steps, she believes, take people back into an intuitive world view, providing the tools to help sensitive people live in an insensitive world. She believes this may be, in the chaotic periphery of evolution, a genetic survival response deep in the limbic system.

56   See G. Uhl, K. Blum, et.al., "Substance Abuse Vulnerability and D-sub-2 Receptor Genes," Trends in Neurosciences, Vol. 16(3), March, 1993, pp. 83-88; E. Gordis, et.al., "Finding the Gene for Alcoholism" (editorial), *The Journal of the American Medical Association*, Vol. 263(15), April 18, 1990, p. 2094, and Kenneth Blum, et.al., "Allelic Association of Human Dopamine D2 Receptor Gene in Alcoholism," *The Journal of the American Medical Association*, Vol. 263(15), April 18, 1990, p. 2055.

57   Erickson, Carlton, in a presentation by the Alcoholism and Drug Research Communications Center (4314 Medical Parkway, Suite 300, Austin Texas, 78756), in Santa Barbara, California, Fall, 1992.

58   Terence Gorski believes that the lumping together of compulsive disorders with addictive disorders is an anathema to clinical practice (Robert Wood Johnson's "Recovery: The Capable Community, a Training Event on the Role of Coalitions in Treatment and Recovery Resources, March, 1993, Woodlands, Texas). Gorski is a "relapse prevention specialist" (see note 165).

59   Descartes, p. 93 - 96.

60   In a private letter, Freud wrote: "The moment a man questions the meaning and value of life, he is sick, since objectively neither has any existence." Kurtz (p. 169) quoting Philip Reiff, *The Triumph of the Therapeutic* (New York: Harper Torchbook, 1968).

61   Freud himself had a relationship with cocaine, and his comments on the effects of the drug are of interest. "I take very small doses of it regularly," he wrote to his fiancee, Martha, in 1884, "against depression and against indigestion, and with the most brilliant success." He sent some to Martha, "to make her strong and give her cheeks a red color." He first expressed his interest in trying cocaine to Martha on April 21, 1884, and by June 18 he had completed his essay on the subject, "Song of Praise," which was published in the July, 1884 issue of the *Centralblatt fur die gesammte Therapie*. In this essay, he describes the effects of small doses of the drug as including "exhilaration and lasting euphoria, which in no way differs from the normal euphoria of the healthy person... You may perceive an increase in *self-control* [italics mine] and possess more vitality and capacity for work ... In other words, you are simply normal, and it is hard to believe you are under the influence of any drug... Absolutely no craving for the further use of

cocaine appears after the first, or even after repeated taking of the drug; one feels rather a certain curious aversion to it." Freud continued to praise cocaine until July, 1887, when he published a final defense of the drug, but thereafter stopped using it, both professionally and personally. He appears to have had no problem stopping. See Ernest Jones, *The Life and Work of Sigmund Freud*, 3 vols., New York: Basic Books, 1953 (quoted in Brecher, p. 274 - 275).

62   By the end of the Eighteenth-century, the earlier Hippocratic concept of "humors" in Western medicine gave way to - and became the ultimate harbinger of - the dualism and reductionism of Cartesian rationalism. While George Eliot's Adam Bede reflected, "That which is essential is hidden to the eye," Western medicine moved toward the exclusion of any process that could not be objectively observed or measured. That which was "hidden to the eye," beyond observation, was discounted, ignored, or denied. Francois Xavier Bichat, the founder of histology (the study of tissue), wrote that "With a few feverish and nervous complaints excepted, all else belongs in the realm of physical pathology." (quoted in Porkert, p. 26.)

But there has developed a profound political dimension to this reductionism and compartmentalization in modern medicine. Physicians have become, in a sense, the "High Priests" of Cartesian culture. Questioning their conservative authority is considered taboo. Although it could be argued that this authority is exercised and experienced across gender, according to Muschinske the sacred political power of physicians is gender-based (p. 140-41). Citing S.B Ruzak (*The Women's Health Movement* (1978) New York: Praeger Publishers, p. 67), Muschinske states that "physicians have historically represented the interest of those in power by offering technical expertise and by assuming the position of 'arbiters of morality and agents of social control.' She (Ruzak) attributed the reactionary efforts on the part of physicians to define Victorian women as helpless and reliant on men as an attempt to restore equilibrium in a society rocking from capitalistic growth, development, and disruption. As doctors became synonymous with authority and science, medicine became a paragon of paternalism in which men established the proper 'place' for women based on biological differences."

The male dominance of medicine is, of course, not uniquely a Western phenomenon. Although in popular medicine as practiced within the family system, women generally are the providers, and while folk healers are of either gender depending upon varying local custom, patriarchal dominance of organized medicine is characteristic of classic Chinese or Greek medicine as it is of medieval European and modern cosmopolitan medicine, in which it has become an extension of the control by men of the bodies of women (See Capra, p. 126).

63   R. M. Zaninelli, B. Porjesj, and H. Begleiter studied the personality variants among nonalcoholic as compared with alcoholic sons of male alcoholics, using a tridimensional personality questionnaire. No statistically significant differences in

the three subscale scores of the two groups were found. ("The Tridimensional Personality Questionnaire in Males at High and Low Risk for Alcoholism," *Alcoholism - Clinical and Experimental Research*, V16[1], February, 1992, pp. 68-70).

64   George Vaillant, "The Alcohol-Dependent and Drug-Dependent Person." Chapter 31 in *The New Harvard Guide to Psychiatry*, edited by Armand M. Nicholi (Cambridge: The Belknap Press of Harvard University Press, 1988), pp. 700-713.

65   John Bradshaw's books (Pompano Beach, FL: Health Communication, Inc.). include *Bradshaw on the Family* (1988); *Healing the Shame that Binds You* (1988), and *Homecoming: Championing the Inner Child* (1990).

66   Alice Miller cast a profound influence on modern popular psychology with *The Drama of the Gifted Child: The Search for the True Self* (originally published as *Prisoners of Childhood*), translated by Ruth Ward (Basic Books of HarperCollins, 1981).

67   See Appendix II for pharmacological references.

68   The length of time an addict uses drugs before seeking treatment has a proportional impact, of course, on the severity of physical symptoms, and this varies with different drugs. People addicted to chronic alcohol use, for example, when no other drugs are involved, generally begin to seek treatment within fifteen to twenty years; heroin addicts typically seek treatment within seven years following the onset of chronic use; cocaine (powder) users begin to seek treatment at four or five years, and crack cocaine addicts are typically beginning to seek treatment by the end of the first year following the onset of addictive use.

69   Although AA and alcohol are used as our example of the Twelve Step model in the discussion which follows, our comments apply to other substance and non-substance addictions as well.

70   Paradoxically, although AA's program of recovery is inherently feminine in its nature, it was born of patriarchal culture (see note 182). As Capra points out (p. 29), the time span associated with the patriarchy is at least 3,000 years, a period so long that we cannot tell if we are dealing with a cyclic process due to a lack of historical information concerning pre-patriarchal eras (see however Riane Eisler's *The Chalice and the Blade*, San Francisco: Harper and Row, 1987). What is certain is that for the past 3,000 years, in Western civilization, and most other cultures, males have determined, through custom, ritual, and legal, political, and religious systems the roles that women do or do not play. (See also Adrienne Rich's *Of Woman Born*, New York: Bantam, 1977).

71   For this, as for other ideas as previously noted, I am indebted to Belle Muschinske (personal conversations).

72   Although alcohol is used as an example in the discussion which follows, the dynamics are the same for any addictive substance or activity.

73   Kuhn was the first to coin the phrase *paradigm shift*, defining it as "a gestalt switch in perception of an ambiguous figure," in *The Structure of Scientific Revolutions* (Chicago: University of Chicago Press, 1962; 1970). Capra (p. 30) defines is as "a profound change in thoughts, perceptions, and values that form a particular vision of reality."

74   In Zen Buddhism, this turning in the deep seat of consciousness is called *satori*.

75   AA says: "With few exceptions our members find that they have tapped an unsuspected inner resource which they presently identify with their own conception of a Power greater than themselves." (*Alcoholics Anonymous*, pp. 569-70).

76   As Alan Watts writes in *The Spirit of Zen: A Way of Life, Work, and Art in the Far East* (New York: Grove Press, 1958), "(*Satori*) is an experience which generally occurs after a long and concentrated effort to discover the meaning of Zen."

77   Alcoholics Anonymous, p. 59.

78   We paraphrase Morris Berman (*The Reenchantment of the World*, pp. 238 - 241), who describes Gregory Bateson's thesis on this subject. Bateson's ideas were published in his article "The Cybernetics of Self - A Theory of Alcoholism." in the *American Journal of Psychiatry*, 34 (1971), 1-18, which also appears as a chapter in his *Steps to Ecology of Mind* (New York: Ballentine, 1972).

79   A primary source of resistance to recovery for alcoholics/addicts is the subjectively incomprehensible prospect of life-long abstinence, the preeminent fear that they will never be able to drink/use again. AA's prescription of "one day at a time" is the response to this.

80   Berman, p. 241. The science of physics is the first direct descendant of Cartesian rationalism.

81   According to Bateson (who is often credited with originally defining the family as an integral *system*), the agenda of any system, including the body, is always *balance*. In answer to the systemic imbalance of Cartesian mind/body dualism, he wrote: "The individual mind is immanent but not only in the body. It is immanent also in the pathways and messages outside the body; and there is a larger Mind of which the individual mind is only a subsystem. This larger mind is compatible to God and is perhaps what some people mean by 'God,' but it is still immanent in the total interconnected social system and planetary ecology." *(Steps to an Ecology of Mind, p. 461.)*

Candace Pert defines "mind" similarly but less esoterically as "some kind of enlivening energy in the information realm throughout the brain and body that enables the cells to talk to each other, and the outside to talk to the whole organism." (Bill Moyers, *Healing and the Mind*, New York: Doubleday, 1993, p. 189).

82   This anecdote is not intended to reinforce the stereotype that all alcoholics are "bar drinkers." Current research presumes two classes of male alcoholics, one of whom drinks outside of the home and the other who tends to drink at home or in isolation. Female alcoholics, due to status insularity and the social stigma attached to female alcoholism, tend not to seek companionship while drinking (see note 19).

83   According to David Steindl-Rast, "I have a strong suspicion that all our various desires in one way or the other mirror the star of our great Desire. Unless there was something good in what we are looking for, we could never desire it. We always look for something good. And there must be something very good in addiction; that is why it is so strong. In addition, addiction must have something to do with our spiritual quest because nothing else so mobilizes the whole personality. And so it stands to reason that in our addiction we can find an aspect of that for which we most deeply long. Mystical experience is the experience of communion and connectedness, and clearly many alcoholics find some elements of this in their inebriation." ("The Mystical Quest, Attachment, and Addiction, *ReVision: The Journal of Consciousness and Change*, Fall, 1987, p. 40).

84   The surrender prescribed here by AA has analogues in the Buddhist ideal of non-attachment and in the Taoist ideal of *wu-wei*. These ideals (Watts, p. 58) teach that the root of possession lies in the desire that things shall not alter in any way. Since this is completely impossible, nothing can be possessed. "Surrender" in this Buddhist/Taoist sense means "not running away from life, but running with it, for freedom comes through complete acceptance of reality." Or, as Jesus said, to be "as the wind that bloweth where it listeth and thou hearest the sound thereof but cannot tell whence it cometh nor whither it goeth." .

85   According to Candace Pert, "Intelligence is in every cell of your body. The mind is not confined to the space above the neck. The mind is throughout the brain and body." (Moyers, p. 188; see also note 81.)

86   Berman, p. 240.

87   R. D. Laing has said: "True sanity entails in one way or another a dissolution of the normal ego, that false self completely adjusted to our alienated social reality; the emergence of the 'inner' archetypal mediators of divine power, and through the death a rebirth, and the eventual reestablishment of a new kind of ego-functioning, the ego now being the servant of the divine, no longer its betrayer."

(R. D. Laing *Politics of Experience*, New York: Ballentine Books, 1968, pp. 144-145).

Or, as Jacquelyn Small describes, "Hitting bottom (for some addicts) is 'the turn' they make toward returning to the source, or coming back to wholeness. It is 'the dark night of the soul' and requires a movement toward the Light to make them feel that life is worth living again. They can never return to the way it was. They have died to the old self and are reborn on a different rung of the ladder." ("Spiritual Emergence and Addiction: A Transpersonal Approach to Alcoholism and Drug Abuse Counseling," *ReVision: The Journal of Consciousness and Change*, Fall, 1987, p. 25 - 26).

From the perspective of Chinese medicine: "The primal language of *Yin-Yang* and *Five Phases* knits together the threads of our personal, social, and transcendent experience. The momentum of transformation is inevitable and inexorable. What exists gives way to what comes after through a process of labor and striving and contending. Our purpose in this process is to become, to change, and to become again - to organize, disorganize, and reorganize. We cannot resist this cellular impulse, but we can participate with greater awareness, appropriately exercising our will (*Water*), determination (*Wood*), passion (*Fire*), generosity (*Earth*), and discipline (*Metal*). The mission of Chinese medicine is to evoke, provoke, and steer change." (Harriet Beinfield and Efrem Korngold, *Between Heaven and Earth: A Guide to Chinese Medicine*, p. 383).

88   See Chapter 7 for a discussion of the phases of recovery.

89   Parallels are often drawn between addiction recovery and adolescent development. A typical assessment made in treatment and recovery circles is that emotional development is arrested at the onset of addictive drinking/using. There is some wisdom in this. The process of adolescent development and recovery are similar patterns, particularly in the individual's need to test things and to become independent. But it seems an excessively linear view to equate the onset of addictive drug use with the arrest of adolescent emotional development. It is more likely that elements of emotional development are thwarted much earlier as a result of scenarios of the unresolved (unvalidated) trauma that is a precursor of addiction. Muschinske suggests that the *pre-cognitive rage* of the child due to original rejection of self by parents is the essential addictive wound. We will argue that this internalization of oppression is the mechanism by which the tenets of Rationalism are also imposed.

Also of significance, of course, is that we speak here in a certain cultural context in which it is assumed that there *was* a child identity preceding the original trauma. For some contemporary children, however, even that experience is nullified by earlier and earlier trauma in the community experience, especially in the inner city, or indeed through perinatal drug exposure.

90   Self-obsession is a typical alcoholic trait. AA asserts: "Selfishness - self-centeredness! That, we think, is the root of our troubles." *(Alcoholics Anonymous,* p. 62).

91   See Bateson's description of interconnectedness (note 72 above).

92   The importance of Wilhelm Reich's work in post-Cartesian epistemology, according to Berman, is that it comes to the "primacy of visceral understanding;" intellect is grounded in affect. While for Freud, the goal of mental health is repression, for Reich, instinctual repression is unhealthy, and promotes a world view that is factually inaccurate. Body and unconscious, in Reich's view, are one (Berman, p. 148-9).

In this regard, it is interesting that *denial*, which is generally viewed as a primary *symptom* of addiction, in fact becomes an incipient *cause* as well. (See section on intervention in Chapter 6) The experience of acupuncture, regardless of the specific points that are applied, is often one of connectedness with ones physical organism.   Directing the attention of chronic alcoholics/addicts to this consciousness of *body* is probably the salient subjective therapeutic mechanism of acupuncture in the chemical dependency treatment setting, as well as a source of the primary resonance between acupuncture and the Twelve Step program.

93   See note 70.

94   The reading of this Step in some Twelve Step meetings has, by group consensus, been changed to "God *as we understood God*," eliminating the gender reference.

95   This is a false theology because it is, of course, impossible. One occupies the field one observes *ipso facto*, and thus is a participant with the thing observed, both casting influence upon it and processing what is observed through subjective experience (see p. 71-73). Sense, which is the mechanism of observation, *is* biological participation by definition despite Descartes' denial of its reality (see p. 46). In the case of vision, for example, what is "seen" *out there* is actually a sensation in the optic nerve in the back of the brain. The struggle of child consciousness with this problem of disembodiment is seen in the adolescent riddle about whether a tree falling in a forest makes a noise if no one is there to hear it.

Capra writes, "The crucial feature of quantum theory is that the observer is not only necessary to observe the properties of an atomic phenomenon, but is necessary even to bring about these properties. My conscious decision about how to observe, say, an electron will determine the electron's properties to some extent. If I ask it a particle question, it will give me a particle answer; if I ask it a wave question, it will give me a wave answer. The electron does not *have* objective properties independent of my mind. In atomic physics the sharp Cartesian division between mind and matter, between the observer and the observed, can no longer be maintained. We can never speak about nature without, at the same time, speaking about ourselves." (*The Turning Point*, p. 87).

96   *"Pass it On:" The Story of Bill Wilson and How the A.A. Message Reached the World* (New York: Alcoholics Anonymous World Services, Inc., 1984), p. 384.

97   See note 31.

98   *Alcoholics Anonymous*, p. 59. In AA, this inventory step is often referred to as "housecleaning."

Referring not to addiction recovery *per se*, but to a more global shift in consciousness, Capra writes (p. 33): "What we need, to prepare ourselves for the great transition we are about to enter, is a deep reexamination of the main premises and values of our culture, a rejection of those conceptual models that have outlived their usefulness, and a new recognition of some of the values discarded in previous periods of our cultural history."

99   See Appendix VI for a list of Twelve Step groups.

100   John Bradshaw is perhaps the most popular proponent of the "Inner Child" movement through his workshops and his PBS television series and book *Homecoming: Championing the Inner Child* (Pompano Beach, FL: Health Communication, Inc.). 1990. See note 65.

101   Steps Five through Nine involve sharing one's personal inventory "with God and another human being," asking God to remove one's shortcomings, and making amends to those one has harmed. *(Alcoholics Anonymous*, p. 59). These steps are often taken with a "sponsor" (see note 22) chosen by the recovering person. Enlightened twelve-step program sponsors often ask the sponsee to include themselves when making their amends, since self-forgiveness is essential to successful recovery.

102   The problem with this conventional bias, that family of origin and trauma work should not be undertaken too early in sobriety, is that many addicts never remain sober long enough to do the work at all! Recent experience at Lincoln Hospital in New York, under the direction of the psychiatrist Mindy Fullilove, has indicated that particularly traumatic events in the lives of women may be addressed early and successfully *so long as adequate program support is in place.*

103   See Gravitz and Bowden (note 10) and Bradshaw (note 65).

104   Notice that this psychic splitting off is not only the inception of the staging ground for addiction, but is also the inception of the fundamental dualism of Exclusionary Rationalism. It is, as noted earlier, the method by which that theology itself is generationally passed.

105   The appropriate therapeutic movement is from the status of *victim* to that of *survivor* of the trauma and abuse of induction into the addictive state. The "Survival Frame" of treating addiction has found preference to the "Disease Frame" partly because of its implicit support for this therapeutic movement.

106   Muschinske writes (p. 27) that "The transmutation of Enlightenment-Modern attitudes and values into a powerful political movement and social structure was generated by the faith in their ideals so inherent to the identities of both country and citizen, no other definition of truth existed." These ideals included "the dominion of man over nature, the certainty of absolute truth, and the belief in the efficacy of scientific rationalization and methods of control as procedures of authority in following material laws." For a further discussion of Enlightenment values, see both Kurtz (pp. 165-169) and Capra (pp. 68-69 and 197-198).

107   See Kurtz's comment on inside/outside paradox in the Twentieth-century (note 25 above).

108   For definitions of "paradigm shift," see note 73.

109   Julian Silverman, "Psychosis and Psychedelics" (workshop, 1971, San Jose, California).

110   Morris Berman, in a further discussion of Bateson's work, calls schizophrenia "not a disease but a systemic network... a Wonderland in which Alice is not free to tell the Queen she is more than a little bit loony." (Berman, p. 230).

111   R. D. Laing, *The Politics of Experience* and *The Divided Self* (Harmondsworth, England: Penguin Books) 1965.

112   Fritjof Capra writes: "The philosophical basis of this rigorous determinism (of Newton's mechanistic view of nature) was the fundamental division between the I and the world introduced by Descartes. As a consequence of this division, it was believed that the world could be described objectively, *i.e.* without ever mentioning the human observer, and such an objective description of nature became the ideal of all science." *(The Tao of Physics*, Boston: Shambhala, 1991, p. 57).

113   "Epimenides'" or the "Liar's Paradox" dates back to the 5th century riddle in which a Greek poses: "All Greeks are liars." Berman (pp. 217-8) discusses knowledge-generated paradox as a function of epistemology.

114   See Gregory and Mary Catherine Bateson, *Angels Fear - Toward an Epistemology of the Sacred* (New York: Macmillan Publishing Co., 1987), p. 21.

115   See discussion of yin/yang theory (note 17).

116   The *scientific method* is the procedure by which "scientific laws" are established; the orthodox view is that this procedure is inductive, which is to draw a conclusion from (objectively discernible) facts. This is not to rule out the role of

intuition in science, for intuitive insights of course have played a major role in scientific discoveries. These intuitive insights, however, are generally of "no use unless they can be formulated in a consistent mathematical framework, supplemented by an interpretation in plain language." (Capra, *Tao of Physics*, p. 31). By comparison, most schools of Eastern thought (upon which Chinese medicine is based) have, at their core, mystical experience. Even among highly disciplined and sophisticated systems of Eastern thought, the intellect is never seen as the source of knowing, but is seen rather as a tool for the interpretation and analysis of mystical (intuitive) experience. According to Joseph Needham (*Science and Civilisation in China* Vol. II., Cambridge, England: Cambridge University Press, 1956, p. 85), this Taoist principle is the basis of Chinese science and technology. The early Taoist philosophers, in Needham's words, "withdrew into the wilderness, the forests and mountains, there to meditate upon the Order of Nature, and to observe its innumerable manifestations." (Quoted in Capra, *ibid.*, p. 34). This is science based upon participatory consciousness (see following note).

117   According to Berman, participatory consciousness is to know things by an act of identification; this is a sensual as well as an intellectual experience, a totality, what Berman calls "sensuous intellect." We've lost that except for the two experiences of lust and anxiety, experiences in which one *becomes* the act, in which it is no longer an "I" experiencing "it." Here the skin loses boundaries; I'm "out of my mind." The essence of original participation is feeling, the bodily perception that there is something behind the experience which somehow represents me and with which I identify. In this "pre-modern" state, subject and object, self and other, man and environment, are ultimately identical (pp. 76-7). This is the holistic world view Bateson spoke of, and it is the "pseudo-holism" achieved by the addict when intoxicated.

118   Carl Jung, *The Undiscovered Self* (New York: Atlantic-Little, Brown, and Co., 1957) pp. 15-16.

119   Robert Bly, ed., *News of the Universe - Poems of Twofold Consciousness* (San Francisco: Sierra Club Books, 1980).

120   Quoted in Carolyn Merchant, *The Death of Nature* (San Francisco: Harper San Francisco, 1989, p. 168 - 169), citing Francis Bacon, "De Dignitate et Augmentis Scientarium," (written 1623), in *Works*, ed. James Spedding, Robert Leslie Ellis, Douglas Devon Heath, 14 vols. (London: Longmans Green, 1870), vol. 4, p. 296.

121   Bly (*ibid.*).

Harriet Beinfield and Efrem Korngold write, "Out of the absolute fissure between self and other is born the problem: other becomes Nature; women; children; people of color. As genders, nations, and cultures we exist in dynamic tension and sensitive ecological balance." (*Ibid.*, pp. 381-382).

122 Merchant, p. 3.

123 It is of interest that the first drug regulation in the United States took the form of attempts to control ethnic and racial minorities, including the first laws against Chinese opium dens in the mid 1800s, marijuana laws directed against Mexican Americans, and heroin laws directed against African Americans in the 1920s. The stigma against inebriation in women reflects the patriarchal view of women as "lifeless objects" as well.

Note again that the addictive system is not stigmatizing or outlawing the *addictive* state but the *intoxicated* state.

124 Cooleridge, a friend of the Wollstonecrafts, offered further evidence of the "dysfunctional" character of Mary's family in expressing his distress at the "cadaverous silence" of the Wollstonecraft children. Others close to the family commented on her father's coldness, cruelty, and intolerance. See Emily Sunstein's *Mary Shelly - Romance and Reality* (Boston: Little Brown, 1989), p. 25.

125 The expectation of the possibility of perfection may lie at the core of addiction (see Marion Woodman's *Addiction to Perfection - The Still Unravished Bride*, Inner City Books, 1982.

Carl Jung has said that *perfection* is a masculine (yang) value whose feminine (yin) counterpart is *completion*.

126 Sunstein, p. 121.

127 Ibid., p. 132.

128 Muriel Spark writes in *Mary Shelly* (New York: E. P. Dutton, 1987, p. 161), that "Frankenstein and his significantly unnamed Monster are bound together by the nature of their relationship...Frankenstein is perpetrated in the Monster. (They are) both complementary and antithetical beings."

129 There is a profound distinction to be drawn between isolation and *solitude*. Henri J. M. Nouwen writes of the movement from isolation and loneliness to solitude in his book *Reaching Out: The Three Movements of the Spiritual Life* (New York: Doubleday, 1975, p. 25): "It is probably difficult, if not impossible, to move from loneliness to solitude without any form of withdrawal from a distracting world, and therefore it is understandable that those who seriously try to develop their spiritual life are attracted to places and situations where they can be alone, sometimes for a limited period of time, sometimes more or less permanently. But the solitude that really counts is the solitude of heart; it is an inner quality or attitude that does not depend on physical isolation. On occasion this isolation is necessary to develop this solitude of heart, but it would be sad if we considered this essential aspect of the spiritual life as a privilege of monks and hermits. It seems more important than ever to stress that solitude is one of the human

capacities that can exist, be maintained and developed in the center of a big city, in the middle of a large crowd and in the context of a very active and productive life. A man or woman who has developed this solitude of heart is no longer pulled apart by the most divergent stimuli of the surrounding world but is able to perceive and understand this world from a quiet inner center."

130   The generic acupuncture protocol we will describe that is used in the drug treatment setting is a departure from the principles and philosophy of traditional Chinese medicine. In Chinese medicine, the utilization of acupuncture involves rigorous patient diagnosis, and the decisions about where to place needles for maximum therapeutic effects are based upon over two thousand years of clinical experience. Paraphrasing David Eisenberg, M.D., from *Encounters with Qi: Exploring Chinese Medicine* (New York: W. W. Norton, 1985, pp. 62-3), acupuncture began with the belief in ancient China that the stimulation of certain points on the body could cure or relieve diseases by affecting the internal organs. It was observed that sensations evoked by stimulation of the surface of the skin always traveled to other parts of the body along definite routes. These routes, or paths, are called "channels and collaterals" or "meridians." By linking the acupuncture points of similar therapeutic effects along identical paths, the Chinese defined the system of meridians.

The meridians are distributed symmetrically over the human body. They are considered conduits for the flow of "blood" and *Qi* ("chi"), which is the fundamental life energy. The meridians connect internally with the viscera and externally with the skin and sense organs. There are twelve major meridians, corresponding to twelve "organs." In addition, there are eight "extra meridians," called collaterals, and a network of minor meridians. (Literal translation of "organs" such as the liver and lung in problematic, since Chinese medicine is not *somatic* medicine [see note 62]. Therefore, "organs" are perceived not as "things" but as dynamic systems. "When viewed in these terms, the body, like the universe, is a complex system of Yin and Yang." [Eisenberg, p. 37]).

In 1955, the French physician Paul Nogier discovered, using an instrument to measure the level of electrical activity on the surface of the skin, that all of the traditional Chinese acupuncture meridians were accessible at points of the ear. Clinical experimentation and research in China soon confirmed this, and both Chinese and "Nogier" ear charts began to appear and find clinical application (see Paul F. M. Nogier, *From Auriculotherapy to Auriculomedicine*, Sainte-Ruffine, France: Maisonneuve, 1983).

131   For ideas in this section, I am especially indebted to Michael Smith, particularly in "Acupuncture Helps Programs More than Patients," presented at the NADA Conference, May, 1993 (available from --.

132   Carol Taub, *The Treatment of Chemical Dependency: A Guide for the Acupuncturist*, a dissertation, SAMRA University of Oriental Medicine, Los

Angeles, CA, Sept., 1988, p. 13 (available from Carol Taub, 1621 Baxter Street, Los Angeles, CA 90026). Taub writes (p. 19) that the effects of this treatment generally include:

1. Reduction of craving for the substance.
2. Reduction of withdrawal symptoms.
3. Marked relaxation, a feeling of well-being.
4. Improved sleep patterns.
5. A "clearer mind" which promotes receptive, rational thinking and therefore enhances the benefits of counseling and group experiences.
6. Stimulation and strengthening of particular organ systems, especially the kidney, liver, and lungs.
7, Improvement in health problems which often accompany long-term alcohol and drug abuse.

As to point location and needling technique (Taub p. 14), "the location where you, the practitioner, feel heat, tingling or where you observe changes in the appearance of the ear should be the point of needle insertion...Needle technique should be quick and painless with a slight twist. It is best to approach the patient with the eight to ten needles in a group, as even the process of removing single needles from packing often increases the patients anxiety."

Michael Smith writes ("Chinese Theory of Acupuncture Detoxification," a NADA publication, [quoted in Taub, p. 12]), "Intense and frequent abuse of chemical substances damages the Jing-Essence. In turn, the Kidney is damaged because it is the organ that stores the Jing. Usually, the yin is deficient, so we may see many empty fire symptoms. Yang deficiency symptoms are also present." (See Appendix III for a complete list of NADA publications.)

Paraphrasing Taub (p. 12-13), a 40 year old person who has been abusing drugs and alcohol shows signs of premature aging indicative of jing depletion -- stooped posture, decaying teeth, and graying hair, a sunken look about the eyes, etc. Often, nervous agitation may be dominant in the persons outward behavior. As a result it has often been assumed that sedation of an excess is appropriate treatment. Therefore some practitioners choose to use strong electrostimulation in their treatment. The results of this type of treatment are usually short and fail to address the underlying jing and yin deficiencies. By contrast, a gentle, tonifying, repetitive treatment is effective in treating even severely debilitated addicts and alcoholics. It has been the experience at Lincoln Hospital that auricular acupuncture is the most effective form of treatment for abusers, both in crisis, and in long-term recovery, and Dr. Michael Smith suggests (with Khunat Ra, "Acupuncture Treatment of Chemical Dependency and Violence, NADA publication, 1985) that the kidney's association with the ear, the fetus-shape and the passive nature of the ear's function are relevant factors.

Ear tacks, or "press needles" should be used with great discretion since the client's daily participation in the clinic process is seen as an essential part of this treatment. Tacks are therefore recommended generally only for clients upon detoxification from nicotine, or if a client is required to miss treatment.

133   Research has shown that drug treatment outcome is related to client retention (see note 6).

134   Clients should, in general, be prohibited from participation in acupuncture only when their behavior threatens clinic safety. Treatment can have a profound effect on behavior, and, when initiated in cases of even the most unruly clients, can have surprising results.

135   There are new considerations when the acupuncture is integrated in a residential setting, or in cases where treatment is "mandated" by law and justice or other agencies (see note 161 below).

136   The use of "detox specialists" has been common in locations such as New York, Minneapolis, and Texas, where the number of acupuncturists is insufficient to meet the demand for services. Laws governing acupuncture vary from State to State. Some States have had no acupuncture laws, and have no restrictions on who may perform acupuncture. In other States, only a physician may perform acupuncture. California, with an abundance of acupuncturists, is among the States that have specific standards governing the practice of acupuncture, and the utilization of detox specialists would require a statute change in these States. Whether or not to have detox specialists, and the degree of training and supervision they should have, is currently a very controversial subject among both State and National Chinese medical professional associations (see Appendix III for a list of associations).

137   For a review of the literature concerning acupuncture and neurotransmission, see Alan Bensoussan's *The Vital Meridian* (Edinburgh: Churchill Livingstone, 1990), pp. 101-126.

138   The catecholamines (norepinephrine, epinephrine, and dopamine), so grouped because of their chemical structure and function, are neurotransmitters that are synthesized by neurons that convert phenylalanine or tyrosine to a compound called L-dopa. Phenylalanine and Tyrosine are amino acids obtained from protein digestion. Following this conversion, L-dopa is in turn converted to dopamine.

139   Kenneth Blum and Michael Trachtenberg, "Neurochemistry and Alcohol Craving," *California Society for the Treatment of Alcoholism and Other Drug Dependencies News*, Vol.13, No.2, Sept., 1986, p. 4.

140   An acetic is vinegar; ester is a compound formed from the reaction of an alcohol with an acid; choline is a nitrogenous member of vitamin b complex essential in synthesis of amino acids, which are essential building block for proteins.

141   It could be a bit mechanistic to suggest that there are different types of serotonic receptors. What appeared at first to be different sub-types of endorphin receptors turned out instead to be one receptor in a constant state of flux, in a constant transformation between particle and wave. Candace Pert says of the endorphin receptors that scientists "see great heterogeneity in the receptors. They have given a series of Greek names to the apparent heterogeneity. However, all the evidence from our lab suggests that in fact *there is actually only one type of molecule in the opiate receptors, one long polypeptide chain whose formula you can write.* This molecule is quite capable of changing its configuration within its membrane so that it can assume a number of shapes.

"I note in passing that this interconversion can occur at a very rapid pace - so rapid that it is hard to tell whether it is one state or another in a given moment in time. In other words, receptors have both a wave-like and a particulate character, and it is important to note that information can be stored in the form of time spent in different states." ("The Wisdom of the Receptors: Neuropeptides, the Emotions, and Bodymind, *Noetic Sciences Review*, 2, 1987, pp. 14-15, quoted in Ernest Rossi and David Cheek, *Mind-Body Therapy: Methods of Ideodynamic Healing in Hypnosis*, New York: W. W. Norton & Company, 1988, p. 210) Rossi and Cheek note that "What is most fascinating from theoretical and practical points of view is how *alternating states of the receptor may be a psychobiological mechanism whereby energy and information could be converted into one another in living systems.*" (p. 211).

142   Monoamines are broken down into smaller compounds by the enzyme monoamine oxidase (*MAO*), which restricts transmission activity. Drugs blocking MAO enzyme activity were being developed in the 1960s for the treatment of depression on the theory that inhibiting the breakdown of the monoamines will result in a greater proliferation of NE, 5-HT, and DA in the system. These drugs are called MAO Inhibitors (MAOI's). There are dangerous side effects, however, due to essential functions of monoamine oxidase, such as breaking down tyramine, which affects blood pressure and is found in certain cheeses, beer, wine, chicken liver, canned figs, etc. Other MAOI side effects include damage to the liver, brain, and cardiovascular system, and, in overdose, hallucinations, fever, and convulsions.

143   Platelets, the source of thromboplastin (necessary to blood clotting), are minute bodies in blood plasma consisting of non-nucleated fragments of the cytoplasm of megakaryocytes (the large, multi-nucleated cell of red bone marrow). Significant differences in blood platelet levels have been found in genetic alcoholism.

144   Essential amino acids are those that cannot be synthesized internally but must be acquired through diet. There are many essential amino acid products currently on the market that are used in addiction treatment (See Appendix II).

145 Charles Carroll, *Drugs in Modern Society*, 3rd Edition, Madison, Wisconsin: Brown and Benchmark, p. 194.

146 Candace Pert writes "We have been looking for the mind, and the question arises: Where is it? In our own work, consciousness has come up in the context of studying pain and the role of opiate receptors and endorphins in modulating pain. A lot of labs are measuring pain, and we would all agree that the area called periaqueductal gray, located around the third ventricle of the brain, is filled with opiate receptors, making it a kind of control area for pain. We have found that the periaqueductal gray is also loaded with receptors for virtually all the neuropeptides that have been studies.

"Now, everyone knows that there are yogis who can train themselves so that they do or do not perceive pain, depending on how they structure their experience. Women in labor do the same thing. What seems to be going on is that these sorts of people are able to plug into their periaqueductal gray. Somehow they gain access to it - with their consciousness, I believe - and set pain thresholds. Note what is going on here. In these situations, a person has an experience that brings with it pain, but a part of the person consciously does something so that the pain is not felt. Where is this consciousness coming from - the conscious I - that somehow plugs into the periaqueductal gray so that he or she does not feel a thing?

"I want to go back to the idea of a network. A network is different from a hierarchical structure which has one top place. You theoretically can plug into a network at any point and get to any other point. A concept like this seems to me valuable in thinking about the processes by which a consciousness can manage to reach the periaqueductal gray and use it to control pain." ("Neuropeptides: The Emotions and Bodymind, *Noetic Sciences Review*, pp. 17-18, quoted in Ernest Rossi and David Cheek, pp. 214-215).

By 1993, Pert was calling endorphins *agents of information* (Moyers, p. 180). "They carry messages within the brain, and from the brain to the body, or from the body to the brain. The old barriers between brain and body are breaking down. The way scientists like to work is to have the immunology department over here and the neuroscience department over there. People from these departments don't talk to each other that much unless they're married to each other. But in real life the brain and the immune system use so many of the same molecules to communicate with each other that we're beginning to see that perhaps the brain is not simply 'up here,' connected by nerves to the rest of the body. It's a much more dynamic process. ... When people discovered that there were endorphins in the brain that caused euphoria and pain relief, everybody could handle that. But when they discovered that they were in your immune system, too, it just didn't fit, so it was denied for years. The original scientists had to repeat their studies many, many times to be believed. It was just very upsetting to our paradigm to find mood-altering chemicals in the immune system - and not just the chemicals, but the receptors as well."

147 U.S. Department of Health and Human Services, "Drug Abuse and Drug Abuse Research: The Third Triennial Report to Congress from the Secretary," DHHS Publication No. (ADM) 91-1704, 1991, p. 11.

148 The receptors are not static, but dynamic. Candace Pert (Moyers, p. 186) describes them as "wiggling, vibrating energy molecules that are not only changing their shape from millisecond to millisecond, but actually changing the way they're coupled to. One moment they're coupled up to one protein in the membrane, and the next moment they can couple up to another. It's a very dynamic, fluid system."

149 If we look for our radical center here, we find ourselves in the eye of the mirror. We follow the dazzling Western "yellow brick road" through the land of the neurophysiological mechanism of mind itself, looking at a process somehow from outside the field to which our interest is drawn, and then realize that the process we view is the very mechanism by which we view it. There is no abstraction. We are in and of the field we describe at each instant.

Recovery is participatory consciousness; recovery is being in the process of our lives. How does it *feel* to be *in* rather than "above" or "behind" or "outside of" this process of thought, to invite into our dualistic dominion the awareness that the conscious attention we have given to these neural substrates has been an activity of these neural substrates?

But, the illusion that we are ever outside of this process is so persistent, so tenacious. I cling to an "I" somehow detached from "it." To let go of this center of "intelligence" (control) would be to lose my footing and my very identity. How, then, would i control thought? How would i continue to exist without the vigilance of an ego to make sure everything is working properly, both inside my skin and "outside" in the realm of my senses?

This fear-based, internalized state of oppression and control, is the addictive template. This fear seems parallel to the codependent fear that drives prohibition, that has motivated the current "war" on drugs, that fuels society's obsessive need to control mind-altering substances, and the disdain in general of mind-altered states of consciousness, of euphoria.

And this is an operational as well as an existential issue. I follow, for example, with sharp interest the conversation about how information flows and gets processed in the "entity" called "brain" and realize that if I knew all about exactly how it works, I wouldn't be able to "work" it any better than someone who has never even heard of a neurotransmitter!

Is it possible to recall child-consciousness, pre-rational consciousness, before the ascent of ego? Is it possible to recall the *sensation of self* as a *trustworthy process* that functions in fact very well without the apparition "I" at the helm? As Alan Watts observed (presentation at Monterey Peninsula College, *circa* 1968), I open and close my hand, but I don't know *how* I open and close my hand except in the sense that I can *do* it. I don't know *how* I do it unless I am a physiologist, and then I can't open and close my hand much better than anybody else. I don't know how I color my eyes, shape my bones, or grow my brain upon which consciousness rests, but I do it - without "thinking."

What, then, is the sensation of experience that what I perceive of as *mind* is actually a function not simply of brain but of *body*? - the sense that i is, as Bateson suggested, immanent - a matrix extending infinitely inward and infinitely outward? - the prospect that my little toe *knows* what I am thinking, and that my actions here in Santa Barbara, California, somehow affect the people in Kansas or South Africa? - that intelligence is replete, and that all things are connected?

Descartes postulated that there was indeed a physical membrane separating *mind* from *body*, and someone raised in the institutions of the West can certainly see how he was led to such a brazen hypothesize, for it feels in my rationalism as though "I" and my body share a relationship not unlike that which the telodendria of the presynaptic cell shares with the dendrite of the postsynaptic cell: *nestling into without touching*. "I" refuses to traverse the cleft and plunge into self. Perhaps in some mysterious fashion, rational man has in fact grown just such a physical membrane. Perhaps Descartes (as Bateson said of Newton with respect to gravity) *invented* rather than *discovered* this phenomenon, but perhaps it has a certain reality just the same. Perhaps the impulse toward healing that we call *recovery* is the bursting in some macrocosmic cisternae of highly specialized and discerning "messenger molecules" which "go to the wall" of this mind/body membrane searching for balance, longing to connect, yearning to open the channel so that the message can get through that *yes*, something is happening "out there" as well as "in here," and perhaps the medium is the message, that "out there" and "in here" are seamless aspects of the same process.

Is this the impulsive craving of addiction, Jung's "low level spiritual thirsting for oneness (with God)?" For here is the core of the addict's isolation. The rift within, the sense of being disconnected and unhealed, produces the yearning for its imagined equivalent outside. We can create, through drugs (and through other things as well), the *sensation* (for the moment) of oneness, of connectedness, of the intoxication of Bateson's "pseudoholism," and we turn to these things partially out of fear of looking within; we can't trust the "flesh" within because we have estranged ourselves from it. We are, so to speak, stuck in the middle, having created the void we most fear.

But with an acupuncture needle at *shenmen*, sympathetic, liver, kidney, and lung, with eyes closed, in the presence of others who share this riddle, we catch for an instant just a glimpse of the possibility of trusting *something* within, something ancient and forgotten, and, in that surprising instant, the gate has opened.

We find ourselves not at the *cure* or "fix" we were seeking, but at the first step in "a journey of a thousand miles," at the end of one adventure and the beginning of another.

150   A single blind placebo research study is currently being conducted in Hennepin County, Minnesota, under the direction of Milton Bullock and Pat Culliton comparing acupuncture with Valium on the effects of acute alcohol withdrawal.

151   Edward Brecher describes this process in *Licit and Illicit Drugs: The Consumer Union Report*. (Boston: Little, Brown and Company. 1972). For a discussion of psychological symptoms that may forebode relapse, see pp. 137-141.

152   See Jeffrey Jonas, M.D., and Ron Schaumburg, *Everything You Need to Know about Prozac* (New York: Bantam, 1991), and Peter D. Kramer, *Listening to Prozac* (New York: Penguin Books, 1993).

153   Barry Stimmell and the editors of Consumer Report Books, *The Facts About Drug Use*, New York: Haworth Press, 1993, p. 285.

154   Weldon Witters and Peter Venturelli, *Drugs and Society* (2nd edition), Boston: Jones and Bartlett, 1988, p. 235-6 .

155   Henry Spitz, M.D., and Jeffrey S. Rosecan, M.D., eds., *Cocaine Abuse: New Directions in Treatment and Research* (New York: Brunner/Mazel, 1987).

156   *ibid.*

157   Michael Kuhar, et. al., "Cocaine Receptors on Dopamine Transporters Mediate Cocaine-Reinforcing Behavior," in *Mechanisms of Cocaine Abuse and Toxicity*, NIDA Research Monograph 88, U. S. Department of Health and Human services, 1988, p. 19.

158   This is a special funding mechanism, varying from State to State, employed by the State in response to the availability of Federal Medicaid dollars matching State dollars which fund drug and alcohol outpatient or day treatment services. In California, for example, this money is available only to State Certified Drug or Alcohol "Medi-Cal" Programs who already have non-discretionary State funding in place, which is used for the match, and services are available only for clients meeting Medicaid eligibility requirements (clients who are under eighteen, over sixty-five, disabled, pregnant, or those with dependent children if they meet certain income requirements). Since maximizing these programs on the State level maximizes potential Federal dollars coming into the State, States are currently doing everything they can to get programs certified, and the numbers

are dramatically increasing. Revision of this system is currently under discussion at the Federal level, partially because Federal Medicaid, an entitlement, is a primary force driving the Federal deficit. For information about these programs in your State, contact the State Alcohol and Drug Department (see Appendix IV, Section B for a listing).

For California readers, or for those in other States which provide public insurance reimbursement that covers acupuncture, note that this is not regular "fee-for-service" reimbursement for which the individual treatment practitioner becomes a "provider" and submits a patient's claim for a specific treatment episode.

159   A residential treatment research project funded by the State of Florida found that patients who completed at least ten days of acupuncture and who do not receive concurrent medications would be ten times more likely to complete a thirty day residential program than they would without acupuncture. See Jay Holder, et.al., "A New Auricular Therapy Formula to Increase Retention of the Chemically Dependent in Residential Treatment" (available from Jay Holder, 3180 Biscayne Boulevard, Miami, FL 33137).

Note that the clinic dynamics outlined in Chapter 4, which take place in an outpatient setting, change in a residential setting where any relapse generally results in expulsion from the treatment program. Not only has acute detoxification already been achieved by clients, but in an extended clean and sober cloistered environment, more accurate assessment can be made. There are more opportunities here for traditional Chinese medicine through diagnosis, but we have lost many of the advantages of the NADA protocol which serve the goal of client retention in the outpatient program where abstinence is not a criteria for program involvement.

160   In a controlled study at Bayview Hunter's Point Clinic in San Francisco, acupuncture has compared favorably with methadone in heroin detoxification. See W. Clark's "Trial of Acupuncture Detoxification (TRIAD): Final Report," (August 15, 1991), available from the California State Legislature. These results also appear in Allyson M. Washburn, et. al., "Acupuncture Heroin Detoxification: A Single Blind Clinical Trial" (*Journal of Substance Abuse Treatment*, Vol. 10, pp. 345-351, July/August 1993; reprints available from Allyson Washburn, Ph.D., San Francisco Treatment Research Unit, San Francisco General Hospital, Substance Abuse Services, Ward 93, 1001 Potrero Avenue, San Francisco, CA 94110).

161   A common pitfall in all programs to which clients come under the urging of criminal or social service authority is that clients and staff alike subscribe to the premise that client attendance and participation is mandated. In the vast majority of these programs, the technical and significant fact is that the client was not *mandated*. The client made a *choice* at some point in the process. The choice may have been to elect treatment in lieu of losing custody of a child, or in lieu of

going to prison, but no matter how unattractive the alternative presented, the treatment was *chosen*. It will be beneficial in such programs if a concerted effort is made on the part of all staff - including the referring officials - to adapt as a primary treatment goal that the client acquiesce to and *own* the choice that was made. This will dispel the "good cop/bad cop" syndrome that can negate any therapeutic movement in programs in which both client and staff have tacitly agreed to the mistaken assumption the client brings that "I am here because I have to be."

The right of the state in fact to mandate drug treatment is a matter of current controversy. For an excellent analysis, from both a public health and a legal point of view, see Lawrence Gostin's "Compulsory Treatment for Drug-Dependent Persons: Justification for a Public Health Approach to Drug Dependence (*Milbank Quarterly*, v.69, n4, Winter, 1991, p. 561):

162   SSI (Social Security Insurance) disability recipients include individuals who have been medically diagnosed as alcohol or drug addicted and/or chronically mentally ill. These individuals are generally required to have a "Protective Payee" to manage their funds, and some outpatient drug and alcohol programs offer these services to their clients. Some clients, depending upon the local Social Security administrative authority, are required to seek treatment as a condition of receiving benefits.

163   For the addict, this creates a queer illusion: it is as though my life is a movie, and the only real person on the set is me, the director (the ego). All others present are objects, here to play out a script. And, I am not only directing; I also wrote the screenplay! The people in my life have a singular collective and conspiratorial identity which I project upon them, possessing no integrity or autonomy as individuals. I must manipulate and control them to keep the movie going; the script demands it. So long as I can achieve this, the focus is off myself.

164   See Anne Wilson Schaef and Diane Fassel, *The Addictive Organization: Why We Overwork, Cover Up, Pick Up the Pieces, Please the Boss and Perpetuate Sick Organizations* (San Francisco: Harper & Row, 1988).

165   The concept of "latent withdrawal," was introduced into the literature by Jerome Jaffe in the edited work of Louis S. Goodman and Alfred Gilman, *The Pharmacological Basis of Therapeutics* (New York: Macmillan, 4th ed. 1970). Other pioneers in relapse prevention treatment include Stephanie Brown, *Treating the Alcoholic* (New York: John Wiley and Sons, Inc., 1988), and Terence Gorski, *Staying Sober - A Guide to Relapse Prevention*, and *Passages Through Recovery* (New York: Harper and Row, 1987; 1989). An important recent contributor to the field is George M. DuWors, *White Knuckles and Wishful Thinking: Breaking the Chain of Compulsive Reaction and Relapse in Alcoholism and Other Addictions* (Seattle: Hogrefe and Huber, 1992).

166   The specific length of time varies depending upon chronicity and intensity of use. The typical three to fifteen day acute withdrawal is longer for the benzodiazapines (see p 105) and for methadone (see p 110).

167   Michael Smith & I. Kahn, "An acupuncture programme for the treatment of drug addicted persons", *Bulletin on Narcotics* XL(1) (1988), 35-41.

168   Although we will discuss program staffing issues at some length in Chapter Nine, it may be noted that persons in this initial recovery phase from six to eighteen months often make the best program counselors because of the intensity of their personal involvement in recovery. Programs utilizing counselors who are in early recovery need especially to have relapse-prevention programs in place for these and all recovering staff members.

169   The work of psychotherapist Carl Rogers, described in his 1951 book *Client-Centered Therapy* (Boston: Houghton Mifflin), can be seen as a counter-cultural reaction against the autocratic Freudian analysts of the 1940s. It represented a shift of power away from the omniscient patriarchal authority of the psychotherapist and toward a humanistic therapeutic movement based upon and trusting in the client's own life process, capacity for growth, and inner experience.

170   Reentry into community is a fundamental goal of treatment, and challenge as well, since the community to which the client is returning is generally an addictive one! This is, of course, why the short-term treatment efforts are seldom effective in long-term outcome. It is also why it is desirable for the treatment provider to have the resources to involve the client's family or other primary social system in the treatment recovery process. These resources may be available either within the program or through creative linkages with other service providers in the community. The early transitional client, always looking for the "quick fix," will come to learn that he or she needs to "stay close to the program" (generally, a Twelve Step program) during the transition period of the first eighteen months or so. The danger otherwise is that "the center will not hold."

171   Step 4 is, "Made a searching and fearless moral inventory of ourselves;" step 5 is, "Admitted to God, to ourselves, and to another human being the exact nature of our wrongs."

172   Empowerment in the sense that we are using the term implies a new and deeper center from which to act - not as one has been taught to act, but as one chooses to act. It also implies elements of self-efficacy, group consciousness, reduced self-blame, and the assuming of personal responsibility for change. (See Lorraine Gutierrez's "Working with Women of Color: An Empowerment Perspective," *Social Work* (March, 1990, pp.149-153).

173   The 37 common progressive symptoms is copyrighted and proprietary information of the CENAPS Corporation. It is reproduced here with the

permission of The CENAPS Corporation. Any further reproduction is specifically prohibited without written permission of The CENAPS Corporation, 18650 Dixie Highway, Howewood, Illinois 60430, 708-799-5000.

174   DuWors, Chapters Four and Five.

175   *Alcoholics Anonymous*, 3rd ed. (New York: Alcoholics Anonymous World Services, Inc., 1976; orig. pub. 1939), p. 45.

176   Anne Wilson Schaef workshop on "The Addictive Society," Santa Barbara, 1988.--For an overview of Schaef's beliefs, see her autobiographical *Beyond Therapy and Science: A New Model for Healing the Whole Person* (San Francisco: Harper & Row, 1992).

177   Anne Wilson Schaef, *Women's' Reality* (San Francisco: Harper & Row, 1981).

178   See references to Kurtz in Part I.

179   Robert Bly, ed., *News of the Universe - Poems of Twofold Consciousness* (San Francisco: Sierra Club Books, 1980).

180   As we have noted, repression of the feminine is implicit in the repression of nature by the White Male system. Robert Bly points out that in the male psyche, attitudes toward women are usually the same as those toward the earth and the unconscious (Bly, *Ibid.*)..

181   Schaef, *Co-Dependence: Misunderstood, Mistreated* (San Francisco: Harper & Row, 1986).

182   Since we are using the AA model to define recovery, this poses a curious paradox. As we have mentioned, at its inception in 1935, AA was a white male society. It was established, and its principles drafted by (and primarily *for*) white males. The book *Alcoholics Anonymous*, in which the program is described, presumes a white male psychology; generic references (as well as all references to God) are always in the masculine gender. Yet, as Schaef here implies, the twelve steps themselves and the organization they have fostered are inherently feminine.

For a less generous critique of the gender implications of the twelve steps, see Charlotte Kasl, "Paths of Recovery," (1991 Monograph, available from Charlotte Kasl, P.O. Box 7073, Minneapolis MN 55407) - or her book *Many Roads, One Journey: Moving Beyond the Twelve Steps* (New York: Harper Collins, 1992).

183   Schaef, *When Society Becomes an Addict*. San Francisco, Harper and Row, 1987.

184   Worthy of celebration for feminism is Gloria Steinem's *Revolution from Within: A Book of Self-Esteem* (Boston: Little, Brown, & Co., 1992), an appeal for the shifting of focus from external to internal referents for healing.

185   A case could be made that romance addiction, which includes addiction to a political or social cause or movement, was the first Modern addiction: the addiction, on the part of its founders, to Rationalism itself.

186   Though the authorship of *Alcoholics Anonymous* is "anonymous", this chapter, as with most of the text of the first 164 pages, was written by Bill Wilson.

187   *Alcoholics Anonymous*, p. 53.

Note the paradoxical juxtaposition of this statement with the title of Kurtz's book, *Not-God*. From the point of view of the implicitly dualistic and mechanistic addictive system, any definitions of God end up being exclusionary, in which any notion of what God is requires as a necessary correlate that which God *isn't*. A non-dualistic and hence inclusionary world view, such as that inherent in the philosophy of Alcoholics Anonymous and of Chinese medicine (see note 17), allows for the immanence of God. As the pre-modern folk adage has it, "there's not a spot where God is not!"

188   *Ibid.*

189   In his book, *The Cry for Myth* (New York: W. W. Norton & Co., 1991), Rollo May claims that the preeminent modern Western myth is Faust. The Faustian landscape has interesting parallels with that of Mary Shelly's *Frankenstein*, the "myth of the addictive state" that we proposed in Chapter 3.

190   Rollo May, personal interview, *circa* 1987.

191   *The Wizard of Oz* can also be seen as an example of an endogenous Western myth. While elements of the story can be traced to the shamanism of Northeast Asia (as well, however, as to Native American culture), wizards and witches are Western, and the story's essential frame is American. As a myth, the story has also been interpreted to provide meaning for gay men in their struggle for identity. See Larry Hermsen's, "Over the Rainbow and Into our Hearts," *The White Crane Newsletter and Journal for the Development of Gay Men's Spirituality*, Number 8 (P.O. Box 170152, San Francisco, CA 94117-0152).

192   Of course, as we move from culture consciousness to a more global consciousness, the East and West are inexorably linked. In his introduction to Richard Wilhelm's translation of *The Secret of the Golden Flower*, Carl Jung framed this linkage in a curious way: "The European invasion of the East was an outrage on a grand scale that has left us - *noblesse oblige* - with an obligation to gain some understanding on the East. This is perhaps more of a necessity than we may realize at the present time."

193   This story is recounted in *Alcoholics Anonymous*, pp. 26 - 7; in Kurtz's *Not-God*, pp. 8 - 9, and in *"Pass it On:" The Story of Bill Wilson and How the A.A. Message*

Reached the World (New York: Alcoholics Anonymous World Services, Inc., 1984), pp. 381-86.

194   *Alcoholics Anonymous*, p. 27.

195   As we have previously mentioned, alcoholism had been discussed in the medical literature as a disease since 1810. Silkworth's opinions and the dominant medical view of alcoholism in the 1930's is described in *Alcoholics Anonymous*, pp. xxiii-xxx, and 571-2.

196   Kasl, *Many Roads...*

197   See Appendix VI for additional information on these recovery resources.

198   Modern civilization faces a number of formidable issues whose resolution is simply not possible within the framework of the old paradigm. The economics of forest economies, land use in South America, displacement of workers in military-related industries, and the inner city economies are examples of problems so demandingly complex that a new world view has become, like recovery for the addict, a matter of survival.

199   See, however, note 102.

200   See note 92.

201   *Alcoholics Anonymous*, p. 27.

202   *Ibid.*

203   R. D. Laing, *Politics of Experience* (NY: Ballentine Books, 1968), 144-145.

204   *Alcoholics Anonymous*, p. 27.

205   Hence one reason for the renewed popularity of Albert Ellis and rational-emotive therapy, which focuses on changing self-talk. According to Benjamin Lee Whorf (*Language, Thought and Reality*, John B. Carroll, ed. Cambridge Mass, 1956. p. 213-14). "We cut nature up, organize it into concepts, and ascribe significances as we do, largely because we are parties to an agreement to organize it in this way - an agreement that holds throughout our speech community and is codified in the patterns of our language."

206   For a helpful analysis of addictive systems, see Anne Wilson Schaef and Diane Fassel, *The Addictive Organization: Why We Overwork, Cover Up, Pick Up the Pieces, Please the Boss and Perpetuate Sick Organizations* (San Francisco: Harper & Row, 1988).

207   As we mentioned in the introduction to this section, for purposes of explanation we will use the fairly common structure of drug and alcohol treatment administration that is in place in California. It is important to note that *the process of accessing the system* is the same, regardless of the way in which the

system may be organized in the reader's locale. That is to say that all expenditure by government of public funds requires some degree of public scrutiny. In California, for example, the mechanism for this is the County Drug and Alcohol Advisory Board. This mechanism may be different in different States, but the mechanism will be there in one form or another, and may be discovered by contacting the local or State agency responsible for administration of drug and alcohol treatment funds. It may be that this mechanism is not organized, but is simply the local or state elected officials.

Whatever form that mechanism takes in the reader's own region, the basic procedures outlined in this section can be applied.

208   In a recent study of acupuncture treating in-custody, substance abusing, mental health patients at the Los Angeles County Jail, clients reported dramatic improvement in the areas of cravings and drug dreams. Unit staff observed in the acupuncture patients calming effects, making patients more relaxed and productive in the program's educational component; a decrease in craving and reduction in depression; a decrease in requests for sleep and anxiety medications, and a decrease of reports of anxiousness and insomnia. (Carol Taub, L.Ac., O.M.D., "Report on Acupuncture Substance Abuse Treatment Adjunct, February, through June, 1993, Biscailuz Intermediate Care, Jail Mental Health Services, Los Angeles, 1993).

A Waco, Texas program reports "consistent improvement in social behavior, cognitive functions, and reductions in ambivalence, delusional pressure, and stress in all of the regular acupuncture patients. Tardive dyskinesia decreased markedly in one previously severely limited patient. Acupuncture seems to effect many aspects of functioning and thereby allow the use of a wider range of conventional therapeutic activities." Hospitalization days dropped from 27 days the previous year to 8. Hours of sleep have decreased from 14 hours to 8 - 10 hours per night. Staff reports that meetings with these residential patients become longer, substantive, and related to "problem solving," and patients are "more motivated," more "fun to be with," and "more at ease," "less violent, less sexually active, and not requiring virtually no police intervention." (Michael Smith, Tom Atwood, and Gloria Turley, "Acupuncture May Prevent Relapse in Chronic Schizophrenic Patients," available from Tom Atwood, 110 South 12th Street, Waco, TX 76701).

For additional information on dual diagnosis, see Appendix XII, Section B.

209   From Belle Muschinske concerning women's treatment programs, in "Prison drug treatment has been ignored but programs are surfacing," *Sober Times*, August, 1992.

210   Los Angeles County District Attorney Gil Garcetti says: "We have expended incredible sums of money on the war on drugs, and we are not anywhere closer to

victory." Once released, drug users are "coming back into the system as people who are continuing to use drugs or are turning to burglaries and robberies to support their habit. ...Society is not being protected under the current system when...a drug user who has committed a burglary or (been involved in) prostitution goes to jail, gets no treatment, and gets back on the street and commits the same crime. That's not protection." ("County Drug Policy Shift Weighed, *Los Angeles Times*, May 17, 1993, Times Mirror Company, p. 1). The same position is stated by Lawrence Gostin in his thoughtful article, "Compulsory Treatment for Drug-Dependent Persons: Justification for a Public Health Approach to Drug Dependence (Milbank Quarterly, v.69, n4, Winter, 1991, p. 561): "The declared policy of a 'drug free America' by 1995, supported by an ever-widening net of detection through drug screening and law enforcement, is a fruitless, impractical endeavor destined to overwhelm the criminal justice system. It becomes virtually impossible to present a credible law enforcement program with an estimated 28 million people having used illicit drugs..."

211   The Drug Policy Foundation is a self-appointed "watchdog" of the Nation's "War on Drugs." Their publications include the *Drug Policy Newsletter*. (Drug Policy Foundation, 4801 Massachusetts Avenue, N.W., Suite 400, Washington, D.C. 20016-2087 - 202 / 895-1634).

212   The reader is invited to do more precise research in his or her own local jurisdiction through the office of the county's administrator. Here are some other revealing recent statistics from Alice S. Baum and Donald W. Burnes, *A Nation in Denial: The Truth About Homelessness*, Boulder, Colorado: Westview Press, 1993, pp. 182-183).. The cost in Minneapolis for the treatment of chronic public inebriates for detoxification, medical, and psychiatric costs is estimated at $15,900 per person per year, and the legal and social services cost $6,940 per person per year. The New York City Commission on the Homeless reports that not-for-profit agencies spend $15,000 to $19,000 per year to operate substance abuse beds, including capital costs as well as operating costs. In Philadelphia, the cost of emergency shelter is estimated at $11.50 per night; detoxification for seven days at $115 per day (medically supervised, non-hospital; in-hospital detox is estimated at $450 - $550 per day); "intermediate" treatment services, including assessment and inpatient or outpatient treatment at $60 per day; long term service for six to nine months (including dormitory inpatient treatment, counseling, life skills and parenting training, and vocational counseling) at $90 per day, and substance-free living with outpatient treatment at $75 per day. According to these estimates, the cost of treatment for an individual would range from $29,800 to slightly over $31,000 for the first year, and would be $27,000 for a second year. On balance, this program also estimated that the provision of effective treatment to sixteen crack-addicted pregnant women so that their babies were born drug free resulted in a savings to the system of more than $1 million (estimating a cost of $100,000 per infant for in-hospital care). The cost of shelter alone in New

York City ranges from $18,000 to $20,000 per year per sheltered single adult, and from $27,375 to $52,000 per year for a sheltered family in welfare motels. A 1988 HUD survey found that the average cost of a night in a shelter nation-wide was $28, or $10,200 per year.

For information concerning the cost of delivering acupuncture-based program treatment, see sample budgets in Chapter 9.

213   See Chapter 9 for specific budget development guidelines.

214   The potential savings, of course, are skewed by two factors. First is that the cost, for example, of housing one inmate in a county correctional facility may be calculated through simple math at $16,000 per year. Removing that inmate, however, from this setting does not save the system $16,000 because much of the expense of operations are *fixed* costs (personnel, building, utilities, insurance, etc.).. The other problem is that in areas where acupuncture has been in fact widely integrated into treatment services for criminal justice populations, such as New York and Miami, we cannot demonstrate real savings to the law and justice systems because of the extraordinary numbers of offenders entering those systems to replace those who recover.

215   See Appendix XI, Section C, for sample criminal justice referral forms used in sending clients to acupuncture-based programs.

216   Puccio, Paul S., "Acupuncture Detoxification and Relapse Service: A Concept Paper," New York State Division of Substance Abuse Services (1991).

217   This research is not yet published as of this writing. For further information, contact NIDA (see Appendix IV, Section B).

218   See "Miami's Drug Court: A Different Approach," National Institute of Justice, U.S. Department of Justice, Office of Justice Programs, NIJ: NCJ 142412 (June, 1993).

219   A detailed description of this urine testing protocol is contained in the article in Appendix VIII.

220   See Appendix III for sources of acupuncture liability insurance.

221   The Lincoln Hospital program has determined that the most effective tea mix is 1 part peppermint; 1 part catnip; 1 part yarrow; 2 parts chamomile; 2 parts hops, and 2 parts sculcap. Herbs may be purchased in bulk and mixed in this ratio, or a similar "sleepmix" may be purchased pre-bagged through Nutra Control, Box 1199, Old Chelsea Station, New York, N.Y., 10011 (212) 929-3780.

222   NADA certification of acupuncturists also requires an internship, a requirement that can be met in any number of existing NADA programs. Sometimes arrangements can be made to meet this requirement in your clinic once it begins. If you live in an area where there are no laws governing the practice of

acupuncture, or where laws allow for detoxification specialists, and if the decision has been made to use detoxification specialists in your clinic, the NADA certification will include training of these individuals.

223   See p 301 for description of seed protocol for infants.

224   Employee assistance programs are operated either in-house or through subcontract by most public and private enterprises who have a substantial number of employees. EAPs typically provide assessment and counseling to the point of referral for a wide range of psychological and behavioral problems that affect job performance, including chemical dependency. Consequently, EAP service providers are constantly on the lookout for new referral sources for the people they assess.

225   This form of Medicaid is to be distinguished from the substance abuse-specific Medicaid funding mechanisms described in Chapter Five.

226   There is danger, however, in having the same individual filling both administrative and clinical roles, particularly in programs who will see clients who have been mandated by the courts, probation, parole, or a child protective services agency. If the same individual who is responsible for reporting client non-compliance to a referring criminal justice agency is also leading a therapy group or doing individual counseling, there is a conflict of interest. Daily urine testing, as described in the article in Appendix VIII can help dispel this conflict. However, it is of premier importance that clinical staff be in a position to advocate fully for the client and to cultivate a the honesty required to accomplish that advocacy. This level of advocacy cannot generally be achieved by a staff person who also has the responsibility of being the "bad cop," the person who interfaces with the referring agency.

227   Clinical supervision such as this is standard in agencies dealing with any level of counseling services. It is typically held weekly, and is attended by all individuals in the program who deal with clients. The Supervision forum provides the opportunity for staff to deal with their own counter transference issues, and to process other frustrations and experiences related to clients.

228   See Appendix XII, Section D for a perspective on counseling in the acupuncture clinic.

229   Urinalysis on site is provided by Syva. This company places the equipment at no charge when numbers of tests warrant it, and then charge for the chemical reagents.

230   *Alcoholics Anonymous*, 3rd ed. (New York: Alcoholics Anonymous World Services, Inc., 1976; orig. pub. 1939), p. 85.

231   See Appendix VII for a list of AA's Twelve Traditions.

232   *"Pass it On:" The Story of Bill Wilson and How the A.A. Message Reached the World* (New York: Alcoholics Anonymous World Services, Inc., 1984), pp. 381-86, p. 368.

233   Acupuncture has been used off and on at the Haight Ashbury Free Clinic in San Francisco, but, existing as it has in the shadow of Western medicine, has never taken the foothold required for its transformative energy to be realized.

234   Some meetings are restricted in membership to individuals addicted to the particular substance which that meeting addresses, such as alcohol; most meetings that are considered "closed meetings" in this sense begin with the announcement that "if you think you may have a problem (with alcohol), you are welcome here." Other restrictions may include gender ("stag" meetings), non-smoking meetings, etc.

235   This is an annotated text of the author's article published February 12, 1993, in Volume 10, No. 1 of the *Journal of Substance Abuse Treatment.*

236   Porkert paraphrases Mao tse-Tung, who called Chinese medicine a "vast treasure trove." See Manfred Porkert and Christian Ullman, *Chinese Medicine - Its History, Philosophy and Practice,* translated and adapted by Mark Howson (New York: William Morrow and Co., 1988), p. 288.

237   *Ibid.,* p. 37.

238   Paul F. M. Nogier describes these events in *From Auriculotherapy to Auriculomedicine* (Sainte-Ruffine, France: Maisonneuve, 1983).

239   There is a degree of controversy about the origins of acupuncture.

240   Reston's syndicated column appeared in the July 26, 1971 edition of *The New York Times.*

241   For a general review of all of this literature, see Bensoussan, Alan (1990). *The Vital Meridian.* Edinburgh: Churchill Livingstone. Works published in Western journals include P.D. Wall's "The Gate Control Theory of Pain Mechanisms; A Re-examination and Restatement," *Brain* 101 (1978), 1-18; Jeans R. Melzack's "How Acupuncture Can Block Pain," *Impact of Science on Society* (UNESCO) 23(1) (1973), 65, and "Acupuncture Analgesia: A Psychophysiological Explanation, *Minnesota Medicine* 57 (1974), 161-166, and Chen Man's "Mechanisms of Acupunctural Anesthesia: the Two Gate Control Theory," *Diseases of the Nervous System* 33 (1972), 730-735, and "Acupuncture 'Anesthesia': A New Theory and Clinical Study, *Current Therapeutic Research* 14(7) (1972), 390-394.

242   Bensoussan, pp. 101-126 (see note 52).

243 See, however, Bruce Pomeranz, "Scientific Basis of Acupuncture," in *Acupuncture: Textbook and Atlas*, edited by G. Stux and B. Pomeranz, Berlin, Germany: Springer-Verlag, 1987, pp. 1-34; J. Katims and J. Lowinson, "Acupuncture and Transcutaneous Electrical Nerve Stimulation: Afferent Nerve Stimulation (ANS) in the Treatment of Addiction," in *Substance Abuse, A Comprehensive Textbook*, edited by J. Lowinson and R. Millman. Baltimore: Williams and Wilkins, 1992, pp. 574-583), and F. Mann, *Acupuncture: The ancient Chinese art of healing and how it works scientifically* (1973). New York: Vintage Books.

That transcutaneous electrical stimulation activates opiatergic pathways was earlier demonstrated by F. Facchinetti, et.al. ("Central and Peripheral B-Endorphin Response to Transcutaneous Electrical Nerve Stimulation," *Progress in Opioid Research: Proceedings of the 1986 International Narcotics Research Congress*, NIDA Research Monograph 75, U. S. Department of Health and Human services, 1986, pp. 555-558).

244 J. Sodipo, & J. Falaiye, Acupuncture and gastric acid studies. *American Journal of Chinese Medicine* 7(4) (1979), 356-361.

245 Carolyn Lane, "Final Evaluation Report: Acupuncture Detoxification Project," Hooper Center, Central City Concern, Multnomah County, Oregon, Alcohol and Drug Program (1988).

246 Michael Smith, "Acupuncture and Natural Healing in Drug Detoxification," *American Journal of Acupuncture* 2, 7 (1979), 97-106.

247 Michael Smith and I Kahn, "An Acupuncture Programme for the Treatment of Drug Addicted Persons,: *Bulletin on Narcotics* XL[1] (1988), 35-41.

248 Bensoussan, pp. 39-41; 109.

249 According to Richard Seymour and David E. Smith in their book *Drugfree* (New York: Sarah Lazin Books 1987), acupuncture arrived at the Haight Ashbury clinic in San Francisco the early 1970s. This is nice symbolism - acupuncture having arrived at both coasts rather simultaneously. Unfortunately, early research on acupuncture at the Haight Ashbury clinic showed that acupuncture was only successful for a certain highly motivated element of the population, and this was a setback.

250 H. L Wen first published his findings with S.Y.C. Cheung in 1973 in "How Acupuncture Can Help Addicts," *Drugs and Society* 2, 8:18.

251 See Bensoussan, 101-126.

252 Michael Smith, "Acupuncture Treatment for Crack: Clinical Survey of 1,500 Patients," *American Journal of Acupuncture* 16 (3) (1988), 241 - 247. Unfortunately, a subsequent NIDA-funded study (Douglas S. Lipton, Vincent

Brewington, & Michael Smith, "Acupuncture and Crack Addicts: a Single-Blind Placebo Test of Efficacy," NIDA Grant No. 1 RO1 DA05632-01 [1990]; available from Narcotic and Drug Research, Inc., 11 Beach Street, New York, NY 10010) failed to meet standards required for publication due to problems with the urinalysis protocols. However, the researchers reported significantly lower positive urine toxicology for acupuncture patients versus controls who remained in treatment for over two weeks.

A more recent study not cited in this original article showed that cocaine-addicted patients on methadone maintenance who received acupuncture at Lincoln Hospital delivered fewer positive urines than a control group receiving weekly psychotherapy. This study also showed that females who received acupuncture had better outcomes than males. (Arthur Margolin, et.al., "Acupuncture for the Treatment of Cocaine Dependence in Methadone-Maintained Patients," *The American Journal on Addictions*, Vol.2[3], Summer, 1993, 194-201).

253 Brecher describes this process in his authoritative book *Licit and Illicit Drugs: The Consumer Union Report*. (Boston: Little, Brown and Company. 1972).

254 Gorski, Staying Sober - A Guide to Relapse Prevention. New York: Harper and Row, 1987.

255 Ted Kaptchuk, *The Web That Has No Weaver* (New York: Congdon and Weed, 1983).

256 Smith, "Acupuncture and Natural Healing in Drug Detoxification," *American Journal of Acupuncture*.

257 John D. McPeake, B. P. Kennedy, and S. M. Gordon, "Altered States of Consciousness Therapy: A Missing Component in Alcohol and Drug Rehabilitation Treatment," *Journal of Substance Abuse Treatment* 8 (1991), 75-82.

258 A. R. Childress, A. T. McLellan, M. Natale, & C P. O'Brien, "Mood States Can Elicit Conditioned Withdrawal and Craving in Opiate Abuse Patients," National Institute on Drug Abuse Research Monograph Series, No. 76, (Washington, DC: U.S. Government Printing Office), 1986. The specific "mood states" in this study that elicited cravings were depression, anxiety, and anger. These same mood states, as well as fatigue, were found to elicit heroin cravings by J. Sherman, et.al., in "Subjective Dimensions of Heroin Urges: Influence of Heroin-related and Affectively Negative Stimuli," *Addictive Behaviors* 14(6): 611-623, 1989.

259 Janet Konefal, "Acupuncture Program Services: Mid-year Progress Report," 1990 (Available from University of Miami, School of Medicine, Department of Psychiatry, P.O. Box 016069, Miami FL 33101). See also "The Miami Success Story: Transforming the Criminal Justice System with an Acupuncture Based Diversion Program," (NADA publication, September, 1990); for an overview of

the drug court program, also see "Miami's Drug Court: A Different Approach," National Institute of Justice, U.S. Department of Justice, Office of Justice Programs, NIJ: NCJ 142412 (June, 1993). A research study, conducted by Temple University has just been completed as of this writing, and publication is forthcoming.

The Miami Drug Court, and its acupuncture-based treatment component, was replicated with similar success in Brower County, Florida, and the Florida State Senate is moving toward replication in all Florida Counties. Las Vegas, Nevada, has implemented a similar model, and many other jurisdictions have expressed interest. Portland, Oregon's drug court/diversion program (PAAC) had success similar to Miami's. In their "Semi-Annual Report for Diversion Drug STOP program (July 1, 1991 - January 31, 1992, by David Eisen, Director), they report that as clients receive more acupuncture and are in group counseling longer, they stay clean and sober longer. In the first two weeks of treatment, 65% of the program participants stayed clean and sober. The clean-and-sober rate was 90% for people who completed the first three months of treatment, which includes two acupuncture treatments per week and two counseling groups per week. At the time of the report, only four out of 164 participants were known to have re-offend.

260   Alex Brumbaugh & Susan Wheeler, "Six Month Jail Demonstration Project: A Preliminary Analysis," 1991 (see Appendix IV for the text of this and of a further study done with female inmates).

261   Brumbaugh, (1992), *ibid.*

262   Patricia Keenan "Treatment for Babies in the Face of the Crack Epidemic," *MIRA: The Quarterly Newsletter of Multicultural Inquiry and Research on AIDS* 5 (2) (1991) (Available from MIRA, 5815 3rd Street, San Francisco 94124). Keenan's protocol for infants involves the application of the herbal seed *semen vaccaria* taped to the infant's ear at *shenmen*, kidney, and brain stem points. The ear canal should be avoided because of its proximity to the lung point. A central aspect of the therapy is the relationship of the mother with the infant. Holding the baby, she presses each point ten times, three times per day, and is asked at the same time to focus her attention on the baby in a loving and nurturing way. The seeds will eventually dissolve. (For further information on perinatal treatment and research, see Appendix VII).

263   Michael Smith, "Raising Healthy Babies for the 90s," 1990 (Available through Lincoln Hospital, Maternal Substance Abuse Services, 349 East 140th Street, Bronx, NY 10454).

264   Since this article was written, the results of this study have been published in "Acupuncture Heroin Detoxification: A Single-Blind Clinical Trial," *Journal of Substance Abuse Treatment*, VOL. 10, pp. 343-351, July/August, 1993.

265 Kate Black has also been providing acupuncture treatment for drug-exposed infants at the Family Addiction Center for Education and Treatment (FACET) in San Francisco since 1990, using protocols based upon Pat Keenan's work. Matu Feliciano at the SITIKE Counseling Center for Addiction, Prevention, and Recovery in South San Francisco, has further developed these protocols. The FACET program was part of a five year perinatal program funded by the Federal Center for Substance Abuse Treatment (CSAT). Since this article was published, acupuncture components have been implemented at a number of CSAT-funded and California State Medi-Cal funded perinatal treatment programs.

266 NAPARE. "Substances Most Commonly Abused During Pregnancy and their Risks to Mother and Baby," *National Association for Perinatal Addiction Research and Education Newsletter*, 1989 (available from National Association for Perinatal Addiction Research and Education, 11 E. Hubbard Street, Suite 200, Chicago, IL 60611, 312 / 329-2512).

267 L Cregler, & H. Mark, "Medical Complications of Drug Abuse, *New England Journal of Medicine* 315 (1986), 1495 - 1500.

268 Paul S. Puccio, "Acupuncture Detoxification and Relapse Service: A Concept Paper," New York State Division of Substance Abuse Services, 1991.

269 Joel A. Egertson, Chief, Government and Constituent Relations Branch, National Institute of Drug Abuse, memorandum dated February 4, 1991, to Ron Weich, United States Congress.

270 Deborah Grossman, National Institute of Drug Abuse (personal interview, 1992).

271 OTI (1990). Summary statement for Application Number: 1 H87TI 00112-0103 by the Office of Treatment Improvement, United States Department of Health and Human Services, to Santa Barbara County Drug and Alcohol Program, cover letter dated September 21, 1990.

OTI (now CSAT [The Center for Substance Abuse Treatment]), in its 1993 funding cycle, reported that acupuncture components in program proposals would not be used as a basis for rejection. In fact, veteran NADA clinician David Eisen was retained by CSAT to review the acupuncture components of several proposals. Requesting funding for acupuncture components was, however, discouraged.

272 Mark Cunnif, Executive Director, The National Association of Criminal Justice Planners, 1331 H Street N.W., Suite 401, Washington, D.C. 20005 (personal interview, (1991).

273 Charles Rangel, Chairman, United States House of Representatives Select Committee on Narcotics Abuse and Control, letter dated July 11, 1990, to Beny J. Primm, MD, Associate Administrator, Office of Treatment Improvement, ADAMHA.

274 U.S. Department of Health and Human Services, "Drug Abuse and Drug Abuse Research: The Third Triennial Report to Congress from the Secretary," DHHS Publication No. (ADM) 91-1704, 1991.

275 Porkert, pp. 13-63; 265-278

276 Ernest Kurtz, *Not-God - A History of Alcoholics Anonymous*, (Center City, MN: Hazleden Press, 1979), p. 171.

277 See M. Bullock, A. Umen, P. Culliton, & R. Olander, "Acupuncture Treatment of Alcoholic Recidivism: A Pilot Study," (*Alcoholism: Clinical and Experimental Research*, 11(3), May-June, 1987, pp. 292-295), and their follow-up of the same study, "Controlled Trial of Acupuncture for Severe Recidivistic Alcoholism, *The Lancet* (June 24, 1989), 1435 - 1439.

This research used sham acupuncture, in which "non-therapeutic" points are used on the control group. A separate study of sham acupuncture has shown that patients are subjectively unable to distinguish sham from real acupuncture, and concludes that sham acupuncture is therefore a valid investigative tool (Arthur Margolin, et.al, "Effects of Sham and Real Auricular Needling: Implications for Trials of Acupuncture for Cocaine Addiction," *American Journal of Chinese Medicine*, VOL.XXI[2], 1993, pp. 103-111).

278 Clark, "Trial of Acupuncture Detoxification: Final Report."

279 There is a "Community Action Commission" or its equivalent in every Congressional jurisdiction. These large "advocacy" agencies, remnants of Lyndon Johnson's "War on Poverty," have the responsibility of representing their communities in the administration of Federal "McKinney Act" and other funds designated for low income recipients such as Senior lunch programs, Head Start, and homeless, including some funds specifically designated for substance abusing homeless. Call the office of your local United States Congressman to find out how such funds are administered in your area.

280 Casa Rosa is among a number of perinatal residential programs funded by the Federal Center for Substance Abuse Prevention. To contact this organization, see Appendix --).

281 See pp. 320-322 for a further summary of this important research. Bullock, M.L., Culliton, P.D., & Olander, R.T. "Controlled trial of acupuncture for severe recidivistic alcoholism." *The Lancet*, (1989, June 24), 1435-439.

282 The recent funding increase for perinatal treatment is, as with most policy funding decisions, fiscally motivated. The cost of a mother having a drug-exposed infant with two children being maintained in foster care due to her untreated chemical dependence is estimated in New York at around $120,000.

283 Proposals that are not funded should not be viewed as failures. There are a multitude of reasons why proposals are not funded which do not necessarily bear on the quality of the proposal, but each proposal submitted to any funding source should be seen as important "seed-planting." Each proposal submitted presents a premier opportunity for educating important members of the community about acupuncture, because the recipients of the proposal are a "captive audience." Most proposals are seriously reviewed, often by committees representing important and sometimes powerful people in the field.

284 See Appendix IV for full text of this report.

285 Foster, K., Chu, A., Adjuluchukwu, D., & Brown, L. S. "The Increasing Need for Primary Health Care as an Integral Treatment Component," in *Problems of drug dependence 1991: proceeding of the 53rd annual scientific meeting of the committee on problems of drug dependence, Inc.*, Louis Harris, ed., (NIDA, 1992, p. 488).

286 Heverkos, H. W. (1991). Infectious disease and drug abuse: prevention and treatment in the drug-abuse treatment system, Journal of Substance Abuse Treatment, Vol. 8, N4, 269-275.

287 NIDA, Drug abuse and drug abuse research: the third triennial report to Congress from the Secretary, Department of Health and Human Services (1991, pp. 87-89).

288 Jarlais, D. C. D., Casriel, C., Stepherson, B., and Friedman, S., "Expectations of Racial Prejudice in AIDS Research and Prevention Programs in the United States," in *AIDS and Alcohol/Drug Abuse: Psychosocial Research*, Dennis G. Fisher, ed. (New York: Harrington Park Press, 1991).

289 NIDA, p. 87.

290 Ibid., pp. 95 and 101.

291 Metzger, D. S., et.al., "The impact of HIV testing on risk of AIDS behaviors," in Problems of drug dependence 1991: proceeding of the 53rd annual scientific meeting of the committee on problems of drug dependence, Inc., Louis Harris, ed., NIDA, 1992, 297-8.

292 Dixie, E. & Roper, W. L., "The New Tuberculosis" (editorial), *New England Journal of Medicine*, v 326 n 10 p. 703, and Goldsmith, M., "Medical Exorcism Required as Revitalized Revenant of Tuberculosis Haunts and Harries the Land," *The Journal of the American Medical Association*, V268 n2, pp. 174-5.

293 P. A. Selwyn, et.al., "A Prospective Study of the Risk of Tuberculosis among Intravenous Drug Users with Human Immunodeficiency Virus Infection, *New England Journal of Medicine*, vol. 320 n9, 1989, 545-551.

294   M. B. Gregg and G. A. Ingraham, "Tuberculosis and Acquired Immune Deficiency Syndrome: New York City," *Morbidity and Mortalty Weekly*, v 36, n 48, 1987, pp. 785-795.

295   J. Elvin, "Tuberculosis Comes Back, Poses Special Threat to Jails, Prisons, *National Prison Project Journal*, V 7, N 1, 1992, pp. 1-4.

296   See Mary K. Ryan and Arthur D. Shattuck's "Treating AIDS with Chinese Medicine," and other publications of the Pacific View Press, P.O. Box 2657, Berkeley, CA 94702.

297   Declaration of the 30th Anniversary, International Convention of Alcoholics Anonymous, 1965.

298   The publication FOCUS: A Guide to AIDS Research and Counseling is an excellent resource available from UCSF AIDS Health Project, Box 0884, San Francisco, CA 94143-0884.

299   NIDA, Drug abuse and drug abuse research: the third triennial report to Congress from the Secretary, Department of Health and Human Services, 1991, pp. 61 - 62),

300   Ross, H. E., Glasser, F. B., & Germanson, T. (1988). The prevalence of psychiatric disorders in patients with alcohol and other drug problems. *Arc Gen. Psychiatry* 45(11):1023-1031, in NIDA, *Drug abuse and drug abuse research: the third triennial report to Congress from the Secretary, Department of Health and Human Services*, 1991.

301   Galanter, M., Castaneda, R., & Ferman, J. (1988). Substance abuse among general psychiatric patients: place of presentation, diagnosis, and treatment. *American Journal of Drug and Alcohol Abuse* 14(2): 211-235, quoted in NIDA, *Drug abuse and drug abuse research: the third triennial report to Congress from the Secretary, Department of Health and Human Services*, 1991, p62.

302   Rosenthal, R. N., Hellerstein, D. J., and Miner, C. R., (1992). "A model of integrated services for outpatient treatment of patients with comorbid schizophrenia and addictive disorders," *The American Journal on Addictions*, 1:4, 339-348).

303   For a review of the research on Chinese medicine and psychiatric disorders, see Alan Bensoussan, (1990) *The Vital Meridian*. Edinburgh: Churchill Livingstone.303 Bensoussan, p. 109. For a non-clinical primer on the application of Chinese medicine to mental illness, see David Eisenberg's "On Mental Illness: Freud's Not Here," in *Encounters with Qi: Exploring Chinese Medicine* (New York: W. W. Norton, 1985, pp. 169-196).

304   Nigram, R., Schottenfeld, R., & Kosten, T., (1992) Treatment of dual diagnosis patients: a relapse prevention group approach, *Journal of Substance Abuse Treatment*, 9:4, 305-309.

305   See Rose Marie Friedrich and Robert Krus's "Cognitive Impairments in Early Sobriety: Nursing Interventions," *Archives of Psychiatric Nursing*, Vol. V, No. 2 (April), 1991: pp. 105-112 (reprints available from Rose Marie Friedrich, R.N., M.A., College of Nursing, University of Iowa, Iowa City, IA 52242).

Bibliography

Alcoholics Anonymous. 3rd Ed., *Alcoholics Anonymous* World Service, New York, NY, 1976.

Bateson, Gregory, *Steps to Ecology of Mind*, New York: Ballentine, 1972.

Bateson, Gregory and Mary Catherine, *Angels Fear - Toward an Epistemology of the Sacred,* New York: Macmillan Publishing Co., 1987.

Beasley, Joseph D., *Diagnosing and Managing Chemical Dependency*, Essential Medical Information Systems, 1990.

Beattie, Melody, *Codependent No More: How to Stop Controlling Others and Start Caring for Yourself*, Minneapolis: Harper/Hazelden, 1987.

Beattie, Melody, *Codependents' Guide to the Twelve Steps*, New York: Prentice Hall/Parkside, 1990.

Beinfield, Harriet and Korngold, Efrem, *Between Heaven and Earth: A Guide to Chinese Medicine,* New York: Ballantine Books, 1991.

Bensoussan, Alan, *The Vital Meridian*, Edinburgh: Churchill Livingstone, 1990.

Berman, Morris, *The Reenchantment of the World*, Ithaca, New York: Cornell U. Press, 1986.

Berman, Morris, *Coming to Our Senses,* Ithaca, New York: Cornell U. Press, 1990.

Black, Claudia, *It Will Never Happen to Me*, Denver: Medical Administration Co., 1982.

Blum, K. *Alcohol and the Addictive Brain: New Hope for Alcoholics from Biogenetic Research*, New York: Free Press, 1991.

Bowden, Julie and Gravitz, Herbert, *Genesis*, Pompano Beach, FL: Health Communication, Inc. 1988.

Bradshaw, John, *Bradshaw on the Family*, Pompano Beach, FL: Health Communication, Inc. 1988.

Bradshaw, John, *Healing the Shame that Binds You*, Pompano Beach, FL: Health Communication, Inc. 1988.

Bradshaw, John, *Homecoming*, Pompano Beach, FL: Health Communication, Inc., 1990.

Brecher, Edward, *Licit and Illicit Drugs: The Consumer Union Report*, Boston: Little, Brown and Company. 1972.

Brown, Stephanie, *Safe Passage: Recovery for Adult Children of Alcoholics*, New York: John Wiley and Sons, Inc., 1991.

Brown, Stephanie, *Treating the Alcoholic*, New York: John Wiley and Sons, Inc., 1988.

Burt, E. A., *Metaphysical Foundations of Modern Science*, 1932.

Capra, Fritjof, *The Tao of Physics*, Boston: Shambhala, 1991.

Capra, Fritjof, *The Turning Point*, Toronto: Bantam, 1982.

Carlton, Peter L, *A Primer of Behavioral Pharmacology*, New York: W. H. Freeman & Co., 1983.

Carson, Richard D., *Taming Your Gremlin*, New York: HarperCollins.

Cermak, Timmen, *Diagnosing and Treating Co-Dependence: A Guide for Professionals Who Work with Chemical Dependents, Their Spouses and Children*, Johnson Institute, 1986.

Cohen, Sidney, *The Chemical Brain*, Minneapolis: CompCare, 1987.

Descartes, Renee, *Discourse on Method and Selected Writings*, translated by John Veitch, New York: Dutton and Company, 1951.

DuWors, George M., *White Knuckles and Wishful Thinking: Breaking the Chain of Compulsive Reaction and Relapse in Alcoholism and Other Addictions*, Seattle: Hogrefe and Huber, 1992.

Eisenberg, David, M.D., *Encounters with Qi: Exploring Chinese Medicine*, New York: W. W. Norton, 1985.

Eisler, Riane, *The Chalice and the Blade*, San Francisco: Harper and Row, 1987.

Ellison, J. M., *The Psychotherapist's Guide to Pharmacotherapy,* Chicago: Year Book Medical Publishers, 1989.

Fingarette, Herbert, *Heavy Drinking: The Myth of Alcoholism*, Berkeley: University of California Press, 1988.

Fitzgerald, K.W., *Alcoholism: The Genetic Inheritance*, NY: Doubleday, 1988.

Gilman, Alfred G., et al, *Goodman & Gilman's Pharmacological Basis of Therapeutics*, New York: McGraw Hill, 1990.

Gerstein, D. R., and Harwood, H. J., editors, *Treating Drug Problems*, Volume I, Washington D. C.: National Academy Press, 1990.

Gitlen, M. J., *The Psychotherapist's Guide to Psychopharmacology*, New York: The Free Press, 1990.

Gorski, Terence T. *Passages Through Recovery*, New York: Harper and Row, 1989.

Gorski, Terence T. *Staying Sober - A Guide to Relapse Prevention*, New York: Harper and Row, 1987.

Gravitz, Herbert L., and Bowden, Julie D., *Guide to Recovery: A Book For Adult Children of Alcoholics*, Holmes Beach, FL: Learning Publications, Inc., 1986.

Gravitz, Herbert L., and Bowden, Julie D., *Genesis*, Pompano Beach, FL: Health Communication, Inc. 1988.

Hubbard, R. L., et.al., *Drug Abuse Treatment: A National Study of Effectiveness*, Chapel Hill: The University of North Carolina Press, 1989.

Inaba, D., and Cohen, W., *Uppers and Downers and All Arounders*, Ashland, Oregon: Cinemed, Inc., 1989.

Jonas, Jeffrey, M.D., and Schaumburg, Ron, *Everything You Need to Know about Prozac*, New York: Bantam, 1991.

Julien, Robert, *Drugs and the Body in Health & Disease*, New York: W. H. Freeman & Co., 1987.

Julien, Robert, *Primer of Drug Action*, 6th edition, New York: W. H. Freeman & Co., 1991.

Jung, Carl, *The Undiscovered Self*, New York: Atlantic-Little, Brown, and Co., 1957.

Jung, Carl, *Symbols of Transformation* Vol. 2, Harper and Row, 1958.

Kaptchuk, T., *The Web that Has No Weaver: Understanding Chinese Medicine*, New York: Congdon and Weed, 1983.

Kasl, Charlotte, *One Journey, Many Paths: Beyond the Twelve Steps*, Harper, 1992.

Kuhn, Thomas, *The Structure of Scientific Revolutions*, Chicago: University of Chicago Press, 1970.

Kurtz, Ernest, *Not God: A History of Alcoholics Anonymous*, Center City MN: Hazeldon Press, 1979.

Laing, R. D., *The Divided Self*, Harmondsworth, England: Penguin Books, 1965.

Laing, R. D., *Politics of Experience*, New York: Ballentine Books, 1968.

Lawson, Gary, *Clinical Psychopharmacology for Non-Medical Therapists*, Aspen Press, 1987.

Lawson, Gary W. & Cooperrider, Craig C., *Clinical Psychopharmacology: A Practical Reference for Nonmedical Psychotherapists*, Gaithersburg, Maryland: Aspen Publishers, 1988.

Lusane, Clarence, *Pipe Dream Blues: Racism & the War on Drugs*, Boston: South End Press, 1991.

Madsen, William, *The American Alcoholic: The Nature/Nurture Controversy in Alcoholic Research and Therapy*, Springfield: Charles C. Thomas. 1974.

Madsen, William, *Defending the Deisease of Alcoholism: From Facts to Fingarette*, Akron, OH: Wilson Brown and Co., 1969

Mann, F., *Acupuncture: The Ancient Chinese Art of Healing and how it Works Scientifically,* New York: Vintage Books, 1973.

May, Rollo, *The Cry for Myth*, New York: W. W. Norton & Co., 1991.

McClure, Mary Beth, *Reclaiming the Heart: A Handbook of Help and Hope for Survivors*, Warner Books.--

Mellody, Pia, Miller, Andrea J., and Miller, Keith, *Facing Codependence: What It Is, Where It Comes From, How It Sabotages Our Lives*, San Francisco: Harper & Row, 1989.

Merchant, Carolyn, *The Death of Nature*, New York: Harper & Row, 1980.

Metzger, Lawrence, *From Denial to Recovery*, San Francisco: Jossey-Bass, Inc., 1987.

Miller, Alice, *The Drama of the Gifted Child: The Search for the True Self* (originally published as *Prisoners of Childhood*), translated by Ruth Ward, Basic Books of HarperCollins, 1981.

Needham, Joseph, *Science and Civilisation in China* , Cambridge, England: Cambridge University Press, 1956.

Palif, Tibor & Jankiewicz, *Henry, Drugs & Human Behavior*, Madison, Wisconcin: Brown & Benchmark, 1991.

"Pass it On:" The Story of Bill Wilson and How the A.A. Message Reached the World, New York: Alcoholics Anonymous World Services, Inc., 1984.

Peck, M. S., *The Road Less Traveled*, New York: Simon and Schuster, 1978.

Peele, Stanton, *The Meaning of Addiction,* Lexington: D.C. Heath and Co., 1985.

Peele, Stanton, *Diseasing of America: Addiction Treatment Out of Control*, Lexington: D.C. Heath and Co., 1989.

Peluso, L. S., and Peluso, E. *Women and Drugs*, Minneapolis: CompCare Publishers, 1988.

Porkert, Manfred, and Ullman, Christian, *Chinese Medicine - Its History, Philosophy and Practice*, translated and adapted by Mark Howson, New York: William Morrow and Co., 1988.

Rich, Adrienne, *Of Woman Born*, New York: Bantam, 1977.

Ricketson, Susan, *The Dilemma of Love: Healing Co-Dependent Relationships at Different Stages of Life*, Pompano Beach, FL: Health Communications, Inc., 1989.

Ridlon, Florence V., *A Fallen Angel*, -- Associated University Press, 1988.

Rogers, Carl, *Client-Centered Therapy,* Boston: Houghton Mifflin, 1951.

Ruzak, S. B., *The Women's Health Movement*, New York: Praeger Publishers, 1978.

Schaef, Anne Wilson, *Women's Reality: An Emerging Female System in a White Male Society*, Minneapolis: Winston, 1985.

Schaef, Anne Wilson, *Co-dependence: Misunderstood, Mistreated*, Minneapolis: Winston, 1985.

Schaef, Anne Wilson, *When Society Becomes an Addict*, San Francisco: Harper Row, 1987.

Schuckit, M. A., *Drug and Alcohol Abuse: A Clinical Guide to Diagnosis and Treatment*, New York: Plenum Press, 1989.

Sivin, Nathan, *Traditional Medicine in Contemporary China* (*Science, Medicine, and Technology in East Asia*, Volume 2), Ann Arbor: Center for Chinese Studies, University of Michigan.

Snyder, S.H. *Drugs & the Brain: A Scientific American Book*, New York: W. H. Freeman & Co., 1986.

Spitz, Henry, M.D., and Rosecan, Jeffrey S., M.D., eds., *Cocaine Abuse: New Directions in Treatment and Research*, New York: Brunner/Mazel, 1987.

Steinem, Gloria, *Revolution from Within: A Book of Self-Esteem*, Boston: Little, Brown, & Co., 1992.

Stimmell, Barry, and the editors of Consumer Report Books, *The Facts About Drug Use*, New York: Haworth Press, 1993.

Vaillant, G. E., The Natural History of Alcoholism, Cambridge: Harvard University Press, 1983.

Watts, Alan, *The Spirit of Zen: A Way of Life, Work, and Art in the Far East*, New York: Grove Press, 1958.

Whitfield, C., *Healing the Child Within*, Pompano Beach, FL: Health Communication, Inc., 1987.

Wilbur, Ken, *The Holographic Paradigm and Other Paradoxes: Leading Edge of Science*, Boulder, CO: Shambala, 1982.

Wilsnak, S. C., and Beckman, L. J. (eds.), *Alcohol Problems in Women*, New York: The Guilford Press, 1984.

Woodman, Marion, *Addiction to Perfection - The Still Unravished Bride*, Inner City Books, 1982.

Index